Praise for Maia Szalavitz

"Maia Szalavitz is one of the bravest, smartest writers about addiction anywhere. Everything she writes should be read carefully—I guarantee you'll have a lot to think about, and you'll know far more than at the start."

—JOHANN HARI, *New York Times* bestselling
author of *Chasing the Scream*

"Maia Szalavitz is one of our most incisive thinkers about neuroscience in general and addiction in particular and her writing is astonishingly clear and compelling. In the timely, important, and insightful *Unbroken Brain,* Szalavitz seamlessly interweaves her moving personal story with her investigation into what addiction is (and isn't) and how we can most effectively prevent and treat it."

—DAVID SHEFF, *New York Times* bestselling
author of *Clean* and *Beautiful Boy*

"Through the lens of her own gripping story of addiction—supported with empirical evidence—Szalavitz persuasively shows that addiction is a disorder of learning, *not* one characterized by progressive brain dysfunction."

—CARL HART, PhD, author of the Pen/E. O. Wilson
Literary Science Writing Award–winning *High Price:
A Neuroscientist's Journey of Self-Discovery That
Challenges Everything You Know about Drugs and Society*

"Of the countless writers out there whose focus is addiction, no one can begin to touch the brilliance of Maia Szalavitz. She is by far my favorite addiction writer, perhaps one of my favorite writers ever. Her passion and exceptional writing talent combined with her exhaustive research, create a book that will inspire, educate, enrage, and entertain. I can only promise one thing: if you read this book, you will never be the same again."

—KRISTEN JOHNSTON, actress, author of the *New York Times* best-selling memoir *Guts*, addiction advocate, founder of SLAM NYC

"As more professionals realize that addiction isn't really a disease, our challenge is to determine exactly what it is. Szalavitz catalogs the latest scientific knowledge of the biological, environmental and social causes of addiction and explains precisely how they interact over development. The theory is articulate and tight, yet made accessible and compelling through the author's harrowing autobiography. *Unbroken Brain* provides the most comprehensive and readable explanation of addiction I've yet to see."

—Marc Lewis, author of *The Biology of Desire*

". . . a new way of looking at drug addiction that offers a fresh approach to managing it. [Szalavitz] writes frankly about her background . . . In a heartfelt manner, she exposes her own fears and pain . . . A dense blending of self-exposure, surprising statistics, and solid science reporting that presents addiction as a misunderstood coping mechanism, a problem whose true nature is not yet recognized by policymakers or the public."

—*Kirkus*

"Anyone who has battled addiction or seen it harm a loved one will gain insights from *Unbroken Brain*, and if it influences policymakers, too, everyone will benefit . . ."

—Associated Press

"Journalist Szalavitz offers a multifaceted, ground-up renovation of the concept of addiction—both its causes and its cures."

—*Publishers Weekly*

"Ms. Szalavitz deftly threads her life story through the book to illustrate the dynamics that put people at risk of addiction."

—*The Wall Street Journal*

"Szalavitz makes a novel and even beautiful proposal. Addiction, she hypothesizes, is a developmental disorder. Specifically, it is a learning disorder . . . [Szalavitz] explores problems with the criminalization of drugs, the place of racism in our culture's treatment of drugs and addiction, and she looks closely and illuminatingly at different treatment methods. There's a lot of news you can use in this book if you or someone you love is an addict."

—NPR.org

Undoing Drugs

ALSO BY MAIA SZALAVITZ

*Unbroken Brain: A Revolutionary
New Way of Understanding Addiction*

*Help at Any Cost: How the Troubled
Teen Industry Cons Parents and Hurts Kids*

With Bruce D. Perry, MD, PhD:
*The Boy Who Was Raised as a Dog and Other Stories
from a Child Psychiatrist's Notebook*

Born for Love: Why Empathy Is Essential—and Endangered

With Joe Volpicelli, MD, PhD:
Recovery Options: The Complete Guide

Undoing Drugs

How Harm Reduction Is Changing the Future of Drugs and Addiction

MAIA SZALAVITZ

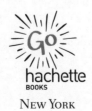

hachette
BOOKS

NEW YORK

Hachette Go, an imprint of Hachette Books
Hachette Book Group
1290 Avenue of the Americas
New York, NY 10104
HachetteGo.com
Facebook.com/HachetteGo
Instagram.com/HachetteGo

First Paperback Edition: August 2022
Hachette Books is a division of Hachette Book Group, Inc.

The Hachette Go and Hachette Books name and logos are trademarks of Hachette Book Group, Inc.

The publisher is not responsible for websites (or their content) that are not owned by the publisher.

Print book interior design by Linda Mark.

Library of Congress Cataloging-in-Publication Data
Names: Szalavitz, Maia, author. Title: Undoing drugs : the untold story of harm reduction and the future of addiction / Maia Szalavitz.
Description: First edition. | New York : Hachette Go, [2021] | Includes bibliographical references and index. Identifiers: LCCN 2021015025 | ISBN 9780738285764 (hardcover) | ISBN 9780738285740 (trade paperback) | ISBN 9780738285757 (ebook)
Subjects: LCSH: Drug addiction—United States—History. | Harm reduction—United States—History. | HIV infections—United States—Prevention—History. | Needle exchange programs—United States—History. | Drug addicts—Health and hygiene—United States—History. | Drug addiction—Treatment—United States—History. | Drug abuse—United States—Prevention—History.
Classification: LCC HV5825 .S948 2021 | DDC 362.290973—dc23 LC record available at https://lccn.loc.gov/2021015025

ISBNs: 978-0-7382-8576-4 (hardcover); 978-0-7382-8574-0 (trade paperback); 978-0-7382-8575-7 (ebook)

Printed in Canada

FRI

10 9 8 7 6 5 4 3 2 1

To Edith Springer

Contents

Author's Note

WRITING THIS BOOK HAS BEEN AN EXTRAORDINARY EXPERIENCE, INVOLVing wrangling hundreds of interviews and thousands of documents, websites, films, and books. Throughout the process, I have been acutely aware that I am the first to try to write the story of harm reduction in America—and painfully conscious of how much I've had to leave out in order to create a book that is readable. The resulting work is at best a first approximation, a place where others can start to understand the roots of this idea—and is in no way meant to be taken as complete or as implying that the stories that had to be left out are less important than those I was able to include. There is so much more to tell!

Many additional specialized works need to be written, particularly to encompass the story of harm reduction outside of the United States and within specific communities. To aid that process, I am creating an archive of interviews and other material, which will be available online for anyone who wishes to dig further. It will initially be at maiasz.com and later have a dedicated site. I hope people will use it extensively. I also want to note that as a person who engaged with this movement from almost the beginning, my work will inevitably reflect my own perspective and not that of either a complete outsider or a movement leader. Again, I would like the book to be a spur to further thought, discussion, and, yes, argument. It is in no way intended as the final word or as the only way to view harm reduction and its origins.

Please be aware as well that some of this book covers clashes between people in harm reduction and those who see twelve-step programs like Narcotics Anonymous as the best way to understand and recover from addiction. This does not mean that harm reduction itself is necessarily incompatible with twelve-step recovery or vice versa. Many of the founders of harm reduction in the U.S. participated in twelve-step programs and some still do. While there are certainly conflicts between aspects of these approaches, there is also room for ecumenical views and a critical aspect of harm reduction is welcoming diversity.

Finally, a note about language. Almost invariably, the terms we use to discuss drugs and addiction are stigmatizing. Research has even found that some of them can directly cause harm by biasing clinicians toward punitive approaches. Consequently, as I did in my previous book, *Unbroken Brain: A Revolutionary New Way of Understanding Addiction,* I have tried to minimize the use of such words and phrases. Wherever possible, I use "person first" language to describe people who use drugs or have addictions, except when doing so becomes unbearably repetitive. Because harm reductionists historically have preferred the term "drug user" to "addict"—in part, to make the point that most people who use drugs actually are not addicted—I have used that term in that way when describing this history. Offensive words like "junkie" are avoided, except when used by people to describe themselves, in quotes, or to illustrate the depth of stigma that people have faced.

The story of harm reduction is multifactorial, multifaceted, multicultural, and multidisciplinary. I hope what you are about to read will whet your appetite as the movement grows.

Introduction

I HAD NO INTENTION OF QUITTING. I'D ONLY JUST BEEN INTRODUCED TO THE glories of shooting speedballs, a seemingly divine mixture of cocaine and heroin. I wanted more. But my friend Dave had decided to kick—and he was about to buy heroin for us, for what he hoped would be his last hurrah before rehab. Unnaturally slim, blond, and dressed like a preppy, Dave's white-bread look meant that he was less likely to be arrested when seeking drugs. I was in his tidy East Village apartment waiting for him to return, sitting on his couch with his girlfriend. She was visiting from San Francisco, where he'd formerly lived, in part to ensure he actually made it into treatment.

And as we waited, she probably saved my life. It was 1986. Despite being a regular reader of two newspapers a day, I had no idea that needle sharing put me at risk for HIV. Dave, who not long afterward became ill with AIDS, was likely already infected. At that time, at least *half* of all intravenous drug users in New York City silently carried the deadly virus: your odds of exposure were fifty-fifty, even more if you shared in some neighborhoods. Thankfully, his girlfriend quickly taught me how to protect myself, which I did from that day forward. Don't share, she advised, but if you have no alternative, run bleach through the syringe at least twice, then rinse at least twice with water.

I didn't know it at the time, but Dave's girlfriend was practicing a philosophy that would come to be known as harm reduction. Back then, it hadn't yet become a political movement, one that currently includes hundreds of thousands of active supporters. Back then, it wasn't supported by hundreds of studies, backed by governments as a key aspect of dealing with drug issues, or taught as an element of public health programs and a viable career path within medicine, nursing, epidemiology, psychology, and social work. It wasn't a phrase found in op-eds and news stories calling for a better way of fighting pandemics. And it certainly wasn't—as it is today—the first real threat and alternative to international drug prohibition and our current failing addiction treatment system.

Even now, the story of harm reduction—and its potential to tame the opioid crisis, mitigate future drug problems, and quell other pandemics—has never been told. That is the task of *Undoing Drugs*. It is a story about how a small group of committed people can change the world—and about the power of a great idea. It is also the story of the rugged persistence of fundamentally bad ideas—and how hard it is to become free of them once they have been widely accepted. It is about how minds change—and how racism can become so embedded in a system of law that it becomes almost invisible, even to those who perpetuate it. It is about how the labels we use for substances shape people's identities—and how that itself can warp law and policy, dehumanizing victims. It is also about how personal, direct human connection and kindness can inspire profound transformation.

When I began writing this book, I didn't know who "Dave's girlfriend" was. In fact, I didn't even know she was his girlfriend: I thought they were just friends. I had only met her once in 1986 and could no longer remember her first name, let alone recall if I ever knew her last. I wanted to find her and thank her for saving my life, but I knew virtually nothing about her.

Once I decided that I was going to try to tell the story of harm reduction, however, I realized I had to do it: lacking critical information about her made writing my own harm reduction origin story somewhat awkward, for one. Far more importantly, of course, I wanted her to know how grateful I am and to find out more about the person who had so dramatically altered my trajectory. I wanted to know how she had come to practice harm reduction so early.

Unfortunately, I had little to go on. I couldn't really recall what she looked like. I had a vague idea that she was a bit older than I was and thought that she was white and might possibly have an Irish name. But that was pretty much it. At the time I met her, I had no idea that the conversation would be one of the most important I'd ever had.

Before we'd crossed paths, I'd been on a pretty clear course toward infection: I was injecting drugs more and more frequently. I didn't even know that sharing needles put me at risk, and I was in a city where I was as likely as not to share with someone who was already HIV-positive. I would spend another two years injecting daily before I recognized that I needed help, sought treatment, and began recovery.

Fortunately, as I dug into the history of harm reduction and its roots in AIDS prevention, I determined that she must have been somehow affiliated with San Francisco's "bleach and teach" programs, which were the first major effort in the United States to try to stop the spread of HIV in drug users by promoting the use of bleach to clean needles. This gave me a place to start.

From even the short conversation I'd had with her, it had been clear that she knew more than most people did about AIDS and drugs. Working at such an organization—or at least knowing someone who did—was pretty much the only way that she would have had the specific information she gave me about how to protect myself.

That would also almost certainly be the only way someone who was visiting New York to get someone else into drug treatment would have known to provide safer injection information in a nonjudgmental and matter-of-fact way. Most addiction counselors at the time would have just given me a lecture about why I should be in rehab, too—not practical information about how to stay alive.

Her empathic approach made all the difference. Once I learned about cleaning my needles with bleach, I became as compulsive about doing so as I was about getting high, which was pretty much as compulsive as an already compulsive person can be. And, once I had this life-saving information, I became compulsive about sharing it.

As a person who'd grown up with the privileges of the white middle class, it astonished me that my country could be so cruel as to let people who use drugs die of ignorance to try to "send a message" to children and prevent them from following our example. I may not have been particularly good at caring about myself at the time, but I certainly cared about my friends. And I didn't think letting anyone die a preventable death was okay.

Simply by becoming addicted, however, I had apparently become a person who didn't matter. The brute fact of this reality astounded me; it infuriated me in a deep part of myself that neither addiction nor depression could obliterate. Though I still carried the self-hatred that had made me susceptible to getting hooked in the first place, I also retained a sense of justice—if not for me, then because no one deserved to be below basic consideration. The mere act of taking drugs that society had deemed illegal seemed to make my friends and others like us, as the Nazis had put it, "life unworthy of life." As the child of a Holocaust survivor, I knew where such ideas led.

I finally succeeded in tracking down Maureen Gammon in 2020; it took about a dozen interviews with people who worked in HIV prevention in San Francisco before I found her. I spoke with a sociologist, whose 1980s research interviews made her insist that her bosses take action against AIDS, rather than just study how it spread. That work had led to the development of the bleach program, which Gammon had helped carry out. I spoke with one of the self-proclaimed witches who did bleach outreach and then helped found San Francisco's first needle exchange. I interviewed an epidemiologist, now a small-batch vintner, who wrote some of the earliest papers on bleach.

Finally, I spoke with Jennifer Lorvick—now a sociologist, then the administrator of the collaborative that created "bleach and teach." Others had suggested that my mystery woman might have been Lorvick herself or Moher Downing, another early S.F. needle exchanger. Lorvick hadn't visited New York at the right time, however. And Downing had purple hair, which would have been a very hard thing for me not to notice, even in the state I was in when I had that conversation.

"So, it was a woman and it was 1986?" Lorvick asked about the person I was looking for. "Yeah, and she was white and that's about all I can remember," I replied.

"Was it Maureen? Was she British?" That was indeed an Irish name. I said yeah, that was possible. And so Lorvick helped me get in touch.

Oddly enough, however, when I finally reached Gammon on the phone, it didn't click at first for her that she was the person I was trying to find.

I gave her the backstory. I told her about the woman I sought, whose friend in New York needed treatment in 1986. At first, she didn't recall any such incident. But I continued the interview, simply hoping to get a few more anecdotes about the early days of AIDS work on the West Coast.

Later in the conversation, though, she casually mentioned visiting New York to see a boyfriend—and thereby helping him get into rehab. She'd been thrown by the fact that I'd said friend, rather than boyfriend. By then, we'd established that the chronology would fit, and it struck me immediately.

I started crying and soon she did, too, as we began to piece our memories together. We were both so overwhelmed that we decided we'd have to continue the conversation after we'd both had more time to compose ourselves.

But it hit her immediately that ours was a story of how change happens and how even the smallest things we do can sometimes make a tremendous difference. And when we talked again, I was reminded of a parable I'd often heard about a child who comes across thousands of starfish stranded on a beach. She tosses them, one by one, back into the sea. Another person comes by and asks why she is bothering and whether she could genuinely make a difference when there are far too many to save. "It matters to this one," she says, as she throws another one home.

This also brought to mind the wisdom of the Talmud, which says that saving one life is equivalent to saving the entire world. These ideas are at the very heart of harm reduction, which takes the perspective that every life is worth saving. Maureen's simple, kind act of teaching me to protect myself allowed me to survive until I was able to recover from addiction and probably allowed me to do much of the work I've done since. Her actions also meant that I was there to cover American harm reduction, from its earliest days until now.

AS WAS THE CASE WITH HIV INITIALLY, THE RISING TOLL OF OUR CURRENT overdose epidemic seems inexorable. Nearly a million people—mothers, fathers, friends, siblings, children—have died of overdose since 1999, and several million more continue to be at risk daily. Before the COVID-19 pandemic hit, many had thought we might be at a turning point, but now it is clear that it was only a plateau before a further rise. Between June 2019 and June 2020, provisional statistics showed a 21 percent increase in deaths, for a total of 81,000 lost. That is the highest overdose toll ever— and epidemiologists expect the data from the rest of 2020 to be even worse.

Today, overdoses kill more Americans annually than guns, cars, or breast cancer. Most of these deaths involve mixtures of drugs, typically including an illegal opioid like heroin or illegally manufactured fentanyl, although recently cocaine- and methamphetamine-related overdose deaths have jumped as well. Meanwhile, journalists and politicians flit from targeting one demon drug to the next, only just beginning to acknowledge the unspoken despair that drives the desire for oblivion.

And as the pandemic has heightened addiction and overdose risk even further, people like me who are knowledgeable about addiction hear frequent pleas from desperate family members and friends. Often, we have little to offer to guide them. In practice, our health care system and criminal justice policies overwhelmingly reject or, at minimum, inappropriately restrict the approaches that have been proven to work. Most of what we do is not only ineffective but actively harmful. For instance, by drastically cutting opioid prescribing in the early twenty-first century without offering alternative care, we have increased disability in many pain patients— driving some to suicide—while escalating overdose deaths even further by pushing addicted people to more dangerous street drugs. Our policies often make things worse.

Fortunately, harm reduction provides reason for hope. Developed and championed by an outcast group of people who use drugs and by former users and public health geeks, it offers guidance on how to save lives. And it provides a way of understanding behavior and culture that has relevance far beyond drugs. Harm reduction is an important guide to all types of policy. It's really a philosophy for living.

The harm reduction revolution has hidden in plain sight. Like the Beatles, it was born in the British port city of Liverpool and ultimately went global. Despite its relative obscurity in the American media, this new paradigm has begun to break through the deadlock of the drug war.

And as fentanyl and similar cheap, easily made synthetic opioids have spread—many of which are hundreds or even thousands of times more potent than heroin—they are irrevocably altering global drug markets. Harm reduction offers the only clear guide to managing the inevitable and potentially frightful future of drugs.

The concept itself is surprisingly simple. Harm reduction applies the core of the Hippocratic oath—first, do no harm—to addiction treatment and drug policy. This takes the focus off of psychoactive drug use itself, which is a human universal, found across cultures, history, and even across species (catnip, for example). Instead, this approach works to minimize the damage that may be associated with substance use. By reframing drug policy to target harm rather than highs, harm reductionists have popularized once-radical ideas and forever altered the debate.

That's because, fundamentally, when protecting life and health is made the measure of success, it becomes difficult to ignore the intense damage done by drug policy itself. Once the negative consequences of policy actions count in evaluating their usefulness—and success isn't just tallied by the amounts of drugs seized or the numbers of people arrested— it is quite hard to avoid concluding that the damage done by prohibition outweighs any benefits the war on (some) drugs could conceivably have. And the harm reduction philosophy can be used to weigh risks in other policy areas where human behavior matters, too.

In essence, harm reduction is radical empathy. The basic idea is that regardless of whether people continue to use illegal drugs or engage in other problematic behaviors, their lives have value. While that may seem obvious and even banal, the reality of our drug laws is that the moral crusade against these substances has repeatedly taken priority over protecting life and health. We must change, indeed, undo our concept of drugs if we are to move forward.

In the name of "sending the right message" about certain drugs, we have caged people for decades, separated them from their children, taken their property, denied them scholarships, medical care, housing, and other benefits, including food. We have deliberately allowed the spread of fatal diseases like HIV by denying access to clean needles and even information about how to reduce risk.

During alcohol Prohibition, the federal government forced manufacturers to poison industrial alcohol—despite knowing that it was being diverted for human consumption—killing thousands. The deaths were the point; they were meant to deter others. Stopping an evil drug from theoretically corrupting children mattered more than the lives of the actual people who were already using it. And right now, we are allowing many more folks to die from illicitly manufactured fentanyl and similar analogs, rather than taking immediate, practical measures that would preserve life.

Outside of the drugs field, of course, harm reduction has a history at least as old as medicine: the Hippocratic oath, first recorded in the fifth century BC, stresses that a doctor's first goal is not to cure illness. Instead, the physician's most important job is not to make the patient worse. It seems that ever since the first humans tried to heal sickness and injury, there were drugs, therapies, and surgeries that were worse than the ailments they aimed to treat, which exacerbated the problem and sometimes even killed the patient.

In other realms, many strategies can also retrospectively be seen as harm reduction. Using shields, armor, and other kinds of barriers to protect soldiers in battle is clearly a way to at least attempt to make a highly dangerous activity less deadly. Seat belts and a whole variety of auto safety devices are other highly visible examples. Physicians wear masks and other protective gear in the operating room—and during the deadly 1918 flu and once again today, we wear them to reduce risk from respiratory viruses.

People who engage in every type of risky activity and industry have devices and practices that are used to temper risk—whether it's space travel, explosive or caustic chemistry research, studying lethal infectious agents, or engaging in risky sports like mountaineering, skydiving, deep-sea diving, or even mainstream sports like football or baseball. And, when it comes to substance use, campaigns like having a "designated driver" to avoid drunk driving and using an experienced "guide" to accompany psychedelic trippers developed decades before the harm reduction movement that would eventually claim them began.

Modern harm reduction arose in response to the AIDS pandemic. It was driven and created both by people who take drugs and by other advocates, public health workers, and physicians who saw the disaster that HIV spread by unsterile syringes could cause. In this book, you'll meet a cadre of colorful activists and groups, all of whom shaped harm reduction and helped it to become a global movement. While there are many scientists and other professionals whose stories should also be told, I've focused here on activists who not only helped create and develop the idea of harm reduction, but also made it into a social and political force. Through their stories, we'll see what harm reduction is, how it works, and how it moved from the fringe to the mainstream.

Among them are:

A driven Puerto Rican activist who stirred up hunger strikes in the Rikers Island jail's AIDS ward and spurred ACT UP to get involved with needle exchange.

A San Francisco consortium of rebels, researchers, and a caped crusader who promoted the idea of cleaning needles with bleach and saved many thousands of lives.

A group of working-class drug users in Liverpool, England, who, aided by doctors and public health officials, devised and publicized the key principles of harm reduction.

A social worker who became known as "the Goddess of Harm Reduction."

The "Needle Eight," whose arrest and trial helped change the law in the epicenter of the AIDS epidemic for drug users.

The Black harm reduction activists who stood up to their own political establishment.

A Chicago man who helped get the lifesaving antidote to opioid over-dose out of hospitals and onto the street—and a Lands' End heiress and a Seattle biker who helped him found the first major national harm reduction organization.

The Black attorney whose powerhouse book created critical new coa-litions between the harm reduction, civil rights, and criminal justice reform movements.

A group of moms facing the current overdose crisis, a mother who fought for the rights of pain patients, the Canadians who founded the most successful drug user activist group in the world—as well as the U.S. activists who are continuing the fight alongside them.

Nearly all of these folks interacted with one another repeatedly—de-spite being spread out across two continents—which makes the story of the movement nonlinear and rather difficult to tease apart. And unfortu-nately, some of these key leaders have died, which makes representing their specific views and personalities even more challenging. The crux of the matter is that harm reduction is a collective idea and many peo-ple have shaped the innovations within it. Some of them, because of the criminalization of drug use, are lost to history because they felt they had to remain anonymous.

I hope to convey here the most critical points and themes in harm reduction and to explore the lives of just a few of the people who devel-oped and spread them in North America and Europe. Please recognize, however, that there are many others around the world who are equally important whom I could not include for reasons of time, space, budget, and simply avoiding narrative overload.

The crisis that these activists faced was acute; their task was daunting. Simply to get the tools that were needed to prevent the spread of HIV in injectors meant challenging an overwhelmingly popular public policy, which had the wholehearted support not only of both of America's two parties but also the media and a large majority of the public.

We now recognize the utter failure of the drug war—in part because of the rise of harm reduction. But to understand the roots of the movement, we must remember just how popular harsh crackdowns on drugs, dealers, and users were in the age of AIDS. When harm reduction was born, even the idea of legalizing cannabis was seen as extreme and radical. In the 1980s and early nineties, more than three-quarters of the population opposed legal weed. The drug war was so uncontroversial that newspapers like the *New York Times* and the major TV networks didn't see taking government money to promote President Clinton's billion-dollar "anti-drug media campaign" and insert its messages into drama and news as representing bias or being used to push propaganda. They just joined right in.[1]

There was almost monolithic agreement—even among the majority of the population who'd smoked pot themselves without apparent disaster—that illegal drugs were a deadly moral peril. This made gaining public sympathy for those we were warning our children against almost impossible. People who'd passed through the "gateway" that the authorities claimed that marijuana would open to "hard drugs" were below contempt.

It was mainstream to see people who used drugs as worthless, disposable, and deserving of every horror, even AIDS. While calling for genocide based on race, ethnicity, or sexual orientation was recognized as evil, calling for the obliteration of drug users was not. Indeed, even now a campaign to kill people suspected of using or selling drugs in the Philippines is euphemized as a "drug war" rather than a crime against humanity.

In fact, one of the things that most infuriated me before I first got tested for HIV was the notion that what would ultimately kill me was my ignorance about how to protect myself, not just the virus itself. This was especially offensive to me for its being deliberate. It wasn't just that people like me weren't being told how to stay safe out of indifference or because of other spending priorities. It was much worse. The information was being kept quiet on purpose out of fear that letting us avoid AIDS might possibly encourage some future children to try drugs. We were useful only to suffer and die as bad examples.

The CDC knew as early as 1983 that people who injected drugs were at great risk—at a time when I hadn't even graduated high school, let alone started shooting up. Until I met Maureen, I didn't know that HIV was spreading rapidly among injectors—not to mention how I might avoid it. It enraged me that almost no one seemed to care whether we even knew about the deadly disease that was targeting us.

It didn't seem fair or right to see anyone as being that worthless. One of the most critical tasks of harm reduction, as a result, is to try to get the public to see that the lives of people who use drugs do have value. There is no need to demonize them to protect children—or declare "war" on inert objects.

The history of harm reduction shows us that there is a better way— and it lies in undoing and dismantling all of our mistaken concepts about the nature of drugs and the people who take them. It began as the world faced an unprecedented epidemic.

one

Facing AIDS

I T'S HARD TO DESCRIBE NOW JUST HOW FRIGHTENING AIDS WAS IN THE LATE eighties and early nineties, before effective treatments existed. Everyone knew that the disease was nearly 100 percent fatal, even as we tried to deny the fact in hopes it would spare the people we loved. We also knew—and just as furiously tried to deny—that as the virus pulled our friends toward inexorable death, the illness itself was often unspeakably grim.

Untreated HIV unleashes an immense catalog of suffering, in countless, varied, lingering, cruel, and often disfiguring agonies. Sometimes it blinds you; sometimes it starves you; sometimes it causes cancer, with lesions, large and small, everywhere. Almost always, there is pain. AIDS can usher in the worst symptoms of every viral, bacterial, and fungal disease possible—as well as some cancers—as the wounded immune system can no longer fight the "opportunistic" invaders and malignant growths it encounters. It is brutal.

Facing this, as I began to learn about harm reduction, I was too terrified to get tested. It wasn't that I worried about my recent risk behavior. After I'd met Maureen, I bleached my works, every time, thoroughly, without fail. However, I was seriously concerned about the chances I'd taken in the few months that I'd shot up pre-Maureen in 1985 or '86.

I'd only been a daily injector for a short while when I learned about bleach—and I certainly wasn't yet shooting up dozens of times a day, as I would be by August 4, 1988, when I finally stopped. But during my active addiction, I had shared needles with at least one person who I found out

later had tested positive. That was the man who'd initiated me into injecting, using his needle—probably in late 1985. I'd gotten hepatitis pretty
soon thereafter, so there was no doubt that I'd shared unsterile works at
least once. And the friend who first injected me had died by suicide, not
long after he got his own HIV test results. I wasn't just neurotically anxious: I had real reason to be afraid.

Consequently, I didn't want to get tested until I knew I had at least
some chance of remaining in recovery if the results were positive. If I was
positive, I knew, there would be a before and an after—and I wanted that
before to be as long as possible.

Then, when I had around two years in recovery, I was assigned to write
my first article for the *Village Voice*—after many, many pitches to many,
many places. Finally, I'd have the chance to make the case for clean needle availability in a major publication, from the perspective of someone
who had injected drugs. Finally, I'd be able to explain why all the arguments against syringe exchange were flawed. At last, I'd be able to show
why people who use drugs deserve a chance at life just like everyone else
does. Perhaps most critically, I'd be able to represent at least one voice
of the people who were most affected and who were rarely heard from in
media debates about the "controversy" over saving our lives.

As I'd been instructed by my rehab, I was attending twelve-step meetings daily. I was also attending weekly meetings of ACT UP—the AIDS
Coalition to Unleash Power. The group was quickly becoming a force to
be reckoned with through its radically creative approach to activism. I
wanted to do everything I could to fight both AIDS and addiction. Ironically, I probably also felt ready to deal with getting tested because I felt
I was finally beginning to make a contribution—and that this, perhaps,
would mean I was worthy of life.

I recognized the paradox of believing that everyone else deserved the
chance to avoid AIDS while feeling that, for myself, I needed to earn that
opportunity. I understood this as part of what psychologists call the "just
world hypothesis"—or the deep-seated, human need to see the world,
somehow underneath all the inequities, as fair. But I was still under its
influence. I thought I might magically not be positive if I could prove
myself worthy. It would take immersion in the harm reduction movement

for me to learn how truly insidious the idea that only some are "deserving" can be.

I made an appointment and visited a run-down New York City Department of Health clinic, located in Chelsea at Ninth Avenue and 28th Street. The date I was given to get my blood drawn was January 16, 1990. The night before, I had had a nightmare about it: I woke up screaming, at least in my head, "I don't wanna die, I don't wanna die, I don't wanna die." I forced myself to get on the subway and show up.

I soon found myself in a waiting room plastered with posters about pregnancy and all kinds of sexually transmitted diseases. While the clinic had clearly seen better days, the warmth of the staff and the beat-up cleanliness of the place pleasantly surprised me. I warned the person who drew my blood that I was high risk because I had been a drug injector and suggested that they take the sample from my right arm, which had fewer damaged veins. A counselor went over some basics about HIV and gave me an appointment nearly two weeks later to receive the results. Back then, clinicians were too concerned about how people might respond to bad news to provide any test results over the phone.

I wrote this in my diary the day after I got the test: "13 days till I either never have to worry about it again or constant nearness of death and slow progressive decline in life quality. Fear. Fear . . . Feel sick from worry. Fear. Don't want to die." Looking back, I still don't understand how I got through those days without relapsing.

But at the time, I knew—regardless of whatever my results would be—that I had to try to make sure that other people who injected drugs at least knew how to protect themselves. To do that, I had to find out the best ways to promote safety—and highlight, in as many articles as I could succeed in publishing, the activism and practices that were already being done to help. I had to learn where the idea of harm reduction came from and why so many others found it so threatening.

NO ONE KNOWS MUCH ABOUT THE FIRST AMERICAN WHO WAS INFECTED WITH HIV by sharing needles. The virus probably began to colonize syringes in New York City in 1975 or 1976, when Jimmy Carter was running for president and Queen's "Bohemian Rhapsody" ruled the charts. But that's the extent of our knowledge. Since men are more likely than women to inject drugs, it's likely that the first to fall ill were male; however, even that isn't certain. We don't know how old these people were, who they loved, what they liked, how they lived.

We don't know whether it was their first injection or their five hundredth, whether they were using a plastic syringe or a glass one or a jury-rigged eyedropper—or how they discovered that they were sick and died. Researchers suspect that the virus traveled first from gay or bisexual men and then to people who inject drugs, but even that isn't confirmed by data.

All we can say for certain is that HIV had spread far enough from needle to needle in New York City that it had also infected three infants born in 1977—either before they were born or during their mothers' labors. All of these babies had mothers who injected drugs.[1] Their cases were only diagnosed retrospectively via searches of medical samples decades later—and their stories and those of their parents are lost to time.

The first known adult who could have been infected by unsterile syringes was a gay man who also injected drugs. This case, too, was uncovered via a historical search of anonymized hospital data. His infection is believed to have occurred in 1979. Nothing more is known about the man himself.

While the first contemporaneously reported AIDS cases in gay men heralded the start of what was soon understood to be a global pandemic, the spread of the disease among people who take drugs was insidious. From the beginning, we were ignored, dismissed, minimized, or neglected. Reporters and historians tracked down some of the gay men whose illness was first known only in the dissociated language of medical journals. Activists made sure gay voices were heard, from day one. Members of the LGBT community told their stories in loving detail, imbuing them with meaning. However, the people with addiction whose disease helped define the new disorder for physicians remain anonymous. Even their activism often went unheralded. No actors or fashion designers or even drug-loving rock stars were holding black-tie benefits to save people who inject drugs from AIDS.

In fact, if HIV at first had infected only people who inject drugs, it might have spread much further into the rest of the population before anyone ever recognized that a new, fatal infectious disease existed. Physicians who wanted to warn the public that babies were being born infected were, at first, repeatedly rebuffed. In 1981, when a pediatrician in the Bronx tried to publish case reports suggesting a new immune disorder in babies whose mothers had injected drugs, his papers were rejected.[2] Indeed, if researchers had paid closer attention to the health of people who shot drugs, the virus might have been discovered years earlier. But, as a writer in *Newsday* put it in 1988, "The average American's sympathy for heroin dependency could fit on the tip of a hypodermic needle and there would still be room for, say, a small airport."[3]

This neglect pervaded both the scientific literature and the media: between 1981 and 1986, there were ten times more research papers on AIDS among gay men than there were on AIDS and addiction. The *New York Times* had at least some coverage of the epidemic among the people it insisted on calling "homosexuals" (they preferred "gay men"), starting in 1982. However, the first mention of AIDS in straight drug injectors in the paper of record didn't appear until 1985.[4]

Later, data from stored blood samples of people in treatment for heroin addiction showed that between 1978 and 1981, the virus had spread well, virally, and undetected among New York's estimated quarter million intravenous drug users. The proportion of injectors who were infected soared from less than 20 percent to over 50 percent in just three years.[5] This pace is easily replicated anywhere that clean syringes are rare because needle sharing is a very efficient way of transmitting blood-borne disease, second only in deadliness per exposure to blood transfusions. In New York, that meant thousands of people were at great risk.

But few seemed to care. A few more dead "junkies"? So what? Drug-war-crazed politicians insisted that addicted people chose their "lifestyle"—along with its high mortality risk. Their crusade demanded a high death toll from drugs to justify the extreme prison sentences, constriction of civil liberties, invasive searches, mass incarceration, and other penalties it imposed. Even recovery groups like Narcotics Anonymous were nihilistic. A commonly heard slogan was "Some must die so that others may live."

At the same time, those who tried to argue that addiction is a disease did so within a social and political context that accepted its criminalization without question. While experts often claimed that we must view addiction as a medical disorder, they simultaneously talked about how it made people into liars, thieves, muggers, and murderers—and why the threat of prison was required for effective treatment. Disease theorists also had to make their case within a coercive and highly punitive treatment system, which typically focused on having patients find a higher power, take moral inventory, and face their "defects of character" by working the twelve steps—hardly a nonjudgmental clinical approach.

In essence, the equivalent of a death penalty for people who take unsanctioned drugs was acceptable and unremarkable before and while AIDS was first hitting the United States. In 1990, the Los Angeles police chief actually proposed to the Senate that "casual" drug users should be "taken out and shot."[6] Few thought about how odd it was that equally or more dangerous substances were advertised and sold legally with quality controls—while it was okay, even admirable, to let users of other substances die to "send a message." Certainly, calling for us to be actively exterminated was seen as a bit extreme—but it was not as far outside the mainstream of politics as it would be to call for the deliberate killing of any other group of people.

This war on certain drugs had begun in 1914, with the Harrison Narcotics Act, which banned nonmedical use of cocaine and morphine and prohibited opium outright. It was escalated by the Nixon administration, starting in 1971, and was further expanded by Ronald Reagan and George H. W. Bush in the 1980s. And it was funded even more extravagantly by Bill Clinton in the 1990s. The drug war was generally viewed as wholly justified because alcohol, caffeine, and nicotine weren't perceived as drugs at all. And questioning it in the late 1980s and early nineties was like attacking motherhood and bashing apple pie. Anyone who did so risked being tagged as a traitor who wanted to hook American children on poison and destroy the greatest country in the world.

Gay rights had become a political cause and a movement long before AIDS hit, blossoming after the Stonewall riots of June 1969. However, it would take the HIV pandemic to spur widespread activism to argue for the inherent humanity and the value of the lives of people who take drugs. That's a core message of harm reduction—and the activists who spread it began to do so as AIDS cases and deaths among people who use drugs began to skyrocket.

YOLANDA SERRANO SUSPECTED THAT THE GRAVE ILLNESS SHE WAS SEEING IN her clients was the same plague that had begun devastating gay men. In 1981, she was working at Long Island College Hospital in Brooklyn[7] as an addiction counselor in methadone treatment. Unlike many methadone counselors, whom patients often visit grudgingly because they are required to do so, Serrano was well liked. Instead of coming just once a month or once a week, some of her clients saw her much more frequently. In fact, people who were assigned to other counselors would often request Serrano instead.

Serrano stood out because she so clearly cared. She wasn't just punching the clock on a job that often paid little more than minimum wage and was almost as stigmatized as its clients. She was the rare counselor who would attend court dates or welfare appointments to guide people through the often-hostile bureaucracy. She knew names and family members and likes and dislikes, not just methadone doses and urine test results.

But more than ever before, the people she treated were sickening and dying. They weren't overdosing or being killed by the typical infections that can result from unsterile injection technique. These folks were withering away, becoming weak, getting one rare disease after another—only sometimes barely recovering for a bit before they began declining again. "It's hard," she told a journalist. "You see people for five years, six years, they start losing weight . . . The whole thing is their braveness. I've not seen one of them who hasn't been brave."[8]

Serrano, who favored oversize glasses and short haircuts, was born in Puerto Rico but grew up an "army brat" all over the United States. By age thirteen, she'd lived in Arizona, Alabama, and Missouri, shunted to the "colored" drinking fountains in the segregated South. In 1961, her family settled down in Brooklyn. Both her parents were driven: her father once held three jobs at the same time, and her mother worked for the New York City Board of Education while she raised two daughters.[9]

Unfortunately, Serrano herself married young and disastrously. When she tried to leave her abusive husband, he broke into her apartment and tried to kill her. Not long afterward, he was arrested, convicted, and sent to prison. By that point, she had two young daughters of her own. "I was the only one in the family who wound up on welfare," she said.[10]

As soon as she could, she began working and going to school, graduating from St. Francis College in Brooklyn and pursuing a career in social services. Before becoming a methadone counselor, she had worked in the narcotics office of the Brooklyn District Attorney and at the Victim Services Agency, with others who, like her, had survived domestic violence or other crimes.[11]

And then her clients began dying, so many, so young. In late 1985, she was invited to a series of meetings held at the New York state agency that oversaw addiction treatment. Under the leadership of a Latino man who had overcome heroin addiction himself, this agency had preferentially hired many others with similar personal experience. One of these employees had become concerned about the lack of a voice for drug injectors in the AIDS crisis. He knew that a state agency couldn't do advocacy, but he hoped to start a group that could. He invited treatment providers, researchers, and other people in recovery to help set the idea in motion. Their first meeting was held on Halloween of 1985 at the state's offices on the sixty-seventh floor of the World Trade Center, with a sweeping view over the Statue of Liberty.[12]

Everyone, including Serrano, agreed that an advocacy group was necessary. And so they decided to revive an organization of former IV drug users and professionals who worked in the addictions field, known as the Association for Drug Abuse Prevention and Treatment (ADAPT). Originally organized in 1979 to try to unite the often-warring advocates for different therapeutic approaches to addiction in order to seek greater funding together, it had not succeeded in bridging those gaps. But the shell left of ADAPT had the critical advantage of having an existing organizational structure, a few hundred dollars in the bank, and the IRS designation that allowed it to accept tax-free donations and get government grants. Before long, Serrano was hired to be its executive director, and a social worker and former drug injector named Edith Springer (remember that name!) became the chair of its board.

By 1986, ADAPT members were providing "buddy" services to people who were ill, visiting them in hospitals, bringing food and soft pajamas, trying to make them feel just a little better. Because one of ADAPT's leaders worked at Rikers Island, members were able to start visiting the city's massive jail almost immediately after the group was revived.

There, they came upon some of the worst atrocities of the epidemic—and began fighting for change. While New York state had recognized that AIDS was a crisis for people with addiction, not just gay men, unfortunately most treatment centers, at first, just buried their heads in the sand.

Consequently, people who injected drugs were actively rejected by nearly all of society's institutions, including those that were supposedly designed to save and serve us. Addiction treatment programs initially expelled or simply refused to admit HIV-positive folks. Many twelve-step support groups shushed discussion of the virus as an irrelevant "outside issue," which should be kept quiet to keep the focus on addiction. When I tried to post flyers about using bleach to clean needles at the methadone program I attended in 1988, I was told it wasn't permitted because that might encourage people to relapse. Even family members were encouraged to reject us: that would supposedly help us to "hit bottom." In reality, it meant that many of us died alone.

Jails, however, didn't have the option of refusing to take prisoners. AIDS hit Rikers Island—which during these years held 10,000 to 20,000 people at any given point—long before the disease was recognized.[13] Brooklyn's SUNY Downstate Medical Center had begun seeing cases of what we now know to be HIV infection by the late 1970s. By 1978, medical staff there had already identified a syndrome of fevers, night sweats, swollen lymph nodes, and extreme weight loss. They called it "Rikers Island adenopathy," and didn't realize it was a new infectious disease.[14]

During the late seventies and early eighties, rates of death among injection drug users soared. People on the street talked about "junkie pneumonia" or, more poetically, "the dwindles." AIDS doctors at San Francisco General Hospital, too, would later recall unexplained fevers that they'd seen start to pop up among drug users in the late 1970s. Emaciated, sickly drug users, however, weren't seen as anything new. Only years later did they recognize that these cases had probably been HIV infections.[15]

When officials did finally recognize that there was an epidemic afoot at Rikers, however, they began segregating the sickest patients. Keep in mind that around two-thirds of the jail's incarcerated population had not been convicted of the crime for which they'd been arrested. They were locked up only because they were too poor to make bail. Due to their poverty, their addictions, and, more often than not, their race, the presumption of innocence was more like an assumption of guilt. These were lives that very officially didn't matter.

Nonetheless, even jaded, drug war–supporting New Yorkers were capable of being shocked by brutal incarceration conditions, once they became known. ADAPT helped organize the men who were being held in shocking conditions. They began a series of hunger strikes in May 1986. One of the leaders inside was thirty-two-year-old Michael Yantsos, whose name should be better known as an early AIDS activist. Born in Queens, he had started using heroin at fifteen, which led to a string of arrests for dealing, theft, and check forgery. His most recent arrest had been in February 1986. Yantsos became one of the first activists to make a difference in the lives of drug users with HIV.

"The wind would come in off the river and it would be a bone-chilling wind," he told an interviewer, describing how the single cells in the jail were freezing in the winter and also unspeakably hot during summer. Rats, mice, and roaches crept about freely; the ceiling leaked so badly that each cell had a mop, despite the potential for misuse as a weapon. The inmates were not even provided with bed linens, just paper sheets.

"Unbelievably depressing," Yantsos said, describing how, around once a week, one of his fellow prisoners would die, often in extreme distress. No pain medication was permitted, regardless of whether people had cancer or other excruciating AIDS-related conditions. Mistakenly giving dying people with addiction drugs that might feel good was somehow worse than letting them suffer extreme pain.

To protest, Yantsos and his fellow activists began refusing food. This is dangerous for people with AIDS: they can easily develop malnutrition as their bodies are already wasting away from the disease. The hunger strikers used their limited phone calls to contact whatever media they could. After a New York *Daily News* photographer and reporter documented the medieval level of medical neglect, a new AIDS ward was rapidly created. And in many ways, it was genuinely better, with more appropriate food, cells, and services. But it was still awful: as late as 1989, nurses sat in an enclosed booth and wouldn't touch the inmates, who were left to bathe and care for one another as best they could.

From early on, ADAPT also began providing legal support, arguing successfully for many people who would otherwise have died in jail to be freed on compassionate grounds. But Serrano and the other members quickly realized that this wasn't enough. Sitting in jails and hospitals and soothing the sick wasn't going to stop the wasting disease; freeing incarcerated people wasn't going to stop those who weren't already infected from becoming ill. Serrano felt she had to do more, even as her own family sometimes felt resentful and neglected. As her sister put it, "She's given her last dollar to them; she's left her bed to go to somebody else's bedside who's dying. She's strong for everybody else."[16]

Still, Serrano wanted to prevent new cases; she had already seen too much dying and that seemed to be the only way to end the crisis. And so the group decided that they would take the fight against AIDS to the streets. It was clear by this point that the virus was being spread by sex and by shared needles. There was no cure, and it was an ugly way to die. At least they could warn people at highest risk that they should avoid sharing needles if at all possible and tell them to use condoms. And so out they went into the shooting galleries of the Lower East Side, Brooklyn, and the Bronx. Starting in 1986, they began teaching every injector they could find to use bleach to clean their works if they couldn't avoid sharing them.

During my own active addiction, I never knew about ADAPT: the small group of people I injected with were much more privileged and mostly didn't use shooting galleries. That meant it was sheer luck that I happened to learn about bleach from Maureen Gammon. And, as far as I can tell from my research, ADAPT itself had learned about bleach from the same place that she had: the group of researchers and activists in San Francisco that employed her. The story of bleach for needles starts with a cache that was discovered behind a brick in the wall of a punk club in the Bay Area.

THE BRICK DIDN'T LOOK MUCH DIFFERENT FROM THE OTHERS IN THE ALLEY beside San Francisco's unlikely punk palace, the Mabuhay Gardens. The club occupied the lower level of a former theatre in a neighborhood then dominated by strip clubs. In some sections, the walls were painted in colors of varied intensity. Some were left bare and were irregular, dusty red, and chipped. Other parts of the masonry were covered in DIY posters for bands like the Dead Kennedys and Circle Jerks, with collages of shocking photos and lettering that looked like it was cut from a ransom note.

But to those who knew what was behind it, this particular brick hid a portal to pleasure—a secret shared by dozens of the Mohawk-wearing, black leather–clad youth with safety pins through their ears. Stashed behind it was a needle, dulled by having been used for many injections. And those who shared the works were instructed to put the spike back in the small space behind the brick once they were done.

When Sheigla Murphy heard about this semi-secret syringe, she was horrified. Murphy was a divorced mother of two young children. She'd been assigned to intensively interview teenage punks in the Bay Area for a research project, which had begun in 1981[17] as a way to understand and better intervene in youth drug culture. When one kid told her about the secret stash in the wall, she had to hold back her emotional response. She wasn't just distressed to have it confirmed that some of her research subjects were injecting, although that was certainly worrisome. What was far worse was that she knew that you couldn't design a better way to rapidly spread AIDS.[18]

Murphy has an easy, kind manner that encourages all types of people to open up to her. One of six children born to an Irish insurance agent and a nurse in California, she got the unusual "g" in her first name because her father insisted on the Gaelic spelling, but didn't want to include *too* many unpronounced letters. (Her name is pronounced as Sheila.)

To find participants for her research, Murphy had begun by hanging around outside the venue, which was a Filipino nightclub that had begun showcasing punk rock. Many of the genre's best-known bands played the "Fab Mab," including Devo, the Ramones, Hüsker Dü, Patti Smith, and Flipper. (The club appears in Jennifer Egan's iconic Gen X novel *A Visit from the Goon Squad*—insults, bottles, and other objects are hurled at a character's band, while spit flies.)

As the colorful, pierced, and sometimes pogoing crowd lined up for shows, Murphy would chat them up, trying to get kids to agree to an appointment for a longer, paid interview. By this time in her life, she was not easily shocked. Her own father had served time for marijuana smuggling after he lost his insurance job; he'd first told the family he'd begun a business to import "organic vegetables." Her ex-husband, too, was in the drug scene. He had been addicted to and sold heroin and then died by suicide in jail. Even though she now looked like the middle-class mom that she was, she had street cred, and the punks let her in.

Nonetheless, when she learned about the syringe in the wall, she was stunned. "It was in a little alleyway and you just pulled this brick out and there was this outfit and everybody would use it and then put it back," she said. Murphy knew that something had to be done, and quickly.

While most of America remained blissfully unaware of AIDS in 1983, Murphy knew about the disease because one of her brothers was gay. Her mother, who worked in the intensive care unit, had also begun coming home from San Francisco's French Hospital unusually affected by her work. Young, beautiful men were becoming emaciated and dying, in staggering numbers. It was also starting to become clear that sharing needles could be a very efficient way to spread the disease. In March of 1983, the Centers for Disease Control (CDC) first listed intravenous drug users as one of the highest risk groups.[19]

"We're just learning that you can get AIDS from sharing needles," Murphy said. "And I'm almost in tears. I mean, these are young kids." She thought to herself, "They're all going to die."[20]

UNLIKE MANY, MURPHY WAS IN A POSITION TO DO SOMETHING ABOUT IT. Determined to help, she went back to her office. It was located on Haight Street, in the center of the city's earlier famous youth scene—that of the punks' parents, the hippies, against whom punk was something of a reaction. At the time, Murphy was a relatively low-level employee in the youth study, but she knew she had to convince the group to take action, so she called a meeting.

The research project she was working on would soon become part of an organization called the MidCity Consortium to Combat AIDS—a collection of agencies that recognized the urgency of the problem among injection drug users and began to work to fight HIV before they were even officially funded to do so.

Initially, Murphy's group's goal had been to try to understand and prevent youth drug use. When AIDS hit, they shifted to trying to determine how HIV spread among injectors. But when she heard about the works at the Mab, she knew it would be unethical to just observe. She couldn't stand by and watch as the kids she had come to know and like contracted and then spread a hideous and deadly disease.

Of course, the most obvious way to prevent HIV transmission by IV drug use would be to provide clean needles. Unfortunately, that was illegal in California, and changing the law would take years at least—if it were even possible. In addition, very little study had been done of how people actually behave while shooting drugs. Treatment providers argued that drug users were too impaired by intoxication to change their behavior. In brief, no one believed that drug injectors would do anything to improve their health unless they quit first—in which case they wouldn't need needles, clean or otherwise.

Moreover, some sociologists also theorized that people who injected genuinely preferred sharing needles. They saw it as a kind of bonding rite, like passing a joint among friends.[21] Those who took this view claimed that even if injectors *could* change their ways despite being impaired, they probably wouldn't, because they wouldn't want to relinquish this important ritual. Sharing was at the core of the IV drug use experience, these researchers suggested. Although there was no data that supported this view—as anyone who injects can tell you, previously unused needles are better because they are sharper—it was soon seized on by opponents of clean needle programs as an unquestionable fact.

Sheigla Murphy knew this wasn't accurate. Galvanized by what she'd found at the Mab, she addressed her bosses and colleagues. She didn't want to see fifteen- and sixteen-year-olds in her mother's intensive care ward. There had to be something they could do. Hospitals and clinics obviously had ways to sterilize and reuse needles—it had been done for years before disposable syringes were invented—and other types of medical equipment were still frequently and effectively sterilized for reuse. Why couldn't a way be found to help drug users clean needles on the street?

MURPHY DIDN'T PULL PUNCHES AT THE MEETING IN THE HAIGHT STREET office. "We need to do something now," she said. While her bosses first discussed the idea of reporting the syringe at the Mab to the health department, they quickly recognized that that would not begin to solve the problem and might make it worse.

The group included John Newmeyer, an epidemiologist who'd been studying drug trends at the famed Haight Ashbury Free Clinic since 1971, when the problems it dealt with more often involved bad acid trips and sketchy speed. (He's also the brother of actress Julie Newmar, best known as Catwoman in the 1960s *Batman* TV series.) There was also John Watters, a motorcycle enthusiast, surfer, and psychologist, who would soon become a leader in research on HIV in drug users. Another member of the team was Harvey Feldman, a medical sociologist. Almost every day, he brought his gigantic mastiff dog, which frequently farted, to the office. It was a motley group—before you even got to the anarchists, witches, and punks who would come to lead the outreach team.

The researchers looked for processes and chemicals used in hospital disinfection that were also available to the public. These narrowed down to boiling water, alcohol, hydrogen peroxide, and bleach. From interviews with users, they knew that whatever they suggested had to cost little, work within seconds, be easy to obtain, and be as foolproof as possible.

This led to a rapid process of elimination. Boiling water was too slow—people wouldn't wait that long before injecting. Alcohol worked more quickly, but it was rejected because people might use drinking alcohol rather than rubbing alcohol, which could cause other problems. Hydrogen peroxide was ruled out because exposure to sunlight and air weakens it.

That left bleach. It was already known to kill HIV—even when diluted by a ratio of ten parts water to one part bleach. It could be rapidly drawn through a syringe without damaging it; the needle could then be rinsed with water. And it was pretty foolproof. Cases of people who had accidentally or deliberately injected small amounts of bleach—more than might be expected to be left over following even a sloppy rinse—were found in the medical literature. While the experience was unpleasant and left the person's breath reeking of a laundry room, it was not fatal.[22] (Though I will stress here, contra Donald Trump, it is still not a good idea to inject bleach!)

And so, at around the time of the first Burning Man in 1986, San Francisco would be introduced to a new superhero called Bleachman—not Alcoholman, Peroxideman, or Boilingman.

LIKE SUPERMAN AND BATMAN, BLEACHMAN HAS AN ORIGIN STORY. THE JUG-headed, red-caped AIDS fighter came from the planet NaClO (chemists will recognize here the formula for bleach). He "didn't have a cure, but he had lots of bleach," the narrator of an endearingly cheesy TV public service announcement intones. And so Bleachman rushed to Earth to help.

In the spot, the superhero, whose head is a white bleach bottle with a ridiculously crooked smile, suggests first that people refrain from drug use. Then he adds, "If you're going to use the drug, you've gotta use the jug." The ad was produced by the San Francisco AIDS Foundation. A local commercial TV station, KRON, soon began airing it late nights along with other, more conventional public service announcements.

Bleachman was the brainchild of Les Pappas, who led communications for the foundation. Prior to putting on the red cape himself, he'd worked on a campaign to discourage needle sharing, simply titled "Don't Share." That had begun in 1984 and consisted of advertising with this message on buses, billboards, and posters targeted to areas frequented by drug injectors. But, as Haight Ashbury's epidemiologist put it, "To counsel, 'Get your own rig and don't share' is often akin to giving 'let them eat cake' advice."[23]

Pappas hadn't set out to be a superhero. The child of an engineer and a bookkeeper, he attended a Catholic school in Boston. He says he feels like he "always knew" he was gay, but unlike many kids in what can be an unforgivingly homophobic milieu, he found friends who were similar as early as high school. He also found alcohol and other drugs early—and had started drinking and smoking cigarettes by the end of middle school. By high school he was on to acid and speed, but he didn't have any significant problems with substances until after he graduated college and moved to San Francisco in the early eighties.

"I didn't start injecting until I got here," he said, describing how he rapidly became strung out on methamphetamine and found himself continuing to shoot up even after he knew it would make him delusional and paranoid. He'd party all night and sleep all day, in what he jokingly described as a "vampire" lifestyle centered around clubs and nightlife.

Pappas was lucky in many respects: for one, he'd seen a poster at the Haight Ashbury Free Clinic that warned about the risk of getting infectious diseases by sharing needles. He said he'd generally avoided it even before that for hygienic reasons. Like most people—including most injectors—he found the idea kind of gross. Far from being preferred, needle sharing is generally done only when there aren't enough needles to go around.

Second, when he realized that he had lost control over his meth use, he was able to get help. Indeed, in 1983, afraid about what his life was becoming, he entered treatment and stopped using. By this time, AIDS was already a clear threat to the gay community in the Bay Area. As someone familiar with the bars and bathhouses, he was already seeing friends become terrifyingly thin, their faces hollowed out. He wanted to do something. He began working in communications—long his career goal—at the newly established San Francisco AIDS Foundation. And that was where he became Bleachman.

Pappas recalls the excitement that was generated when he put on the costume and went with outreach teams to the streets. The first time, he said, "It was such a rush." As he continued to do it over the course of

several years, he felt like he got a sense of what it was like to be a celebrity, because he was usually greeted so enthusiastically. "People would be
drawn to this . . . a huge, colorful superhero coming in the worst streets in
the worst neighborhoods. It was like, what is going on?" he said.

Occasionally, some injectors who were paranoid and high got hostile—
and at least once someone punched the costume's head. But typically, the
response was positive, especially when he used a mock-up of a giant needle to demonstrate how to use bleach. "When they realized what it was,
they kind of fell in love with it," he said. Used to being ignored or actively
rejected, San Francisco's drug users were moved to see that someone had
gone to the trouble to make them a superhero of their own. More than
once, years after he'd taken a Polaroid in full costume with someone on
the street, he'd see that the same person would still have the photo among
their limited possessions.[24]

WHEN I WENT TO GET THE RESULTS OF MY OWN HIV TEST, MY MOTHER AND
the woman who was then my "sponsor" in twelve-step programs accompanied me. I wanted to ensure that if it all went wrong, I wouldn't easily
be able to run out and buy heroin. I also, of course, desperately needed
emotional support.

The appointment was at the same place in Chelsea, at 1:30 on January 30, 1990. I would be seeing the same counselor. I had been in utter
hell for nearly two weeks of waiting: more nightmares, lots of moments of
lying awake and literally shaking from my terror of death. I kept looking
at the bruise on my arm from where the blood had been taken, which, of
course, reminded me of why I used to have marks there in the past.

But as soon as the counselor entered the small room where they gave
the results, I could tell it was going to be okay: she was smiling. By the
time I got back out to the waiting room to tell my mom and my sponsor,
they were both in tears. At lunch with them afterward at the nearby art
deco Empire Diner, I soothed myself with savory chicken soup followed
by a vanilla shake.

After a week or two of being unexpectedly paralyzed, even somewhat
distressed by the idea that I had a future again, my reprieve gave me re-

newed motivation. Since I'd been spared, I wanted to learn everything I could about HIV prevention for IV drug users. I needed to know how to keep others from suffering the fate I'd only narrowly avoided. I was already determined to use whatever talent I had in writing to try to increase understanding of addiction and improve our policies related to it. Now I knew that fighting for needle exchange would be critical to those goals.

First, of course, I'd continue working on my story for the *Voice*. Then I'd pitch other stories about these ideas to as many major publications as possible. But to do so effectively, I had to learn as much as I could about where the idea for needle exchange and the harm reduction philosophy behind it had developed. That would require a visit to the United Kingdom, where harm reduction advocates had already gone beyond distributing needles and were actually providing heroin itself to those who were addicted. It had all come together in Liverpool.

two

Undoing Powerlessness

I HALF EXPECTED TO FIND THE HAPPIEST HEROIN USERS ON EARTH AT DR. JOHN Marks's medical practice. At the time I visited in the early nineties, he was prescribing both heroin and cocaine at the Halton Drug Dependency Clinic, in Widnes, a suburb of Liverpool in the Merseyside region of northern England. It seemed like pharmaceutical paradise.

The drugs were free or close to it. They came courtesy of the U.K.'s universal health care program, the National Health Service. Clean needles, of course, were also available for injecting, but cocaine and heroin were available in smokable form as well. It was at this clinic—and at the syringe exchange started in the city in 1986—that the international harm reduction movement began. When I got there, it was hard for me to believe it was real.

For someone in twelve-step recovery as I was at the time, it was also terrifying. The very notion that people could function while still taking the drugs they wanted completely contradicted the idea that total abstinence was the only way to fight addiction, which is what I'd been taught. Though I was already starting to be skeptical of these absolute claims, I needed to see for myself.

I walked into the low brick building, which was unmarked and unremarkable in the surrounding gritty working-class neighborhood. The waiting room was like any other, a bit worn perhaps, but nothing like the carceral, chair-free, and armored chamber where I'd stood in line at the methadone clinic I'd attended in New York. Here on Chapel Street, some people received methadone and others heroin, sometimes both. They seemed to be treated without condemnation or contempt—unlike in the U.S.

And they looked utterly ordinary. Marks's patients were mainly in their twenties through fifties. They were a bit more haggard than a typical group you might see at a general practitioner's office, with more visible injuries and disabilities. But some of this could have been due to the wearing effects of low socioeconomic status alone—and they were certainly in better shape than typical street users.

Basically, the folks I saw looked little different from other locals I'd seen coming and going outside. They didn't seem ecstatic—nor did they seem impaired. One woman, with long, dark hair, had a prosthetic arm and hand that was quite realistic looking. Another, a bleached blonde, was sitting nearby with her toddler. And when the first one casually detached the limb and set it on a table, the child stared in complete shock, stunned that an arm and hand could come off that way. I'd later learn that the patient had lost the limb due to injecting tablets that were meant to deter injecting—instead, they'd caused many similar injuries among drug users.

I spoke with Sinead (not her real name), who was thirty-seven at the time. With long, dark brown hair, green eyes, and a smattering of freckles across her face, she was dressed in a hot pink top and black pants. Although she was a patient herself, she also worked at the clinic.

"I smoke a gram of heroin a day," she told me matter-of-factly. While she'd used both cannabis and heroin frequently before she sought treatment, she'd quit the weed after a year or two on prescription heroin because it started making her paranoid.

Before treatment, Sinead had supported her habit by smuggling heroin from Turkey into the U.K. She'd spent seventeen years on the street, in and out of jail. In fact, it was a probation officer who first brought her to Dr. Marks: she was incredulous to learn that she could satisfy the conditions of her probation by getting legal heroin, even if she had no desire to quit.

"I can live a normal life now," she said, describing how receiving the prescription had changed everything. No longer did she have to deal with the intense stress of international smuggling or with unreliable sources or customers; no longer were her days filled with fear of arrest or worries about withdrawal.

"Most people where I live don't even know that I'm a drug user," she told me. "I bought a house and a car and everything. I have a mortgage like everyone else has now. I have a daughter. I can show her all the things in life, make sure she has lots of activities like swimming and dancing and gymnastics. I don't think it's enough just telling your kids, 'Don't take drugs.'"

At the clinic, she'd been hired as a sort of case manager, doing administrative work and helping others find the stability and relief that she'd discovered. She'd had the job for three years when I interviewed her—a first in her history of legitimate employment. When we talked, she did not seem at all intoxicated—nor did her life appear to be one where she was underperforming or stuck in some odd middle position between addiction and recovery. She just seemed . . . fine. And this was possible because taking a steady, regular dose of heroin—or any opioid, really—at the same time each day means that tolerance impedes impairment, so much so that most people can even drive safely.[1]

Another Marks patient reported a similar experience. Her addiction had begun young. After running away from cold and neglectful adoptive parents, she began injecting at fifteen. She supported her habit by selling heroin to sex workers. "I never went on the game myself," she said. Like Sinead, she had been brought to Marks's clinic by a probation officer, who told her she could avoid jail by getting treatment.

And like Sinead, she eventually got a job at the clinic, first as a volunteer and then as a paid staffer. "I saw how the script transformed people's lives, just like mine," she said. "Suddenly, they weren't getting arrested all the time. It wasn't that constant round of shoplifting and prison . . . Suddenly, you can regulate your life."

DURING MY OWN ACTIVE ADDICTION, A PLACE WHERE I COULD BE PRESCRIBED pure, medicinal cocaine and heroin seemed like a pipe dream. Back then I sometimes thought that if only I were able to get what I needed without fear of police or economic catastrophe, I'd be able get on with my life.

That's why my first attempt at treatment had been with methadone—an opioid itself that, when taken in stable, regular doses, relieves withdrawal without producing a high. It hadn't seemed to help me—for reasons I now understand, but then did not. As a result, I eventually sought drug-free treatment in rehab.

And, in the few years since I'd become abstinent, I had been re-educated to see such a situation as a form of hell. Maintenance on drugs like methadone—let alone heroin or cocaine—could never be part of "real recovery," I'd been taught. Instead, these drugs would create a kind of misty limbo or chemical purgatory. They would prevent people from "hitting bottom" and, consequently, from finding their way to the heaven of a more authentic and connected abstinent life.

None of what I saw at Marks's clinic scanned with those claims. No one who was addicted was supposed to be able to have a decent life unless they gave up all drugs entirely. Smoking marijuana was supposed to inevitably lead to relapse into worse addiction—it wasn't supposed to just taper off when someone got paranoid. You weren't supposed to be able to smoke heroin every day and care for your child and hold down a steady job. True, the patients I met were not living lives of total joy. Some were not stable and still used street drugs—just as I'd seen at the methadone clinic back home. But those who had stabilized weren't living lives crippled by addiction or muted by maintenance, either. They seemed to have the same issues everyone else does. And those who continued other drug use were at least at reduced risk for overdose and diseases like HIV.

I interviewed Marks, who has a red beard and an appetite for provocation. The son of a doctor from North Wales, he had no special interest in addiction when he was hired to take over another physician's practice in Merseyside in 1982. "I was as straight as they come—wife, mortgage, three kids, and a cat," he said. "They basically said to me, 'You're the new boy—you can have the junkies.'"[2]

His predecessor had been doing maintenance prescribing for many decades. And so Marks began seeing patients who were already being given heroin and sometimes cocaine. Quietly, like Sinead, these folks had been going about their lives for years, hidden in plain sight.

He particularly recalled a dockworker named Sidney, who'd been on heroin for decades. At the time in his fifties, he was working and happily married, with kids. Sidney and most of the rest of the holdover patients seemed little different from those he was treating for far less stigmatized conditions. "There were maybe a few dozen lads, the occasional girl who came in and got their pot of junk. Workers, bargemen, all walks of life really," Marks said.[3]

He was highly skeptical about the whole concept at first. "I thought giving out junk was crazy—I thought we were supposed to be getting them off this stuff," he said. But when the Thatcher government announced that it had funding available for researchers seeking the most cost-effective ways of managing drug problems, Marks decided to apply for it. He hired a researcher to compare Widnes with a nearby town called Bootle, which did not have heroin prescribing. "When we started, I fully expected to find our problem would be worse in Widnes because we were giving out bloody heroin," Marks said.[4]

What the research found, however, was a surprise. In Widnes, crime rates were lower, with far fewer people needing to steal to support their habits since they got their drugs from the National Health Service. Even more counterintuitively, the rate of new addictions seemed to be reduced as well. As Marks put it, "Let's say you're an addict with a one-gram habit. It costs about a hundred quid a day. Having to go out and steal the whole thing is risky and time consuming. What's much more efficient is to find new users and sell to them . . . Any corporation would dream of having salesmen as motivated as a serious addict recruiting new users to get their own fix. It's the ultimate pyramid selling operation."[5]

By reducing the financial pressure on users to deal, prescribing can also help reduce drug initiation and cut the supply available on the street, Marks argued. Sinead's story is evidence of this: when she got a legal supply, she stopped smuggling heroin into the U.K. And other patients discussed similar experiences, like stopping dealing when they got a prescription. Rather than attracting dealers to the community, prescribing seemed to deter them, the local police said.

And, as Marks continued his practice, he began to think more deeply about the nature of addiction. He saw that when people truly wanted to stop, they often did—regardless of whether treatment was provided or not, regardless of what type of treatment they got and whether they attended self-help groups. Research confirms this, in fact, showing that most people who have diagnosable addictions eventually stop or cut down to a level that doesn't cause problems, without any help whatsoever, not even a support group.[6]

"Motivation appears to me to be all," he said, allowing that there were likely some exceptions. Mostly, though, he thought that if people wanted to stop, they did—and if they didn't, they carried on. He didn't see his job as a doctor as moralizing about this: instead, it was to reduce harm.

I asked him about the overwhelming feeling that many people with addiction have of being compelled to use, even when they recognize that it is harming them. "I think there are repetitive behaviors that people voluntarily choose to pursue, called habits, and that they involuntarily choose to pursue called obsessions or compulsions," he said.[7] But even though some people behave compulsively around drug use, he argued, it's the compulsion that is the problem, not the drug.

In response, I described my own experience using and how, toward the end, I hated cocaine particularly, but couldn't stop myself from injecting it and couldn't hold a job. He said, "If you'd never seen cocaine, heroin in your life, how do you know that you'd be any different? You might have been just as much of a zombie."

My mind was blown. Since I knew that I had indeed had obsessive and compulsive symptoms long before I ever tried drugs, I wasn't fully able to answer him. Nonetheless, I also knew that my drug use had worsened my mental health and that his implication that I had complete control over it was inaccurate. But I began to think about addiction far more broadly—and realized that there was a great deal to be learned from harm reduction, beyond AIDS and clean needles.

AT FIRST, THE LIVERPUDLIANS DIDN'T EVEN HAVE A NAME FOR WHAT THEY were doing—they just put together measures that seemed like common sense to fight AIDS and to improve the health of drug users. Their work was heavily influenced by the drug policy of the Netherlands, where needle exchange was actually invented and where the overall approach was even sometimes described as "harm reduction." But Liverpool went further: their innovations were also rooted in early twentieth-century British drug policy, which allowed doctors to prescribe drugs like heroin to people with addiction.

In essence, the idea of focusing policy on reducing the health consequences associated with drugs wasn't new. What was unique to Liverpool was the founding of the international harm reduction movement. And while many of its ideas were originally pioneered by the Dutch, it was primarily the British who packaged and sold the concept to the rest of the world.

Famously, the Netherlands had first officially recognized, way back in the time of bell-bottoms, that cannabis is less harmful than other substances—and that arresting young people for it can do more damage to their futures than the drug itself. In response, in 1976, the Dutch government created a quasi-legal market for cannabis so that youth who used wouldn't have their lives derailed by arrests, prosecution, and prison. Cannabis, while technically still illegal, would thereafter be "tolerated" by the government and has ever since been openly sold in "coffee shops," most notably in Amsterdam.

An additional harm reduction idea also drove this strategy: the Netherlands aimed explicitly to prevent cannabis users from being exposed to more harmful "hard" drugs through contact with black market dealers, who often sold more than one product. Research later showed that separating out the cannabis market does reduce the so-called "gateway" between marijuana and other drug use that, ironically, Americans have often cited as a reason to oppose cannabis legalization. Regardless, Dutch levels of cannabis, cocaine, and heroin misuse are and have remained lower than those in the U.S.[8]

People who used drugs themselves were also critical to the development of the Netherlands's drug policy. In fact, it was drug users who invented needle exchange. They were supported by Dutch drug policy reformers, who had realized early on that the problems with prohibition went far beyond cannabis. A group of such activists began helping to organize people who used drugs like heroin to fight for their rights.[9]

And so, by 1981, a Dutchman named Nico Adriaans had founded the first "Junkiebond" or Junkie's Union. A heroin injector himself, he wanted to reclaim that stigmatizing word, much as gay people have done with "queer." His group invented and started needle exchange that same year—before the HIV virus was even discovered. They were based in the port city of Rotterdam.

At the time, there was an especially bad local outbreak of hepatitis B. That infectious liver disease is not ordinarily fatal, but in the early eighties, around half a dozen users in Rotterdam had died from it. From Adriaans's perspective as an injector, it was obvious that providing clean needles would work to prevent blood-borne disease. And so, the group started handing out sterile syringes—in exchange for disposing of used ones when possible.

The Rotterdam Junkiebond had previously held demonstrations and even once successfully occupied a local alderman's office, demanding a meeting. They were angered by his advocacy for a new law that would imprison drug users and forcibly treat them. After he agreed to meet, that plan was dropped. Adriaans and his colleagues also spread the idea of users organizing to other cities. At their peak in the early eighties, there were about forty junkiebonden in cities in the Netherlands and three in West Germany—and they also had a coalition to allow them to collaborate with one another.[10] At least some—including one in Amsterdam—are still operating.

As later harm reductionists would also find, significant participation by active users is essential to better treatment and policy. Basically, it's extremely difficult to change people's behavior if you don't know how and why they do what they do and what they see as their alternatives. This applies far beyond addiction, whether you are talking about safer sex or getting people to wash their hands or recycle. If you don't know what motivates folks and what obstacles they face when trying to change, it's almost impossible to make a lasting difference in what they do.

Because their perspective is so helpful, Dutch junkiebonden continue to be provided offices and other support by municipal and national health agencies. Direct collaboration with active users allows public health workers to take the pulse of the current drug scene—and to intervene more effectively and humanely if new problems arise. The policy fits well with

Dutch culture: the nation prides itself on being pragmatic. They see this work as just another way to protect health. And pragmatism is at the heart of harm reduction, which requires dealing with the world as it is, rather than as you wish it might be.

Consequently, Adriaans's work with the Junkiebond meant that when HIV was discovered, the Dutch already had needle exchange. They expanded and scaled up rapidly in response to the threat, particularly in Amsterdam, which had the largest population of drug users. At the same time, health authorities also made methadone more accessible—even providing doses from a roving bus—with the idea that any time an addicted person used methadone instead of street drugs, it would reduce risk.

All of this work had a profound influence on Liverpool's harm reductionists. But their own country's history of drug policy was also critical. That was what allowed Marks to prescribe not only methadone—but heroin and cocaine as well. Without what became known as the "British system" of drug control, what he did would not have been legal.

The story begins at the turn of the twentieth century, when drugs like cocaine and opiates had already become widely available and sold over the counter. When addiction and overdose rates rose, it became clear that there was a need to regulate this trade. Consequently, some doctors began to treat addicted patients by simply providing stable, regular dosages of their preferred drugs. This allowed many of them to become healthier and more productive—in contrast to spending their lives chasing down irregular supplies. Such prescribing was seen as medically appropriate to prevent severe withdrawal and to allow the patient to lead "a useful and normal life," as one physician put it.[11]

Formalizing this policy with a government report in 1926, Great Britain took a radically different direction than the U.S. did at that time. Here, in the twenties, a series of Supreme Court decisions made prescribing simply for the "comfort" of people with addiction illegal—jurisprudence that haunts pain treatment and addiction care to this day. (See chapter seventeen.)

In the U.K., however, prescribing continued. And, the "British system" seemed to be quite successful at keeping addiction to cocaine and heroin medically contained for decades. Until 1964, the number of British people who were addicted to these drugs in the whole of the U.K. was estimated to be less than 350—both numerically and proportionally, a far smaller group than in the U.S. at the time. Soon, however, the worldwide explosion of youth drug use—influenced in part by Liverpool's Beatles— overwhelmed everything. Then, sensational stories of doctors profiting from selling drugs to these new, young customers became a scandal, with headlines like "Doctors who trade in misery," "Dr. Death," and "Victims of the Pusher Doctor."[12]

Due to this apparent failure, by the early 1980s, Great Britain had re-stricted prescribing to a small number of specialty clinics. Then, in 1984, they went even further. A government report based on American ideas recommended abstinence as the superior treatment. In response, nearly all of the clinics in the U.K. stopped most long-term prescribing, including that of methadone, which was the most frequently used medication.

Afterward, they permitted only short periods of tapering doses, rather than indefinite maintenance. Later research would show that this was a deadly policy change, which may have doubled the death risk for people whose methadone had been stopped.[13] Harm reduction had been replaced by harm production. In Merseyside, however, some doctors continued to prescribe the old-fashioned way. That's why Marks had been able to learn through his practice that it worked. Ordinarily, being somewhat of a med-ical backwater would be a problem. But in the case of Liverpool and harm reduction, it was an advantage.

And so while the Dutch invented several key harm reduction prac-tices, it was the British who began the movement that brought the idea to the rest of the world. That work would start with Liverpool's needle ex-change and Marks's prescribing. It would ultimately win support from the great and good who managed national and local health policy, while being driven and developed by a group of working-class activists. The spark that lit the fire in Liverpool was a terrifying HIV outbreak in a not-so-distant Scottish city.[14]

EDINBURGH, SCOTLAND, HAD A GREAT DEAL IN COMMON WITH LIVERPOOL in the 1980s. Both northern cities were facing economic collapse, as

industrial jobs moved south or out of the U.K. entirely and unemployment became commonplace. Not coincidentally, each had also developed
a massive heroin problem in its working class, with Edinburgh's scene
eventually becoming infamous worldwide, via the film based on Irvine
Welsh's novel, *Trainspotting*. But in part due to luck and in part due to
innovation, Edinburgh became an example of what *not* to do to fight AIDS
among drug users—while Liverpool became a world leader in prevention.

As jobs and hope fled and austerity policies cut social services in the
eighties, doctors working in the poorest neighborhoods of Edinburgh began to see unprecedented numbers of injuries and infections in people as
young as sixteen. Such problems were far more typical of older injection
drug users. But now, teens were starting heroin injecting earlier and in
greater numbers than ever before.

In response, city officials cracked down. Police began increasing drug
arrests. Local pharmacists started refusing to sell syringes to anyone who
appeared at all likely to be an illegal drug user. One medical supply company that had previously been reliably permissive ceased sales entirely.
To make matters worse, around the same time, the only local program
that provided methadone treatment closed, leaving most of its patients
to return to street drugs. All of these events combined created an optimal
environment for HIV to spread: fewer needles shared by a larger number
of people, most of whom were in the same small social network.

The first evidence of this unhealthy situation was again an outbreak
of hepatitis B, which led physicians to take blood samples from drug users. Stored, these samples would later help them identify how HIV had
spread, too—and the lightning speed at which it could infect an IV drug–
using population.[15]

Even before testing for HIV became available, local hospitals had
begun seeing weird cases of pneumonia, other unusual infections, and
swollen lymph nodes among young, otherwise apparently healthy people. Some even died, mystifying their doctors. After the first test for HIV
was developed, one concerned physician tried it out on patients known
to have injected drugs. He was horrified to find that at least 60 percent
of them were positive. Then he looked back at the stored hepatitis samples—and what had happened became all too obvious. The disease had

spread explosively just after the needle supply was radically cut, metha-done prescribing ceased, and arrests jumped.[16]

To get the word out, he published an article about the outbreak in the U.K.'s most prestigious medical journal in February 1986. On cue, the national media descended en masse. Edinburgh was soon labeled "the AIDS capital of Europe." Journalists began following the brave medic who'd uncovered the problem into the grotty housing estates of the city, watching as young, otherwise ordinary-looking heterosexual couples in-jected together.[17]

Almost immediately, the entire country recognized that this was no longer a distant threat—and that the U.K. could face a massive hetero-sexual pandemic if something wasn't done to stop the spread among drug users. Indeed, by 1987, there were some 1,200 cases of HIV in injectors in Edinburgh, with 300 heterosexually transmitted infections and even twenty-five infants born with the virus.[18]

Studying the outbreak, a committee on HIV set up by the Scottish government came to what is even now in the U.S. a somewhat shocking conclusion. In 1986, they wrote: "Prevention of the spread of the hu-man immunodeficiency virus (HIV) must take priority over any perceived risk of increasing drug misuse."[19] That still-radical idea that saving lives is more important than stopping drug use would become the foundation of harm reduction.

Critically, just 200 miles down the highway from Edinburgh, Liver-pool shared basically all of the socioeconomic and drug supply factors that had put its Scottish counterpart into such peril. But at the time of the outbreak, Merseyside had yet to see a single locally contracted case of HIV among injectors. Health authorities and activists saw an opportunity to put what they would soon call harm reduction into practice—if they could act quickly and radically.

three

Undoing Addiction

T HE FIRST WORD NEARLY EVERYONE USES TO DESCRIBE ALLAN PARRY IS charismatic. With a soft voice, curly dirty blond hair, and a rock star's boyish charm, he has an almost uncanny ability to persuade. Intelligent, savvy, and headstrong, he would be among the first international ambassadors of harm reduction. He grew up working class in Liverpool and began his drug use in his early teens—but would spread the gospel far beyond the city on the banks of the Mersey River.

Unusually for a British person, Parry found abstinence and recovery in a Christian rehab in the late seventies or early eighties. He became so enthusiastic about spreading the good news, in fact, that he moved to the United States and began working his way up through Billy Graham's evangelical ministry. Although he eventually lost faith and returned home, he'd honed his salesmanship skills while trying to win converts—a talent he'd soon put to work in the service of harm reduction.[1]

In the spring of 1986, Parry attended a lecture on AIDS. He had recently been hired by the Merseyside health authority to work with drug users to try to prevent the spread of HIV and provide public information. His bosses had invited a public health expert from San Francisco, who had galvanized them at a prior meeting, to speak in Liverpool. The speaker, a gay man himself, offered two key lessons. First, he said that effective prevention could not work without authorities genuinely partnering with affected communities. Top-down commands and directives uninformed by people with direct personal experience would fail. And second, the best way to fight HIV in injectors was to provide clean needles. Bleach alone wasn't enough.[2]

Given the disastrous outbreak in nearby Edinburgh, Parry immediately decided that Liverpool needed a syringe exchange program, like those in the Netherlands. He knew how dire the situation had become in New York and San Francisco—and rapidly recognized that the barriers to providing clean needles in the U.K. were much lower. In the U.S., syringe sales and possession were both criminalized in the eleven hardest hit states, including New York and California—and this was a huge political roadblock.

In contrast, public health agencies in Liverpool could simply take action for themselves. There was no similar law to stop them. And, since Parry had recently been hired by those authorities to fight HIV, with their support, he began to make plans. He'd been selected for his job in part because of the ties he had to former and active drug injectors; his knowledge of that community and its needs would be essential to the development of harm reduction.[3]

With direct input from drug users and government funding, the city could have a syringe exchange program—modeled on the Dutch programs—up and running within months. There would be, at least on the city level, no need to fight politicians before they could start their work. And so they got on with it.

On October 24, 1986, a friend and colleague of Parry handed out the first syringe of the day as the U.K.'s earliest needle exchange officially opened its doors. The young man who received the works was another of Parry's friends, whom he'd invited as he spread the word among local injectors that he knew from his past. That first client showed the program's nurse his tracks and offered up a used needle, which was deposited in a medical waste container known as a Sharpsafe. Then he was provided with brand new supplies. Initially, six syringes were allowed per customer—even if they had none to return.[4]

The exchange occurred in what had previously been a bathroom behind a reception area, complete with sink and toilet. The restroom was a half a flight of stairs up from the entrance to the Mersey Regional Drugs Training and Information Centre on Maryland Street, the agency that Parry ran. The location—if not all of the plumbing—was ideal.

The building was next to the city's methadone clinic on Hope Street, which was helpful given that returning to drug use is common in addiction, even during treatment—and also simply because the site was known to many of the local users. As the exchange grew, John Marks would take over this clinic for a time and then return to his prior post in the suburbs. All the while, he continued to advocate for increased medical prescribing to reduce harm from street drugs.

Also, fortuitously, the exchange was located in the Georgian district, a once-and-future upscale area between the city's modernist and traditional cathedrals. In the 1800s, when around a fifth of the world's goods moved through Liverpool's port, gentry and leaders of industry occupied these elegant townhouses. But by the 1980s, at night some of these streets transformed into a stroll for sex workers. Reaching them would be essential to help the needle program prevent HIV, since many injected drugs and might pass the virus to each other or to customers.

One of Parry's smartest moves was his plan for dealing with the press. "The media tended to be sensationalist, and we were very aware that they could cause problems if they dealt with the issue wrongly," he said. Consequently, in a clever bit of jujitsu, Parry and his bosses contacted the most popular local tabloid before they even began work.

"We said, 'We're going to set this scheme up, but we'd rather you didn't actually do anything on it till it had been running for a few weeks and you'd have something to report about.' And the deal was if they left it for a few weeks, they'd get an exclusive, we'd tell them first and they could get the credit for announcing it."[5]

That deal allowed Parry time to use his charms on the reporter and editors before they went with their first impressions and ran screaming headlines about the horror of giving needles to junkies. Critically, he was able to get them to recognize and emphasize the importance of the threat of AIDS, which was not difficult given the reports out of Edinburgh. Since journalists tend to be herd animals, the initial coverage set the tone for later reporting.

And so, right from the start, harm reductionists recognized the media's power. They could see that, because fearmongering had for so long been used to bolster the war on drugs, making any change would also require at least implicit if not explicit media support.

Another group that had to be consulted before the exchange became operational was the police. Here, the Liverpudlians simply got lucky: in many areas, law enforcement is the biggest obstacle to syringe exchange. But the head of the local drug squad had just been appointed after a career in homicide. "I had zero experience in drugs policing," he said.[6] This was, in fact, an advantage: it meant he hadn't picked up the typical prejudices and preconceptions that can come from being a narcotics cop.

To support the program, he agreed not to station officers outside the needle exchange, which would obviously deter people from attending. Instead, he instructed police to publicize it, handing out flyers and referring those who were not being arrested directly to the program: it was in no one's interests to risk the spread of AIDS. Law enforcement in Liverpool also continued a policy of "cautioning" most people they caught for simple possession, rather than arresting them. This meant that—at least for their first offense—they received a verbal warning and, if they were willing, referral to treatment or services like the exchange as appropriate.

Due to the Edinburgh crisis, national health officials were also seeking the best ways to prevent the spread of HIV in drug users. As a result, Liverpool's syringe exchange would become part of a national study of programs in several cities, which examined their effects and tried to determine whether or not they worked.

By December 5, 1986, 105 people had visited Hope Street, receiving 1,618 syringes and returning 1,297 of them.[7] The exchangers neither expected nor demanded 100 percent returns: they recognized that the lives of people who use drugs are often messy and that running around with used needles isn't always a good idea, particularly if they may contain deadly viruses.

The number of visitors more than doubled by the end of March 1987—to 318. Visits continued to escalate sharply over the next several years, until the exchange, its affiliates at local pharmacies, and its outreach workers were believed to be in contact with at least 70 to 80 percent of people who shot drugs in the region.[8] By 1989, there were sixteen exchange sites in

Liverpool, as well as 200 pharmacists willing to exchange or sell syringes and at least 1,500 participants.[9] And there were still no locally acquired cases of AIDS in IV drug users.

Meanwhile, Parry continued to work his spell on the opinion makers, leaders, and drug treatment teams in Merseyside and beyond. Russell Newcombe, the research psychologist who conducted the research on John Marks's clinics, described attending meetings with Parry, among audiences who were primed, even excited, to oppose him.

"I'd be standing outside, having coffee before the meetings, and they'd be going 'This guy, Allan Parry, has come from the health authority to persuade us about setting up needle exchanges in our area. We're going to give him a really hard time and take him to pieces.'" No one liked the idea that workers would be giving out needles in their neighborhoods. They were baying for blood.

But after Parry gave his lecture, there was a sea shift. In fact, the strongest opponents often emerged as the biggest converts. "They'd all be patting him on his back, shaking his hand, and falling at his feet," said Newcombe. "He just had this power to influence people."[10]

THE RESEARCH PSYCHOLOGIST HIMSELF WAS SOON AMONG THE BIGGEST OF Parry's believers. Newcombe didn't know that he was naming an international movement when he published the 1987 article that ultimately did so. But he suspected that Parry and his other colleagues were on to something big. If anyone could change drug policy and the way drug use was seen, he thought, they could. He also thought that if anywhere was open to making such change, Liverpool in the mid-1980s was.

A confluence of factors had made Liverpool unique. For one, the region was a hotbed of radicalism due to rapid de-industrialization. Riots had destroyed at least one neighborhood. Local government was led by the far left—not just garden variety Marxists but self-proclaimed Trotskyites. Known as Militant Tendency, they took control of the city council in 1983.

Such was the economic despair of the time that Militant drew tens of thousands of people to its loud, frequent marches and demonstrations. Its slogan was "Better to break the law than to break the poor," and the council deliberately outspent its budget, trying (but ultimately failing disastrously) to wring the rest out of Margaret Thatcher's austerity government.[11]

Unemployment was at depression levels: a full quarter of adult men were without work[12] and the situation was even worse in some neighborhoods, where an unbelievable 90 percent of working-class youth were jobless.[13] This made it ripe territory for a drug crisis—and, conveniently, there was a surplus of heroin associated with the 1979 fall of the shah of Iran and the Russian invasion of Afghanistan that same year. By the early eighties, authorities estimated that Merseyside had around 20,000 heroin users,[14] including about 12,000 who injected their drugs.[15] Roiled by Militant, the city seemed to have rare space for radical new approaches.

Ironically, however, it would be the conservatives who wound up giving harm reduction its support. Militant—for whom Parry had previously worked—opposed methadone and needle exchange on the grounds that they would stymie the revolution. "We are anesthetizing the revolutionary ardor of Liverpool's youth," one Militant councilor told the Liverpool *Echo* in 1986, explaining his opposition.[16]

Newcombe had himself grown up as a working-class lad—though he was not originally from Liverpool. He had paid for his higher education by selling speed—and discovered he wanted to do research related to drugs. That's why he'd come to Merseyside. By the late eighties, he was looking for a way to characterize the work that he, Parry, and Marks were doing in simple, understandable language. The key was to get people to quickly understand the commonalities that linked needle exchange with other compassionate approaches to drug users, like maintenance treatments.

The phrase that they landed on to convey this was *harm reduction*. Newcombe's 1987 article, published in the U.K.'s trade journal for the addiction field, would be the first to put the term on the map. The piece was supposed to be headlined "High Time for Harm Reduction." However, the actual print version said, "High Time for Haim Reduction." The error reflected the relative obscurity of the publication, which did not have a big budget for proofreading—and it was only corrected retrospectively when the article became widely cited as the movement grew.

In his piece, Newcombe noted that primary prevention had clearly failed to stop thousands of young people from taking heroin. Since this was the case, he wrote, these youth should not be sacrificed "to the many preventable problems (e.g., overdose, infections, organic damage, accidents) that can occur because of lack of knowledge of safe use procedures."[17] Despite the fact that such measures would undoubtedly be controversial, he argued that the spread of AIDS required that harm reduction be both tested and studied, and, if effective, expanded.

Newcombe here identified what would become a critical part of the movement. From the start, because its proponents had to fight at every turn for acceptance, harm reduction needed empirical support. This meant that while harm reductionists would not hesitate to take bold action when they believed it was needed to save lives, a research component was typically embedded in the work from the very beginning. Newcombe authored many of the earliest publications demonstrating that Liverpool's needle exchange was working as intended and did not encourage new users to take up shooting drugs.

And once harm reductionists began using the phrase, it turned out that simply having a name for what they were doing was transformative. The harm reduction "brand" took a group of policies that seemed different on the surface and wrapped them up in simple phrase. The concept showed not only what united these approaches, but it also suggested other strategies that could be tried. Knowing that the overarching goal of policy was reducing harm meant weighing risks in context: it meant recognizing how they are interrelated. For example, in one sense, cutting the needle supply in Edinburgh had been a success: there were indeed far fewer needles circulating in that city after the crackdown than there were before. Overall, of course, it had been a disaster. What mattered was not the number of needles, but the number of HIV infections, and cutting the needle supply had dramatically increased the spread of the disease.

Harm reduction offers a new way to think about drugs, one that forces policy makers to think about the broader implications of their actions, rather than simply trying to stop one substance or danger after another. Focusing on harm also necessarily means caring about the lives of people who use drugs—not just trying to end all use, regardless of the effects of such policies on individuals and communities. "Undoing" the relentless focus of drug policy on drugs in itself rehumanizes such policy. And harm reduction provides a roadmap for reform. One reason that this approach is so powerful is that it has the capacity to make policy makers confront their values.

The goal of a "war on drugs" is simply stopping substance use; in contrast, the goal of harm reduction is making people's lives healthier and better, regardless of their choice to take or not take substances. And when you put it that way, prohibition and other harmful policies start to lose their luster.

As a result, by allowing people to reconceptualize the "enemy" in drug policy, harm reduction changed the debate forever. By giving a name to this new way of seeing and elaborating the concept, Liverpool's harm reductionists started the international movement. And, by emphasizing conducting research on its efforts, harm reduction created an enormous intellectual obstacle for its opponents. After all, if studies show that a policy doesn't reduce harm, it can't be part of harm reduction. And how can you oppose a policy that works?

ANOTHER KEY FIGURE IN THE MOVEMENT—AND THE ONLY ONE WHO WAS PUBlicly open about being a current injection drug user, right from the start—was Peter McDermott.[18] A high school dropout and the son of two assembly line workers, he had gone to back to school not expecting to be employable. However, he was pleasantly surprised when he applied for an academic job and was actually hired as a researcher at Liverpool University.

Unfortunately, once inside the office of the Hope Street drug clinic where he had been assigned to analyze data from patient records, he ran into a doctor who had previously prescribed him methadone. McDermott was honest about the fact that he was still on medication. Within twenty minutes, he'd been fired and escorted out to the street.

A drug addict couldn't be trusted in a research position with access to records, he was told. The fact that he was in treatment didn't matter—apparently, that made it worse. Although the experience dashed his hopes of getting a straight job, the rage he felt about the stigma of addiction helped propel him to become one of the architects of harm reduction.

McDermott had been an obviously bright child, but he constantly got into trouble. "At age thirteen, I came across a copy of William Burroughs's *Junky* and that was quite a determining influence," he said, promptly citing the French Marxist philosopher Louis Althusser to explain.

"What Althusser says is that one of the ways that we create our identity is through texts. It's a process he calls ideological interpellation or hailing—we are hailed by a text and the process is akin to hearing a shout in the street. The text hails us and we turn round in recognition. So reading a book—picking up *Junky*—it was that sense that someone's calling you and I had no other ambitions than to do drugs."

Drugs fascinated him because he liked the idea of being able to control his mood and emotions; they also seemed glamorous. Eventually tiring of being disciplined by teachers—which could involve caning at the time—he dropped out and spent his early adulthood on welfare or unemployment, robbing drugstores and injecting opioids and cocaine.

"I was a fairly inept criminal," he said. "In 1975, I got arrested for forging a prescription. So, I went to treatment and what's the treatment? I'm addicted to these tablets and we'll give you some of those tablets. Not only do I not have to forge scripts, but I can go to different doctors and get ten a day."

The loose British system of prescribing that had fallen out of favor in the rest of the U.K. was still hanging on in Liverpool. Eventually McDermott settled on an injectable methadone prescription: injecting the drug provides a rush as it is administered, unlike the oral version typically used in treatment. Later, he became a patient of John Marks and received heroin. But ultimately, he decided that he preferred injectable methadone because its effects last longer. Being able to take it less frequently allowed him greater freedom.

Over time, McDermott's life became less chaotic and his street drug use rare. Without constantly having to chase down a supply, without going up and coming down every few hours, his life had more room for other pursuits. He went back to school, ultimately receiving a master's in sociology. Then, he'd gotten that research job, although prejudice meant that he didn't keep it for long.

So, while many early harm reductionists would reveal their personal experiences of drug use only when they were long in the past, McDermott was one of the few who was "out" about being a current methadone patient and sometime illegal drug injector, right from the start. He began working at the needle exchange next door to the Hope Street clinic that had fired him. He was soon debating Parry, Newcombe, and Marks about what harm reduction should be and what addiction is.

People who use drugs, he argued, deserve the dignity, respect, and right to self-determination that should be the birthright of all human beings. They need to be at the center of harm reduction—and to be able to work in the field and get paid at least as well as everyone else when performing comparable jobs.

And addiction, McDermott contended, is much less of a determinant of people's behavior than many of those who see it as a disease claim. The disorder can constrain people's decision-making to some degree, he said, but added, "I think that those choices are rational and conscious to a much greater extent than we like to give credence to."[19]

In their arguments, John Marks would take this position to the extreme, contending that even when people are addicted, drug use is almost always a choice.[20] In some circumstances—say, if there are cops around or they have to show up in court—addicted folks often do refrain. In others, they clearly exhibit bad judgment and take risks to pursue their high. But that doesn't necessarily mean that they couldn't have behaved differently or made better decisions. According to Marks, the choices of addicted people were typically as free—or as constrained by circumstance and brain chemistry—as anyone else's. Although Americans tend to see the idea of addiction being freely chosen as support for criminalizing drugs, he took the opposite view. Punishment and moral condemnation, he contended, were simply not effective ways to reduce harm.

Within harm reduction itself, there was and continues to be ongoing debate over just how free the choices of people with addictions are. At one end of the spectrum, people like Marks argued that addiction practically didn't exist.[21] Sure, there was what the Liverpudlians called "chaotic drug use"—where people's using results in damage to health, family, and productivity, as well as problems like homelessness and crime. But even that, they claimed, was mostly chosen, in the context of the economic and social circumstances of users' lives and depending on what they knew about how to reduce harm. Given better options, this group argued, they could improve.

Closer to the center, others, like McDermott, acknowledged that addiction is real and could significantly impair choice, as evidenced by continued use despite undesired consequences. However, he said, this didn't mean that people were completely enslaved by drugs. Instead, harm reduction could help them make better—and freer—decisions over time.

The position at the other extreme that both McDermott and Marks were reacting against, of course, was the abstinence view that addiction means total powerlessness over drugs. The idea that addicted people have essentially lost their free will is part of the American concept of addiction as a disease, which I'd been taught as absolute truth in rehab and twelve-step programs. While many harm reductionists had reservations about seeing addiction as wholly chosen, nearly all agreed that the condition didn't entirely abolish individuals' abilities to control their own lives, either.

Indeed, if people with addiction were truly "powerless," syringe exchange and opioid maintenance could not possibly have the positive results that were seen in the data. And if, as the research and the experience of practicing harm reduction showed, addicted people did have the ability to choose, they needed to be treated humanely, just like everyone else. Drugs didn't turn adults into robots or children; addiction didn't make people into some kind of subhuman automata without any ability to make good choices. Therefore, it was not acceptable to treat these fully equal human beings as if they were toddlers or animals whose behavior could be changed only by coercion, manipulation, or force. Harm reduction showed that there was a better and less paternalistic way.

McDermott, in particular, also had little patience for my initial concerns about maintenance being a trap for people, which might prevent them from achieving an even better outcome through abstinence.

"Well, that's me, isn't it?" he responded. "Effectively, for the last fifteen, twenty years, people have enabled me. If that's true, I am as dysfunctional as you get. I've constructed my whole life around the legit-imization of what I do. I work in drugs. I stand up in front of people who work in the drugs field and tell them what they should do. That's why I got into this game in the first place. It was a very conscious, quite political thought. The alternative's dying for too many."[22]

THE ELEMENTS THAT WOULD DEFINE HARM REDUCTION WERE ALL NOW PRES-ent in Merseyside—and were beginning to be refined and publicized. At the core were people who take drugs—in the spirit of "nothing about us without us," the mantra of rest of the disability rights movement. Practice was based on nonjudgmental compassion or, as harm reductionists came to call it, "meeting people where they're at." This was meant both psycho-logically and physically. To reach the most marginalized groups, workers have to go out into the community and partner with those who are there, not just expect people to come to them and do as they are told.

Essentially, the harm reduction philosophy offered the tools and infor-mation drug users needed to reduce risks—whether that meant needles or maintenance medications like methadone or heroin itself. It encour-aged change through collaboration, accessibility, and kindness. For policy makers, it suggested a new way to shape their decisions—and not just in relation to drugs.

When a policy is meant to affect drug use or any high-risk behavior—whether in extreme circumstances like a pandemic or in more ordinary situations—focusing on reducing harm can lead to better outcomes. For example, if you are trying to fight obesity, telling people to cut back on fat makes sense—unless they simply replace it with sugar. Harm reduction forces policy makers to focus on outcomes that matter, rather than on cutting specific risk behaviors without understanding their context, which can wind up causing more overall damage.

"What we had was a new 'high concept' theory—something that you could pitch to your manager or your funder in a few brief sentences and have them get immediately what was different about this and the common-sense logic behind it," McDermott explained. It wasn't that harm reduc-tion itself was new. Instead, proponents brought together many ideas from several countries and varied academic disciplines, including history and sociology, not just medicine and psychology. Most critically, they didn't just talk about their ideas, but put them into action.

"For the first time, we had a radical theory that was backed up by actual practice," he said. "It was not simply someone saying that this was how you should do it; we were actually doing it, and anyone who was interested could come along and see for themselves whether it worked or not and make up their own mind."[23] To bolster that, they collected data and published results as well. And, by immediately putting their theories to the test, they were able to gain much needed scientific credibility.

The Liverpool harm reductionists recognized that given the means and the information, drug users will tend to protect themselves and their loved ones—just like anyone else. Moreover, they didn't see addiction as a disability that impairs people so completely that they lose all responsibility for their actions and behaviors. Instead, they treated people who take drugs as individuals, able to make meaningful choices in the contexts in which they lived—and, they showed that what they did worked to fight AIDS and improve health.

Much of the genius of harm reduction is in its "branding," McDermott argued. Harm reductionists took a complex policy argument and narrowed it down to a catchphrase that was easily understood and seemed like common sense. Who could oppose reducing harm? This straightforward simplicity could unravel years of drug war indoctrination. Instead of viewing "fighting drugs" as the most important goal, harm reduction offered what is to most people a higher moral value: saving lives. It flipped the arguments over drugs and morality on their heads.

THIS VIEW OF ADDICTION WOULD SOON START TO SHAKE THE FOUNDATIONS OF the drug treatment and policy establishments. And as the fear of AIDS grew in the U.K.—and the mediagenic Allan Parry kept up his campaign of persuasion on radio, TV, and in the papers—the national health authorities took notice. The working-class group that had shaped harm reduction and put it into practice gained continued support from the middle- and upper-class health officials and doctors who had hired them.

In fact, as harm reduction and needle exchange expanded in Mersey-side, the authorities who had originally proposed it as policy—including the regional director of public health and his colleagues[24]—continued to support and promote it. In this quest, they managed to win over no fewer than three different men who'd been knighted by the queen. One of them was a close enough friend of then–prime minister Margaret Thatcher that she would typically pick up the phone when he called.[25]

This high-level advocacy helped the U.K.—unlike the U.S., where Congress rapidly passed laws to block funding for needle exchange—to genuinely protect public health. On March 29, 1987, the British government's Advisory Committee on the Misuse of Drugs released a report supporting harm reduction, which was clearly influenced by Liverpool's strategy. It stated, ". . . we have no hesitation in concluding that the spread of HIV is a greater danger to individual and public health than drug misuse. Accordingly, services which aim to minimize HIV risk-behavior by all available means should take precedent."

And soon, national and international interest in harm reduction became so great that Parry and his merry band of rebels began to be overwhelmed by media and site visit inquiries from health professionals interested in copying it. This further exploded as they began applying the concept to drug use at raves, which were then sweeping across the country, along with MDMA (ecstasy) in what became known as the Second Summer of Love. Some of the earliest measures to reduce risk—like being sure to stay hydrated and not overheat—were promoted in pamphlets and comics written by the Liverpool group and often designed by an artist colleague in Manchester.

But the constant stream of visitors began to disrupt their work. They worried that it might interfere with their clients' willingness to use their services. They were also expanding rapidly. The bathroom that had been originally used for the needle exchange once again became a public toilet. Now, needle swaps took place in a bigger room, along with other medical services. The group had taken over the whole building.

To cut down on the number of research visits and help spread their ideas more efficiently, the group decided to start a journal. Known first as the *Mersey Drugs Journal*, it was published bimonthly, starting in January of 1987. Before long, it had subscribers from around the world—and was reaching hundreds of influential researchers and practitioners. Reflecting this, in 1989, its name was changed to the *International Journal of Drug Policy*.

Many of those who seemed most hungry for information were in New York, where AIDS was still spreading among injectors, virtually unchecked. Indeed, by February of 1988, Parry and McDermott had been featured in the *New York Times*, in an article that mentioned harm reduction for the first time in the paper of record. The piece described their work, saying, "'harm reduction' is the watchword here, not only for the clean-needle program but in Liverpool's drug policy generally."[26]

The *Times* noted that since the exchange had started two years earlier, 2,000 injection drug users in Merseyside had been tested for HIV. Only a dozen were positive—and not a single one had been infected locally. The contrast between the two cities was striking. By 1988, thousands of drug injectors were already infected and at least hundreds were dying or already dead in New York. Far from stopping or even stabilizing, transmission of the virus among this group, their sexual partners, and during their pregnancies was increasing.

Parry had been interviewed by the *Times* when he visited the city. And that trip would irrevocably alter the history of harm reduction in America. While in Manhattan, he met Edith Springer, a social worker who would soon become one of the most influential people in the history of the movement. At the time, she was working alongside Yolanda Serrano, chairing the board of ADAPT and distributing bleach kits to fight HIV. Springer was already practicing a version of harm reduction, although she didn't know then that that was what it was called.

But soon, she'd do far more. When pressed to identify a single person who is most responsible for the spread of harm reduction in the U.S., nearly everyone who knows the history of the movement says her name.

four

The Goddess of Harm Reduction

EDITH SPRINGER OPENED HER HARM REDUCTION TRAININGS WITH A VIDEO originally aimed at preschoolers. It was a musical number from *Sesame Street*, which premiered in 1988. In it, Ernie, the round-faced Muppet, has a problem. He wants to learn to play saxophone, but every time he tries, he simply squeaks. His problem isn't just inexperience. It is instead that while playing, he refuses to put down his beloved rubber ducky, even for a second. His character, after all, is defined by his deep attachment to that duck, which appears in his own signature song.

This newer, jauntier tune, however, has a series of eighties celebrity cameos—from Paul Simon and Danny DeVito to Barbara Walters and Phil Donahue. And all of them advise him, in various tones, to "put down the ducky, if you want to play the saxophone." Critically, however, they also strongly reassure him that he doesn't have to give ducky up entirely or forever. And their gentle approach works.

Springer used this as a metaphor to introduce harm reduction. She'd tailor her presentation to specific audiences—which could include everyone from outreach workers at needle exchanges to drug counselors, psychologists, social workers, AIDS professionals, doctors, and even law enforcement folks. She was helping create and sell an idea, after all, that had relevance to pretty much anyone who interacted with people who use drugs or engage in other risky behaviors.

She'd often break the ice with the infectiously tuneful video, typically bringing along her own yellow rubber duck that someone, at some point, would inevitably squeeze and make squeak. In a completely nonthreatening way, the clip and the prop would get people to think about their strong attachments to the things they use to cope, including, of course, drugs.

She'd start by asking for responses to the video. Then she'd bring out the commonalities in the reactions. Often, someone would mention the fear that giving up a beloved coping tool would be unendurable. She'd note how twelve-step programs address this with the idea of giving up the substance for just "one day at a time."

She'd explain, "What this is really acknowledging is that people change in stages and people generally don't leap from one behavior to either eliminating that behavior or taking on a new behavior in one fell swoop. Okay. The reason I use this video is because everybody understands this concept from the littlest kid all the way up to most professionals."[1] Her combination of humor, empathy, and sensitivity to the needs and reactions of specific audiences made her extremely effective, so much so that a colleague began calling her the Goddess of Harm Reduction, and the nickname stuck.[2]

Her road to goddesshood began with a chance meeting with Liverpool's Allan Parry, in the warren of low-ceilinged downtown offices that housed the drug research institute in Manhattan where she worked. Her boss had been too busy to meet with someone whom he seemed to see as some random guy from Liverpool, so he asked Springer to speak with him instead.

Parry was introduced as a former addict who was visiting to share his AIDS work and learn about New York's response to the virus. Shaking his hand, Springer responded that she, too, had been in recovery for many years. With a devilish glint in his eye, he smiled and replied in his soft Liverpudlian accent, "Recovery? Where are your bandages?"

Within an hour, he had completely altered her view of addiction and begun the conversion that would soon make her one of America's most important proponents of harm reduction. At first, though, she was in tears. "He kept putting me down and putting me down for my belief system," she said. "I cried because I thought I was a good worker and I wanted to be." She soon recognized, however, that he was right. Most of what she had been trained to do simply didn't work.

The February meeting had probably only occurred because her boss hadn't known about the revolution Parry was leading in Liverpool. Springer, whose curly hair was prematurely white and who has a bright smile and an old-time Brooklyn accent, was transfixed.

At the time, she was working as an AIDS education trainer at the research organization that had become the nexus for AIDS work related to IV drug use in New York.[3] Her job was initially to teach basic information about how to work with people with HIV to social workers, counselors, and others who needed to know. It would soon evolve into training people in harm reduction—and, eventually, training other trainers.

Parry told Springer about what he and his colleagues were doing in Liverpool. She couldn't believe what she was hearing. They were giving clean needles to addicts! They were prescribing heroin! They were even prescribing cocaine! And it wasn't illegal: in fact, their work was paid for by the British National Health Service. It was astonishing.

Springer hadn't known anything about the response to AIDS in Europe, but she was all too familiar with the inadequate strategy of the United States. After all, she was part of ADAPT, the tiny group led by Yolanda Serrano. And they were pretty much the only activists doing bleach and teach and trying to fight for the lives of the quarter million IV drug users in New York, which was the epicenter of the American epidemic.

Along with Serrano, she visited the AIDS ward at Rikers Island every Sunday afternoon. They were often accompanied by a doctor,[4] in order to help get compassionate release for people who were incarcerated there. To maximize their odds of winning, they'd tell the inmates to look at Springer while the doctor listed symptoms. If she nodded, they'd say they had that symptom, if she shook her head, they wouldn't. But more and more sick people were arriving each day.

Most evenings, Springer, Serrano, and their colleagues would also go out after work to some of the city's bleakest neighborhoods, often in the Bronx and Brooklyn, to hand out bleach kits and try to teach people to avoid getting and spreading the virus. At first, she'd been a bit afraid. It had been a long time since she herself had injected drugs. It felt awkward to approach people in the garbage-strewn lots and abandoned buildings without heat or power, which were lit mainly by candles and the flickering of lighters hitting bottle caps, spoons, and cigarettes. There were needles and other unsavory debris scattered underfoot, and bare, often stained, mattresses randomly strewn around. But she pushed through her fear and was soon affectionately known as "the little Jewish lady."

"They saw that we were trying to help them and they treated us very well," said Springer, "and they were terrified of AIDS, but they had no belief in themselves that they could change. That's the part that got me, how they felt about themselves."

The injectors began to welcome Springer, Serrano, and the other outreach workers. They would even go out of their way to protect ADAPT members by walking them back through the dangerous streets to the graffitied, crumbling subway stations with their shrieking and irregular trains. Protection was all they had to offer: they had almost literally nothing material to share.

At ADAPT's very first meeting, a researcher had mentioned the bleach education work being done in San Francisco and suggested that they should do the same in New York.[5] In the Bay Area, MidCity had found out how to source pocket-sized containers for bleach from plastics companies; they knew that no one was going to lug jugs of Clorox around. They'd figured out that the most efficient way to fill them up to prepare them for distribution was to use a turkey baster. On the East Coast, ADAPT at first scrounged the plastic bottles used to provide take-home methadone doses from clinics, which were conveniently the right size. However, they were a tiny organization of just a few dozen active members faced with the task of reaching tens of thousands of people.

Moreover, bleach is far from a perfect intervention to prevent HIV. For one, it just makes needle sharing safer; it doesn't completely stop it and thereby eliminate the risk of blood-borne disease entirely. Only giving out clean needles could do that, which is why Springer was so excited to learn that this was already being done in the U.K. But despite the fact that the city was experiencing the world's biggest AIDS epidemic among drug users, syringe exchange remained illegal in New York.

And unfortunately, Springer already had close, personal experience of AIDS. Like Serrano, she'd seen it in her clients before it even had a name. She'd been recruited to her current job by a gay friend with whom she'd worked at a methadone program. He'd taught her to how to become a trainer and lead groups educating people about HIV. He also had co-created the pioneering AIDS workshop for gay men, known as "Eroticizing Safer Sex,"[6] which had helped countless men stop going through cycles of celibacy interspersed with sprees of high-risk sex. He had recognized that the same binge pattern found in addiction relapses also occurred in gay men who had tried to take a total abstinence approach to sex during the HIV epidemic. It was unrealistic to expect perfect celibacy. Far better to know which activities were riskiest and be able to act to reduce risk accordingly. He was also a member of ADAPT—but had become terminally ill by 1988.

Springer was helping care for her friend, visiting him in hospitals while taking on work that he was increasingly unable to do. Springer did not want to see the disease take any more of her people. She wanted a way to do prevention better.

Now Parry was challenging everything she thought she knew about drugs. And that was a lot, both in her personal and professional life. Springer's own heroin addiction had begun in the sixties, after her then-husband—whom she'd met at an anti-war demonstration at Hunter College—returned from Vietnam. A friend introduced her to the drug: she wasn't scared of it because the horror stories she'd heard from authorities about marijuana and LSD had been falsified by her own life experience. Why should she trust that what "the man" said about heroin was any more accurate?

Springer had had a difficult early life. Her mother was so physically and emotionally abusive that she left home at fourteen, refusing to take any more beatings. She got an apartment and a night job by lying about her age and managed to make it through high school. Her earliest experiences of drugs were in the East Village hippie scene: she lived on St. Mark's Place, where things were happening. Then, however, came heroin.

To quit, she'd entered methadone treatment. At the time, abstinence was viewed as the only real recovery, so she eventually tapered off and stopped the medication. She got her degree in social work from New York University in 1982. And during her training, she was steeped in American ideas about how the treatment of addiction must be harsh and demanding. She was taught that recovery required complete abstinence from everything other than caffeine and nicotine, for life—even though this absolutist philosophy didn't seem right to her.

Nonetheless, for many years, she'd tried to convince both herself and her clients to stick with it. Meanwhile, she watched as treatment failed, by its own standards, far more often than it succeeded. It was demoralizing. She knew that she was not the only one who was struggling. In fact, one reason Springer had left drug counseling and clinical practice was her conflicts with management. She was constantly being told she wasn't tough enough; like Serrano, she seemed to get along with the clients almost suspiciously well. Compassion, her bosses seemed to think, was wasted on addicts. If they weren't humiliated and broken and shamed enough to "hit bottom," they'd never change. Springer didn't agree, but she didn't know of a real alternative.[7]

Parry provided one. He told her about how doctors prescribed methadone, heroin, and cocaine in Liverpool, without demanding even an attempt at abstinence, never mind shaming them. He told her that they had nurses who taught safer injection techniques and cleaned wounds without judgment—and that if people wanted to inject their prescribed drugs, they were provided with sterile needles to do so.

And, he said, they had proof that it all worked. People's lives got better, not worse when they had pure pharmaceutical drugs rather than contaminated versions. Crime went down; health improved; family lives were revitalized. What she'd been taught about addiction simply wasn't true. It didn't inevitably escalate into chaos simply because people had drugs in their system. Instead, many patients eventually got bored when doctors provided the drugs they wanted. When they no longer had to spend most of their days chasing money, dodging police, and tracking down dealers, they began to have lots of time on their hands. That gave them space to think. It allowed them room to get on with their lives. In this less frantic state, if they needed services or counseling, they would often voluntarily seek them, without coercion. Under the British National Health Service, of course, health care was free.

The new information Parry provided shattered any remaining belief Springer had in the American treatment system. She had been told again and again that the disease of addiction was progressive, a position taken by the American Society of Addiction Medicine. That meant that addicted people who continued to use any drugs would always get worse. But that wasn't what Parry said was happening in Liverpool—and it wasn't what she'd really seen on the streets or in her practice, she realized. Parry's ideas made much more sense. "He decimated the disease model," she said.[8]

Now Springer cried not just because her core professional ideas about addiction had been demolished—she also cried because she knew that Parry was right and because he'd articulated something about the work she was already doing with ADAPT. She could see that when injectors were taught about using bleach to clean needles, they could and often did change their behavior. They weren't broken robots in the ever-increasing thrall of their disease, unable to make any healthy choices. They could get better, if they had the means and support to do so—even if they didn't quit drugs. It stunned her. "I was just floored because he was saying they were doing the things that we had dreamed of," she said. He had a name for the work, too—and it was harm reduction.

Before long, Springer was visiting Liverpool to see for herself. She stayed with Parry and his wife. On the last day of her first trip, she got down on her knees in their living room by herself before she went to bed. She wasn't religious. But as she knelt near the couple's incongruously elegant silk couch, she swore that she would spend the rest of her life bringing harm reduction to America. And one group training, sometimes just one person at a time, she did.

IN SOME VERSIONS OF HER TRAININGS, SPRINGER WOULD START WITH A different exercise. She'd make a list of substances on a whiteboard and ask participants whether they had used any drugs in the past twenty-four hours, telling them that they shouldn't respond until all the drugs had been listed if they didn't want others to know what they had used. At the end of the list, she'd add coffee and sugar, which usually prompted dissent.

But then she'd talk about her own coffee use and how she couldn't start her day without it and how grumpy she was if she didn't get her morning joe. At the time, coffee was believed to be harmful (it now is seen as beneficial to health, or at least neutral), so she'd talk about how she continued to use it despite that risk. She'd talk about people who kept drinking coffee even when it made them jittery or caused insomnia. And then she'd discuss how this type of obsessive behavior despite harm is viewed with other addictions. Today, in fact, addiction is defined by authorities like the National Institute on Drug Abuse as compulsive behavior that recurs despite negative outcomes, regardless of whether substances or compelling activities like gambling are involved.

Before long, she'd have her trainees recognizing that their own normal human experience is more similar to than different from that of "those" people, whom society stigmatizes for having "drug problems." They'd start to learn that substances like caffeine, alcohol, and nicotine are different only in the fact that they are legal, not in any sort of objective moral superiority or specific safety profile. In fact, bans and harsh policy aimed at particular drugs have always been related at least as much to the kind of people who are seen as the primary users of the substance as they are to the harm associated with the drug itself.

Springer was drawing on a long history of drug policy research when she made these points. For example, the penalty for coffee possession under the reign of Sultan Murad IV of the Ottoman Empire in the seventeenth century was beheading—some accounts say the sultan himself wandered the streets in disguise and did the killing himself from time to time. For a first offense, running a coffeehouse was punishable by a beating; a second offense would have you sewn into a bag and thrown into a river. But the sultan wasn't concerned about coffee "intoxication" or its health hazards; instead, he was worried—as many Western rulers would be at various times as well, with reason—that coffeehouses were meeting places for the types of people who would foment revolution. Under his rule, however, while alcohol was prohibited, cannabis was legal, as was private consumption of opium.

Meanwhile, in Persia during the same century, tobacco smoking could result in a sentence of having your lips and nose cut off—or being forced to drink molten lead or be burned at the stake.[9] In terms of public health harm, of course, smoked tobacco kills about half of its long-term users, while coffee now seems to have overall health benefits. But both are drugs with potentially harmful side effects—as is alcohol. The drugs that are legal do not have that status because they are less harmful than illegal drugs. They are legal simply because their users and sellers had the power to influence lawmakers.

Unfortunately, these facts can be hard to see in a world where we are constantly taught otherwise, either implicitly or explicitly. This was the reality Springer and other harm reductionists would have to wrestle with, over and over and over. It is why we must "undo" the idea of drugs as a useful category. Legal and illegal psychoactive substances have various risks and benefits; their regulated or prohibited status is not based on a rational determination of their comparative dangers, but on historical biases and contingencies. Failing to recognize the contexts of various behaviors and their purposes can lead to narrow policies that increase harm by pushing people toward more dangerous ways of coping.

WHEN A PRACTICE IS SO CULTURALLY ACCEPTED THAT IT IS LITERALLY WRITTEN into law, it becomes hard not to view it as somehow "natural" or even ordained by God. In fact, it becomes difficult to see it at all, especially when the body of related law has lasted over 100 years and is embedded in virtually all aspects of our culture—from music, film, TV, journalism, literature, and art to schools, science, medicine, and government. This is how the distinction between legal and illegal drugs has become in the U.S. and, due to our influence, in most of the rest of the world. It is the air we breathe, the water in which we swim, unable to see the way it directs us and shapes the way we think. Harm reduction had to first uncover the hidden history of drug laws and the truth about how drugs affect behavior in order to begin to make change.

Most people don't consider why some substances are so acceptable that they aren't even considered drugs—despite the fact that alcohol, nicotine, and caffeine are all psychoactive, have addiction potential, and can be lethal. Nor do they give much thought to why others—some far less harmful—are the subject of intense propaganda. Our indoctrination into these ideas is literally part of the grade school curriculum, billed as "drug prevention." Every time we say phrases like "alcohol and drugs" it is reinforced, implying that alcohol is not a drug and somehow belongs in a different classification.

When such language and ideology shape our thinking—and Americans simply accept the idea that "illegal drugs are evil"—allowing people who take such drugs to die to "send a message" that drugs are dangerous becomes tenable and unremarkable. Think about that for a second: we don't accept the death penalty for crimes other than the most extremely depraved murders (and even then, many view it as immoral). But we deliberately make it more likely that people will die of poisoning and spread infectious diseases when it comes to the nonviolent crime of taking certain substances.

This means that we value the lives of people who take these drugs less—and even celebrate their dehumanization as part of sending an anti-drug message. Stigmatizing illegal drugs and, by extension, the people who take them, is seen as crucial to prevention. This idea is very hard to undo and dissect because it is so rarely stated explicitly and seems unbelievable when stated baldly. Harm reductionists were among the first to do this.

So how did we get to this place? For one, American drug policy has, until very recently, been fully embraced by both political parties. As a result, when people do consider drug laws at all, they tend to figure that some wise medical authority like the Food and Drug Administration (FDA) or a Congressional expert committee sat down one day and decided that our three legal substances are the safest and the rest carry unacceptable risks and therefore must be banned. In other words, while the laws might seem odd in this area, surely some smart people must have had good reason to make them.

If only! For many folks, these questions arise first when they smoke marijuana, which about half of Americans do at some point, regardless of its legal status. Many then realize that it would basically be impossible to come up with a scientific justification for banning a substance that literally has no humanly consumable lethal dose (cannabis) while allowing one drug that regularly causes overdose death and liver failure (alcohol) and another that ultimately kills around half of its long-term users (cigarettes).

Before the harm reduction movement took off, however, it was hard for those who sought change to get public attention to focus on the arbitrary nature of drug policy. As far back as the late twentieth century, historians and academics had demonstrated that drug prohibitions have overwhelmingly become law with a large assist from racism and/or anti-immigrant panic.[10] However, this information remained confined to the academy and to those lay readers who were curious enough to seek out the few books and articles that did exist. The tumult of the sixties led to some reconsideration of the question of which substances should be permitted—but the backlash against the hippies and everything associated with them managed to completely reverse all of the momentum that was gained by the 1980s.

What harm reductionists soon learned was that the history of anti-drug laws is a history of media and politician-driven panics, some of which were linked to real harms associated with drugs and others that were drummed up for purely political purposes. The only exception is the creation of what would ultimately become the Food and Drug Administration, beginning with the Pure Food and Drug Act of 1906. This was driven by widespread adulteration of food and the complete lack of labeling information, safety, and purity standards for medical drugs. The agency created a scientific system for regulating and controlling these risks within medicine. The same systematic thought, however, was never put into regulating nonmedical substances.

In fact, prohibitions of drugs for nonmedical use have always occurred piecemeal and with goals purportedly related to specific chemicals, not with a real eye to the bigger picture. No one ever sat down and decided that the only recreational drugs Americans should ever be allowed for all future history are alcohol, tobacco, and caffeine—but there's no regulatory pathway by which anything else could become legal, only a system for criminalizing new substances. And that system has almost always been used more to fight culture wars and attract eyeballs than to create sensible and effective policies.

As former Nixon aide John Ehrlichman told a journalist in a 1994 interview:

> We knew we couldn't make it illegal to be either against the war or black, but by getting the public to associate the hippies with marijuana and blacks with heroin, and then criminalizing both heavily, we could disrupt those communities. We could arrest their leaders . . . Did we know we were lying about the drugs? Of course we did.[11]

Harm reduction upends this use of drug policy in part, by making its cruelty and absurdity visible. By focusing on harm rather than arrest numbers or the morality of certain kinds of consciousness-alteration, it brings attention to just how badly these laws fail to protect life and health. Consequently, in order to "undo" drugs in the public mind, harm reductionists needed first to teach what they'd learned about history and sociology. Many of the founders of the field were educated as sociologists, anthropologists, ethnographers, and criminologists—and this was no coincidence. The analysis that those disciplines provide shaped harm reduction from the start.

From history, the key facts are these. First, the reasoning behind the drug laws in the U.S. cannot be extricated from our history of racism. And since the U.S. has long dominated world drug control policy and its enforcement, this means that our racist views have influenced almost everyone else's.

Here it is clear that these laws were passed by using racism to stoke fear about drugs—and then using panic about those drugs to justify racism against the groups of users that had been targeted as threatening. For example, even seemingly respectable papers like the *New York Times* published stories with headlines like "Negro Cocaine Evil" and "Negro Cocaine Fiends Are a New Southern Menace," which drummed up support for measures like the Harrison Narcotics Tax Act, passed in 1914.[12] Around the same time on the West Coast, major papers ran stories of "Chinamen" seducing innocent white college women in degenerate "opium dens," again calling attention to the evils of these "narcotics."

Dr. Hamilton Wright, who has been called "the father of American narcotic laws,"[13] said in his lobbying that "one of the most unfortunate phases of the habit of smoking opium in this country [was] the large number of [white] women who have become involved and were living as common-law wives or co-habiting with Chinese in the Chinatowns of our various cities."[14] He also warned that cocaine unduly encouraged "the humbler ranks of the Negro population." The idea was that through these drugs, the people that racists feared and hated would corrupt and defile innocent white women and children.

The Harrison Act of 1914 wasn't originally intended as a complete prohibition—it only banned sales and use of opiates and cocaine for nonmedical purposes and taxed medical sales. But because opium and heroin were seen as having no medical use and cocaine was only permitted in limited instances for facial surgery, the result was basically complete criminalization.

As a leading historian of drug policy, David Musto, put it in his classic work *The American Disease: Origins of Narcotic Control*:

[These drugs] were widely seen as substances associated with foreigners or alien subgroups. Cocaine raised the specter of the wild Negro, opium the devious Chinese, morphine, the tramps in the slums: it was feared that use of all of these drugs was spreading to the "higher classes."[15]

Even alcohol Prohibition, which passed in 1919, was associated with racism and anti-immigrant sentiment: the Ku Klux Klan was a leading supporter of the measure, and its membership overlapped significantly with that of the Anti-Saloon League, one of the biggest "dry" pressure groups.[16] And it didn't involve only anti-Black racism: many white Protestants felt their power was threatened by rising numbers of immigrants from Germany, Ireland, and Italy, as well as Eastern European Jews. Prohibition was seen as a way to take back control. Although there were certainly numerous supporters—especially women—who believed banning alcohol would protect families and reduce violence, the politics of prohibition were much more complicated.

Moreover, the leading proponent of marijuana prohibition, which was beefed up in the 1930s, was Harry Anslinger, who was notorious for his hatred of Blacks, Mexicans, and jazz music. His fight for a strict federal ban on the drug was rife with claims that weed, too, would seduce white women and lead to widespread insanity among previously pure white youth—despite the fact that the cannabis plant had a long international and American history of medical use.

Before promoting the criminalization of marijuana, Anslinger had worked as an alcohol prohibition enforcer and hadn't seen cannabis as particularly problematic. But once he became the first commissioner of the Federal Bureau of Narcotics in 1930 and his bureaucratic power rested on having a huge menace to fight, he ignored the twenty-nine of thirty doctors he interviewed[17] who said it wasn't harmful enough to ban. He then publicized any violent crime or case of disturbing behavior that he could that might be even remotely linked to weed.

When all was said and done, by the time Nixon and later Reagan needed a way to stir up racist fear without being too explicit about it, they could raise the specter of drugs and call for renewed war on them. By the 1960s, illegal drugs had been firmly linked in the American mind with poor, Black, and brown criminals—and the stereotype of the "addict" as a lazy, devious, and violent sociopath mapped perfectly on to the racist stereotypes many whites held about those groups. With a compliant media, it was easy to blame violence and poverty on drugs—and not the socioeconomic circumstances that actually do lead people to problematic relationships with substances. It was also easy to spike fear that the evil drugs used by poor Black and brown people would soon be coming for innocent white babes.

EDITH SPRINGER'S TRAININGS MIXED BASIC INFORMATION ON HOW OUR UNSCIentific laws made harm reduction necessary with much more practical and detailed material on how to do it, which was the meat of her work. For those with the intellectual interest in understanding the background, she provided sources and greater depth; for everyone, she offered fundamental grounding in harm reduction technique.

For example, Springer often focused on the stigma and shame associated with addiction, which are often barriers to change. Citing the work of sociologist Erving Goffman, she discussed how he defined it and why it matters. "Stigma is spoiled identity," she said. "And if there's anybody whose identity is spoiled in this country, it's drug users. They're like the bottom of the barrel as far as everybody's concerned. Even their own families, even they treat themselves that way. They've internalized it."[18] That was what she'd seen at work in the self-abnegation of the people she distributed bleach to in shooting galleries—and she had also seen it in herself.

"I looked at my own case," she said, "I felt so stigmatized that I felt that I wasn't any good. And then, when I finally realized that there was nothing wrong with me—that I was struggling with a problem, and I was doing the best I knew how—I began to meet myself where I was at and get better."[19]

In her teaching, Springer also aimed to be highly responsive to the needs of her audience. This is essential in harm reduction if you are to genuinely help people achieve their own goals or, as she memorably puts it, "honor people's druthers." She didn't just preach attunement; she practiced it. This proved to be crucial because, given the widespread public support for the drug war during the 1980s and nineties, she more often than not encountered anger and rejection in response to her message. And so, when she was speaking to groups like drug counselors and other treatment staff who were quite likely to be hostile, she used exactly the same strategy of being compassionate and respectful that she did with drug users. "I would treat them the way I'd treat the client," she said.

Springer would start by identifying with the counselors—and with their genuine desire to help others. "This is what you've been taught, and you've been taught this all along, and you believe this and you mean well for drug users," she'd insist sincerely. Next, she'd talk about her own work in the field and how frustrated she'd been when she worked as a counselor and constantly faced failure after failure after failure. She'd put herself in the place of her pre–Allan Parry self.

She'd talk about the incredible frequency of relapse and continued drug use, about the distress she felt because she so often had to confront

clients for being "noncompliant" and how the system they worked in had
made both groups feel hopeless and suspicious of each other. But then,
she'd discuss how, from a medical perspective, real progress is often hidden by the abstinence model.

For instance, if someone stops spending all his money every weekend
on crack, but still smokes a joint once or twice a month, this doesn't count
as a victory in traditional treatment. From the abstinence point of view,
that person is "still using," is "not in recovery," and hasn't gotten any better
because he isn't abstinent from marijuana, even if he has stopped taking
the substances that were most unhealthy for him.

When an abstinence counselor sees someone like this returning to a
healthy weight after having been malnourished from the crack binges and
even going back to work, these changes aren't seen as significant. Because
the only measure of success is total abstinence, any improvement is seen
as unreliable and shaky at best, so long as any drug use continues. This
is because, in the dominant American model of addiction, "progression"
of the disease is seen as inevitable, which means that the now apparently controlled marijuana use will ultimately spiral back to chaotic crack
addiction.

The result is that counselors must focus constantly on what's wrong,
not what has improved. And, not surprisingly, this tends to cause conflict and distress. In this all-or-nothing view of recovery, nothing is almost always going to be the most common outcome—and both clients
and counselors are rarely going to feel like therapy is working. Springer
emphasized how this perspective could make what was already a challenging, underpaid, and low-status job into one that almost guaranteed
cynicism and burnout.

By recognizing the counselors' own frustrations and issues with their
work, she was often able to dodge much of the resistance that nearly all of
us feel when we are told, "You're doing it wrong." Instead, she allied herself with the people she was teaching, showing that she was on their side.
They weren't failing their clients; the system was failing them. They had
been misled, just like she had been. But there was a better way, which she
would teach them. Her gift was to teach harm reduction without tears—or
at least with fewer of them than she'd personally experienced.

Sometimes she'd show a short documentary about Liverpool's success called *Taking Drugs Seriously*. In one section, John Marks stands in a British bar and declares, "This is a licensed drug dependency unit called a pub." He picks up a beer, which he labels "a sample of its wares," and then shows some ampoules of heroin, noting that when people have access to regulated doses of pharmaceutical heroin, it does far less physical harm to the body than alcohol does.[20] Like Springer's own experience with Allan Parry, the video often radically altered people's perspectives. It showed that most of their basic assumptions about drugs and the people who take them were simply wrong.

Indeed, when, after a few years, Springer decided to use heroin again, she was open about it. "I thought that people needed role models," she said, just as people who are abstinent do. For Springer, one secret to managing her consumption was sheer stubbornness. She was totally committed to proving the naysayers wrong; to showing that it was not impossible to be a top-notch career woman and activist who was also a heroin user. "My real drug of choice was work," she explained. Regardless of how she felt or whether she might suffer withdrawal, the job came first. "If my drug use had gotten in the way, I probably would have stopped it," she said.

Over the course of her decades-long career, Springer worked out that she trained, on average, 2,000 people a year—a minimum of 30,000. She was constantly traveling, across the U.S. and internationally. Many of the people she trained were trainers themselves, who in turn trained hundreds to thousands of others. Her trainees and other colleagues—whom she introduced to harm reduction personally—include nearly every major figure in the early movement in the U.S., as we'll see in coming chapters. It is with good reason that she is known as harm reduction's "goddess."

five

ACT UP and the Johnny Appleseed of Needles

"**J**ON PARKERRRRRRRR CANNOT WALK ON WATER/BUT THAT'S NOT WHAT he does . . ." A guitarist sang these lyrics into the microphone, strumming along to accompany himself. The young musician was playing at a small café-bar on the Lower East Side. I knew him from twelve-step meetings; I was a fan of his music and had come to hear it sometime in late 1989. It was just before I decided to get tested for AIDS. I had been in recovery for just over a year.

The song has a melody that will stick in your head even after just one hearing—and I loved it immediately. But listening to it also made me happy because I had been looking for a way to get in touch with Parker —and it turned out that my musician friend knew him. Parker had been profiled on the front page of the *New York Times* on November 20, 1989. The paper of record had labeled him "the Johnny Appleseed of needles."

"I tell you his name because he is only just one man/Who like many others simply takes a stand," my friend sang. The song was titled "The Ballad of Jon Parker." It takes the form of classic folk, describing Parker's activism, which involved doing needle exchange in cities up and down the East Coast and trying to get it legalized.[1]

After getting Parker's contact information, I scheduled both an interview and a time for me to shadow him as he exchanged needles in New York City. Parker was trying to make needle exchange programs like those in Liverpool a reality here—and he was just about to engage in an important act of civil disobedience intended to help make that happen. It would come together through connections made between Parker, Yolanda Serrano, and ACT UP, the gay-led AIDS activists who seemed to be the only people who could get results fighting government inaction. I would cover it for the *Village Voice* and *Spin* magazine as I began my career in freelance journalism.

Jon Parker is not how most people would picture a Yalie, but at the time we spoke he was an extremely unlikely graduate student at the Yale School of Public Health. Known in his former life as the "Rexall King" for his propensity to rob pharmacies, the blond former boxer with a thick South Boston accent had been arrested during his active addiction at least thirty times, with twenty convictions.[2] One of seven children with an absent father, he recalled shining shoes at age nine to make money to help his mom feed the family. An arrest for theft got him two years in reform school when he was thirteen—and there he began injecting speed. By fifteen, he'd moved on to heroin. His love for opioids and other choice pharmaceuticals soon made him into a compulsive drugstore robber.

Due to these sprees, he spent much of what would normally be his high school years incarcerated. Unsurprisingly, upon release at nineteen, he immediately returned to his old ways, rapidly getting re-arrested. This prompted a judge to give him a chance to get treatment before sending him away for five to seven years.[3]

Here, Parker's life took a turn. He had earned his high school equivalency diploma in prison, and after completing treatment, he did well enough at Hampshire College to get into Yale Medical School. But in one of his classes, his old and new worlds collided.

That collision would set him on a course that led to America's very first underground needle exchange—and helped spur the legalization of the practice in many of the states where syringe possession was criminalized. It also ultimately resulted in a collaboration with ACT UP in New York, which would help make syringe programs legal here.

Parker was motivated in part by anger, sparked by an offhand comment by an AIDS expert. In the early 1980s, a guest speaker had been lecturing on the then newly discovered disease. Gay men, he said, were organizing to protect themselves and were clearly capable of changing their behavior in the face of an epidemic. But drug users were a lost cause: all they wanted to do was get high, and unless they kicked their addictions, there was no hope for them.

Parker found that he couldn't just sit there. He stood up, disclosed that he had been an injector, and said that the instructor was wrong. People like him did care about avoiding HIV infection. The real problem was that—unlike for gay men—the materials that injectors needed to stay safe were not only inaccessible, but illegal in the hardest hit states. He decided that he had to do something to change that.[4]

By 1985, he had founded what he called the National AIDS Brigade, with chapters in Boston—initially dominated by his old friends from the neighborhood—and in New Haven, which included a larger contingent of medical and public health folks. They started giving out needles, which were often obtained from states like Vermont where they could legally be purchased. They rented a storefront on York Street in New Haven as a base. All of this work began interfering with his studies: he was asked to leave the medical school after failing the first part of his medical board exam three times. However, he found a way to transfer to Yale's School of Public Health, planning to write his thesis on needle exchange research.

He also decided that he would get arrested in as many of the eleven states that banned needles as he could, each time planning to bring a challenge against the local laws. Because he'd begun visiting a girlfriend in New York regularly, in July of 1988, he began distributing syringes there, starting on 125th Street in Harlem. The following month, he was arrested while handing out works in the Mission Hill area in Roxbury in Massachusetts, setting up his first trial to challenge the law. Sometime thereafter, he met Yolanda Serrano, who told him that ACT UP might be interested in needle exchange.[5]

By November of 1989, Parker estimated that he'd given out some 50,000 needles. He'd developed a grueling weekly schedule for his work, with stops in New York City; Providence, Rhode Island; New Haven; Philadelphia; Boston; and Jersey City. The AIDS Brigade now had some sixty members and was supported by donations and Parker's earnings from driving a taxi.

Before long, he was tagged as the "Johnny Appleseed of needles," which is more apt than you might think. Appleseed, who spread the fruiting trees across the early U.S. in the early to mid 1800s was not planting them so that people could have a virtuous fresh-fruit-filled diet. The goal was actually to make liquor.[6]

BY THE LATE EIGHTIES, SERRANO AND ADAPT HAD BECOME CONVINCED THAT needle exchange was necessary and bleach and teach was not enough. New York City public health authorities had dithered over the issue for years. As early as 1985—before even Liverpool had acted, when only the Netherlands had any programs at scale—a brave city health commissioner had proposed a syringe program. But he was soon crushed by politics.

His boss, Mayor Ed Koch, who was running for re-election at the time, was attacked for even entertaining the idea. His opponent called it "harebrained." Unenthusiastic in the first place, Koch slammed on the brakes. He said needle exchange was an idea "whose time has not come and, based upon the response, will never come."[7]

But ADAPT had other plans. Several years and around 8,000 new HIV infections later,[8] the crisis was even more acute. By late 1987, the city's new health commissioner, Stephen Joseph, had convinced the mayor to at least allow a pilot study, given the enormous death toll and continuing growth of the epidemic. However, even after seemingly endless negotiations over the tiniest details, the plan seemed to be permanently stalled.

Serrano got fed up. In January of 1988 she was quoted in the *New York Times*, saying that if the city didn't move forward, ADAPT would start doing needle exchange itself. "The argument that this is going to encourage drug abuse is ridiculous," she said. "We're one of only 11 states restricting needles, yet we have the highest rate of drug abuse in the world anyway."

In the same article, the city health commissioner admitted to the paper that AIDS was spreading like "wildfire in minority neighborhoods . . . and no one is really addressing the issue." And so ADAPT's board voted to move forward if the pilot remained stalled, regardless of the fact that they might be prosecuted and could lose their funding and tax-exempt status. They had to act "to protect the public and save lives," Serrano said.[9]

Grudgingly, the Koch administration agreed. It took until September for the city program to finally start. The one location that was permitted was beyond inauspicious. Close to the notorious lockup known as "the Tombs," adjacent to the criminal courts and rife with police activity, the exchange was set up in a tiny office in the back of the health department building. This former X-ray room at 125 Worth Street was about as far from a physically welcoming place for people who were illegally injecting drugs as you could imagine. But at least it existed.

Serrano, along with Edith Springer and the small community of AIDS activists in New York who were then focused on injection drug use, had done all they could to push for it. The activists were not happy about the location. They were not pleased that it was a mere research project, only allowed to enroll 400 people, with just half of this group permitted to have needles. They were angered that in order to participate, people had to prove that they were on waiting lists for treatment. And that the program carried photo ID requirements.

However, the harm reductionists knew that it had to succeed at least nominally if they were ever to get beyond a pilot. And so, despite their weariness with bureaucratic bickering and rule setting, they knew they had to help it have the best possible shot. Any lack of follow-through or perceived problems would be a ready excuse to dismiss all future efforts. They couldn't let that happen.

ADAPT's main challenge was this: how could they get active drug users—even those motivated enough to put their names on a treatment waiting list—to come to the forbidding headquarters of the city health department? Most had had negative or even traumatic experience with the court system and the jails: not surprisingly, this area had become a section of the city that they often deliberately avoided. No one wanted to be in a place that was heavily policed, where you had to go through a metal detector and a possible search to get in the door. Moreover, on top of everything, city officials weren't allowed to advertise the existence of the program in any way. Still, ADAPT would not be defeated. They would make it work. Somehow.

On the first day, the exchange had just two customers, both recruited by ADAPT. They had the required paperwork, proving that they had been turned down by a Brooklyn treatment program. And not only did these two determined men have to deal with being right near the courts and the Tombs, they also had to get past police barricades that had been set up to deal with protesters.

Law enforcement and parent groups had threatened to turn out because they saw needle exchange as an outrage and surrender in the war on drugs. The city's Black leadership was particularly incensed, viewing the program as a cheap substitute for what was truly needed, which was more treatment. This anger would only grow and reveal the complex ways that race and racism affected harm reduction (see chapter seven).

But this time, the protesters didn't materialize. Serving as the equivalent of pro-choice "clinic escorts" who protect women seeking abortions, ADAPT had twenty members marching outside, just in case. They shouted, "Free needles save lives" and "Save the addict, save the child," referring to the fact that the vast majority of the hundreds of children infected with HIV in the city at the time were born to couples in which one or both partners had injected drugs.[10]

Though they had made it over the first hurdle, Serrano knew that the program needed more participants if it was going to be viable. She and Springer kept pressing, urging people at shooting galleries and those turned away from treatment to attend. They helped them get the documentation they needed and kept encouraging them to visit the site, with only marginal results. Fortunately, by this point, Serrano had built a strong relationship with the health commissioner, who had become seriously committed to the project. People needed help with transportation, she insisted. It took a little while, but eventually she convinced him to let them use his official commissioner's car for that purpose.

"We took the car and the driver to shooting galleries, put people in it and drove them to 125 Worth Street and that's how the people got to the syringe exchange," Springer said.[11]

Most of the time the counselors employed at the exchange to help participants get into treatment sat around waiting. But the clients who did show up were pleasantly surprised and grateful. One man, who injected cocaine and lived in a shelter on the Bowery, already knew he was HIV-positive. Still, he kept attending. He didn't want to infect anyone else while he waited for rehab. "The way I live is a nightmare," he told the *Times* after receiving a needle and a bleach kit. But the staff "really seem to care," he said.[12] The coverage failed to highlight that this incredibly downtrodden person was regularly going through a serious hassle not for himself, but to spare others.

Although it would never be as effective as a community-based needle exchange, ADAPT's efforts helped keep the pilot project from being a complete washout. For one, it got more than half[13] of the 250 people it ultimately enrolled into treatment. Second, contrary to opponents' fears, it didn't spur a new generation of youth to take up injecting because it now had the approval of City Hall.

But probably most importantly, it was the early shutdown of this program by newly elected mayor David Dinkins in February of 1990 that spurred the ACT UP to challenge the state laws against syringe possession.

SERRANO LOOKED FOR ALLIES WHEREVER SHE COULD FIND THEM. TRADITIONAL addiction advocates, like treatment providers and concerned parents, weren't at all enthusiastic about her cause. And so at some point, probably in 1989, she decided to try to make the case for needle exchange on the floor of ACT UP. At that time, the group's Monday night meetings were usually held in the Great Hall at Cooper Union, where Abraham Lincoln had once spoken against slavery. Up to 600 people would attend. The meetings were at once raucous and serious—at once chaotic at the edges and (usually) controlled up front where the speakers were.

By then, ACT UP New York was the most powerful AIDS activist group in the world—and they would become some of the most effective activists ever in the U.S., period. For Serrano, the leader of a much smaller organization trying to fight AIDS in drug users, ACT UP was one of the few groups she could turn to that might realistically be willing to help.

The meetings operated under Robert's Rules of Order, with minutes kept and read back and a strict, clear agenda. The agenda listed specific times for the various caucuses and groups planning particular actions to speak to the floor. People who wanted to suggest a new action, create a new caucus or committee, or work in coalition with ACT UP could sign up to get on the agenda. Then they had a few tightly scheduled minutes to make their case.

Serrano used her time to demonstrate how to clean a syringe with bleach, calling for ACT UP to join with ADAPT in support of the city's beleaguered needle exchange, which was still open at this point. She stressed the risk to IV drug users and the urgent need for better prevention in this group.

ACT UP, then near its peak of power, had been founded in 1987 by playwright Larry Kramer, out of sheer rage. Kramer, who had also helped found Gay Men's Health Crisis (GMHC) in 1982, didn't play well with others. Once GMHC was up and running, he had rapidly become impatient with its focus on caregiving and institution building, rather than activism. So he started a new organization, which would be "united in anger and committed to direct action to end the AIDS crisis," as ACT UP's mission statement put it.

These two pioneering AIDS groups and the differing roles they played would provide a critical lesson for harm reductionists. From their experience, harm reduction leaders learned that both insider and outsider organizations are needed to effectively change policies. Collaborative and service-focused groups (like GMHC) are necessary to work with the establishment as much as possible and get government and charitable funding to help people in immediate need.

But radicals who yell on the streets and take over government offices (like ACT UP) are also required to keep the pressure on and to respond rapidly to harmful ideas or policies. Without both, the insiders can get co-opted and activists can be ignored; when they work together, however, the results are powerful.

This kind of division of labor by organizations, however, posed an issue for needle exchange. When illegal, syringe exchange is an unusual hybrid of service and direct action. Exchanging needles to help prevent HIV is quite clearly service work: it means getting prevention tools to people who need to be protected and getting potentially contaminated syringes off the street. But getting arrested for needle distribution is civil disobedience, which is obviously direct action. The question of which kind of work to emphasize and when has always been critical for both AIDS activist groups and harm reductionists.

Early on, this service dimension led to some wariness about ACT UP participation. Fortunately, one of the members who saw Serrano's presentation was Richard Elovich, a gay performance artist and former IV drug user. He'd previously worked as a secretary for both Allen Ginsberg and William Burroughs. With deep-set, intense eyes—somewhere between hazel and brown—he had short, dark brown hair, which had begun receding. At first, he was hesitant about whether needle exchange should be part of ACT UP's work. Seeing the needles used in Serrano's demonstration had been disturbing to him, a visceral reminder of his own past.

On the other hand, he liked Serrano and recognized her clear passion as an activist. And then, not long after her presentation, Elovich had an experience that resolved his ambivalence. Anthony Fauci, who led the federal government's AIDS research efforts, had spoken at a meeting at the New York Academy of Medicine, which is located on the edge of East Harlem. Elovich attended as a representative of ACT UP's powerhouse Treatment and Data Committee. Leaving the subway to get to the meeting, he passed a methadone clinic where he'd once been treated, reminding him again of his past.

At the talk, someone asked Fauci why clinical trials excluded IV drug users. Airily, the government's top AIDS official dismissed the people who were at that point the biggest group infected with HIV. They were a "noncompliant population," he said—the implication being that it wasn't worth the effort to try to get people who use drugs involved in testing the only medications that could potentially save their lives.

"When I heard Fauci say that, I just became enraged," Elovich said. He responded from the audience, saying, "There's no such thing as a noncompliant population. I'm part of that population." And that was the first time he came out publicly as a former IV drug user. It was also when he realized that ACT UP must do more to fight against AIDS in people with addiction.[14]

But this would be a significant struggle. While ACT UP tried to be diverse, the reality was that it was mainly led by well-connected white gay men. A 1989 survey of its membership found that 90 percent of its members were men and 78 percent were white.[15] Most of the IV drug users who were becoming ill, however, were poor Black and brown people. And some ACT UP members, struggling for their own lives, were not eager to take on an additional fight for another stigmatized group.

Moreover, not only was needle exchange a potentially entangling service commitment, it was also a lightning rod for racial tension. The city's first Black mayor had made shutting down the pilot program into a major cause. Eliminating it and preventing future exchanges from opening had been one of his key campaign promises. Keeping that promise was one of the first actions he took upon being inaugurated.

AFTER REALIZING THAT **ACT UP** NEEDED TO ACT ON ADDICTION, RICHARD Elovich arranged to meet Jon Parker on one of his Saturday visits to New York. At this point, some of Parker's work was carried in a single room occupancy (SRO) hotel in Williamsburg in Brooklyn. It was located right near a clattering elevated subway line. Up a flight of stairs were rooms smaller than many prison cells with shared bathrooms and a small common area with a battered table. Everything was dingy and beaten down, even the furniture.

Parker would bring rotisserie chicken or other food, and word of his presence, as well as the appetizing smell, would quickly draw people out of their rooms. Before long, his visits were eagerly anticipated by the residents, most of whom injected drugs. Many were also either HIV-positive or already sick with AIDS. They'd store their used needles in bottles or other containers in their rooms and bring them out to swap for new ones. Their gratitude and concern for Parker was visible and almost overwhelming, in part because they were so shocked to find that anyone cared, let alone enough to risk arrest to help.

"If you see needle exchange happening, it's no longer an argument," said Elovich. "You totally get it when you see it. And when I saw what Jon was doing, I completely got it." Within about a week, he'd proposed the idea on the floor of ACT UP. An official committee to do needle exchange was soon formed.[16]

Like Elovich had been initially, I was also a little anxious about seeing needles myself. In treatment, we had constantly been told to avoid "people, places, and things" that might remind us of drug use and "trigger" a relapse. I could see how this was important, particularly during my first year or so of recovery. I'd completed an inpatient rehab in September of 1988 and had then spent three months in a halfway house in Mesa, Arizona, near Phoenix. It had been good to be away from the temptations of New York at that point.

But by early 1989, I was twenty-three and eager to get on with my life; I wanted to be a journalist and wanted to spread better information about AIDS and addiction in order to help others. (I was also determined to avoid the cliché of becoming an addiction counselor.) I returned to New York and began pitching articles about addiction and AIDS everywhere I could, while I completed my education at Brooklyn College.

Since I'd been told that recovery required it, I dove into twelve-step meetings and attended at least daily. I constantly felt like I wasn't cool enough for the East Village groups, which were attended by many famous eighties musicians, artists, and writers. But I kept going. I was also still furious that so little was being done to stop the spread of HIV among IV drug users—and so when I heard about people like Parker, I wanted to bring greater attention to them.

On March 4, 1990, when I had arranged to meet Parker and report on his work, he had already begun his collaboration with Elovich and ACT UP. The city had shuttered the pilot program on Valentine's Day. Consequently, they were already planning an arrest to challenge New York's needle laws.

With this group, I went back to the streets of Bushwick, where I'd once bought heroin. I was extremely anxious about being near drug use and sales, but I was committed to my recovery. I was also committed to proving the naysayers wrong: I wasn't just some automaton who could be "triggered" by seeing heroin or needles into unthinkingly using them. Besides, I was there to work, to report on needle exchange for a major publication, which meant the world to me. My adrenaline ran high, but I didn't experience craving. Instead, I was deeply moved.

At an intersection in the bleak industrial streets of Bushwick, where I'd more than once crouched down to hide inside a car while a friend went out to buy, Parker was soon surrounded by people. "Sometimes I feel like I'm in a park with breadcrumbs and all the pigeons come out of nowhere," he told a journalist from *Newsday*, who, to my slight dismay, was also along with the group to report.

We watched as people came by to get works. Often, they had the green/gray pallor that can be a side effect of injection drug use—regardless of their natural skin tone—but not always. White, Black, Hispanic, women, men, and transpeople, few were unrepresented, besides those under twenty-five or so (new, young users were rarely connected enough to have heard about the fledgling exchange). There was an occasional mom pushing a baby in a stroller or carriage, lots of people on crutches or walking with canes, and a few in wheelchairs.

What was almost universal was gratitude and surprise. When people who injected drugs realized what Parker and the others were doing, their eyes would light up. Many warned the volunteers about getting arrested; Parker told them he was willing to take that risk. For people who tended to be shunned even by their own families, people whom others tended to physically avoid like the plague, the idea that someone would not only seek them out but risk his freedom for them was incredible.

Parker, whose hair was eighties-style curly up front, with a long rat-tail braid down his back, treated his clients respectfully, instructing them not to share any injecting equipment. That meant not just the needle, but also the spoon or the "cooker," usually a bottle cap, which they used to dissolve and sometimes heat up the drugs in. When we went up the steep, uneven stairs of the SRO in Williamsburg, he was welcomed and greeted warmly.

Like the Liverpudlians, Parker and the other activists deliberately courted the press, particularly the daily papers like *Newsday*, which could run stories rapidly. They wanted the publicity so that the police would have to either visibly arrest them or choose not to enforce the needle law for public health reasons, which would be de facto decriminalization and might lead to legislative change.

With that in mind, for a story that ran on March 2, they told *Newsday* that Parker and ACT UP would be handing out needles on March 6 at the corner of Delancey and Essex Street on the Lower East Side.[17] Then they informed the local police precinct and also sent out a press release to the rest of the media.

WHEN I GOT TO THAT CORNER ON THAT DAY, JUST BEFORE NOON, THE STREETS were unusually packed, especially given the weather. It was during New York's miserable early spring, complete with occasional snow, cold rain, sleet, and the dreaded "wintry mix," which led to piles of graying, melting slush. Different groups were coalescing on two of the four corners of the broad intersection, not far from where Delancey Street carries traffic from Brooklyn across the Williamsburg Bridge into Manhattan.

Dozens of ACT UP demonstrators had taken up positions on the southeast corner, carrying signs and shouting slogans in support of needle exchange. On the northeast corner, around thirty red-bereted Guardian Angels marched. Known primarily for their vigilante anti-crime patrols of the subways, the group was staging a counterdemonstration, shouting "No drugs! No needles!" and loudly rattling chains. Many police officers were on each of the active corners, particularly focused on keeping the Angels and ACT UP from getting too close to each other.

I was with a pack of journalists, which included quite a few TV crews. In court testimony, we'd later be described as the biggest media crowd one ACT UP defendant had ever seen or, more succinctly by another, as swarming "like locusts."

We passed the ACT UP demonstrators from the east and then crossed Essex Street to get to where we knew the real action would be. There, in front of a Chemical Bank, on the southwest corner, Elovich, Parker, and other activists were attempting to set up a folding card table. Elovich carried a sign that read "Needle Exchange." But they had barely gotten the table unpacked and had just begun to pull out needles to distribute when the police moved in to arrest them. I was caught in the middle of the chaos, watching as the cops pulled the activists away.

One of them, a tall, gray-haired nurse wearing the white cap from her uniform, did not look like she belonged. She got separated from the rest of the group by the media just as the police began making arrests. She'd only heard about the demonstration the day before and had joined ACT UP by coming to the strategy meeting they'd held at Katz's Delicatessen just a few minutes earlier. In the confusion, she began shouting that she had clean needles and was able to toss some bleach kits to some locals who waved their hands at her, seeking works. Then she, too, got arrested. It was all over in minutes.

This arrest, however, would be the first blow to New York's criminalization of needles and a key event in stopping the spread of HIV among our drug users. Nearly every second of those few minutes would be debated during what became known as the "Needle Eight" trial, which paved the way for legalization of effective needle exchange in the city. It would be more than six months, however, before the activists got their day in court. And I would be there to cover the story.

six

The Trial of the Needle Eight

N EW YORK CITY HEALTH COMMISSIONER STEPHEN JOSEPH WAS NOT KNOWN as a friend of ACT UP. Their founder, Larry Kramer, once disrupted one of his speeches by standing up and shouting "Liar." The group often wheat-pasted posters around the city, some stating, "Stephen Joseph has blood on his hands," stamped with what looked like a bloody handprint. Others called him "deadlier than the virus." He'd received death threats—late at night, at home. He'd clashed with the group on many issues, most notably on the question of mandatory reporting of AIDS cases.[1] In response, while leading the health department, Joseph had members of the activist group arrested more than once.

But several years after his contentious stint in city government, in April of 1991, ACT UP's former nemesis was in the witness box. He was voluntarily testifying on their behalf—not as a complainant against them. He wore a full beard and sideburns, brown tinged with distinguished white at the sideburns and in a large patch below his lips. He looked like a wise medic from an earlier time, perhaps one of the Smith Brothers of cough drop fame. He sat in the cramped and drably functional criminal court as the ritual legal language was recited, agreeing to tell the whole truth and nothing but. Because the activists had been charged with misdemeanor needle possession, which carries a sentence of up to six months in jail, the trial was held in front of a judge, rather than a jury.

Judge Laura Drager had shoulder-length, curly brown hair, parted in the center, and a thoughtful but no-nonsense manner. Her courtroom's only decorations were an American flag, a standard-issue large, round office clock, and a gold-colored but obviously plastic "In God We Trust" sign. Although drug war money had flown copiously to police for arrests and to expand jails and prisons, funding for the courts to process the increasing caseload had been neglected, and it showed.

The trial was held only steps away from the site of the now-shuttered pilot needle exchange program. But finally, the eight activists—dubbed the "Needle Eight"—who'd been arrested for trying to do needle exchange in reaction to that closure, were getting their day in court. One of the defendants, Boston's Jon Parker, had been acquitted of a similar charge just two months earlier—the charismatic Allan Parry had visited from Liverpool to testify in his defense.[2]

Now Parker sat with the ACT UP defendants along the left side of the courtroom, laughing and joking during breaks. One of them was Dan Keith Williams, a thirty-three-year-old Black, gay graphic designer. He had found being arrested as part of ACT UP quite a different experience from the way men of color were typically treated by police. He'd been driven to participate in needle exchange because of what he called the "denial" and lack of action he'd seen on AIDS and drugs in the African American community.

The others were Elovich; the nurse, Cynthia Cochran; and several people who had volunteered at the exchange. These included Kathryn Otter, a transwoman who'd overcome a drug problem, despite being abused in treatment because of her gender nonconformity; Gregg Bordowitz, a gay HIV-positive filmmaker and former drug user; as well as two lesbian activists, Debra Levine, a theatre director, and Monica Pearl, an editor and author.

Stephen Joseph's presence alone testified to the importance of the case. He'd been before the same judge with some of the same ACT UP members previously—including Elovich—but not by choice. Earlier, in one of their actions against him, eleven activists had taken over his office and refused to leave until police dragged them away. Joseph then had them charged with criminal trespass. In the resulting trial, ACT UP had tried to convince Judge Drager that their occupation of Joseph's office had been necessary to preserve public health. They'd relentlessly questioned the health commissioner under oath for a full two days. But the judge didn't buy their arguments. While not doubting the activists' sincerity, she ruled that "moral conviction is not a defense to criminal action."[3]

In April of 1991, however, here were some of the same people in front of the same judge, once again attempting to use the "necessity" defense. Now, though, Joseph was on their side. He was also no longer the city's health commissioner—he'd resigned when Mayor Koch's term ended. And after how ACT UP had behaved toward him personally, his presence itself spoke volumes.

During his three hours on the stand, Joseph gave a brief history of public health, describing how otherwise criminal actions were sometimes required to save lives. One of the founding stories of epidemiology, in fact, involves such an act, he noted. In 1854, a cholera epidemic was ravaging London, killing more than 600 people and sickening many more. Prior outbreaks of this deadly diarrheal disease had killed thousands of British people since cholera was first reported in England in 1831.[4] At the time, the periodic epidemics that routinely routed cities were believed to be caused by "miasma," which refers to dirty or contaminated air.

But John Snow, a doctor who also pioneered the use of anesthesia, thought differently. He suspected that cholera was caused by filthy water. In London at that time, wells used for drinking water were often located adjacent to cesspools that collected waste. He theorized that it was these contaminated wells that were making people sick.

Snow discovered a clear geographical pattern in the epidemic, Joseph told the court. Most of the people who became ill lived near a pump on Broad Street and presumably got their drinking water from the closest source. To prove the connection between the disease and the pump—and this is why he is seen as a founder of epidemiology—Snow mapped cases and interviewed people about their water use. He found infections among those who drank from the well and their family members. But families who didn't get their water from Broad Street didn't get sick. Snow later located the original source of the well's contamination, which was a woman who'd unwittingly washed her sick baby's diaper at a cesspool that drained into the well.

Although it would normally be illegal to vandalize a public water source, Snow got permission from skeptical local authorities made desperate by the epidemic. They allowed the pump's handle to be removed on September 8, 1854—despite the jeers of passersby who wanted water from it. This action helped end the epidemic.[5] ("Pump day" is now celebrated—at least by some epidemiologists and their students—as a holiday. A replica of the pump now stands where the original did, outside a pub now named for Snow.)

Under questioning by the defense, Joseph drew parallels between Snow's actions and those of the needle exchangers. Like Snow, the activists had recognized an important public health problem. Like him, they'd been moved to try to stop the spread of a disease by eliminating a key source of infection.[6]

Because Mayor Dinkins had shut down the city's pilot program, and because the risk of HIV among IV drug users was so great, the group's actions were appropriate, he said. He described how important clean needles were to HIV prevention and discussed how providing them could also serve as a "bridge to treatment."

In addition, Joseph testified about an idea that is critical to both harm reduction and public health. "Don't let the best be the enemy of the good" is how it is typically expressed, based on a concept first elaborated by Voltaire. What this phrase means for harm reduction is that only aiming for the best possible outcome—say, people being completely drug free and, therefore, not sharing needles—can interfere with achieving real progress, such as saving lives.

In this case, policies that demand abstinence and criminalize needles can actually kill those they seek to protect by exposing them to AIDS. Requiring that people suddenly change everything in their life can prompt resistance or even backfire; this is a core message of Edith Springer's work and a key principle of harm reduction.

And it is now backed by research on numerous behaviors ranging from quitting smoking, treating eating disorders, and increasing exercise to recycling and other environmentally sound practices. For example, nicotine replacement therapies that do not require immediate abstinence, like gums and lozenges, roughly double the quit rate for cigarette smoking—and e-cigarettes may be even more effective. In terms of many eating disorders, requiring immediate cessation of the harmful behavior is rarely effective and can even worsen bingeing—while approaches that allow for small, positive changes that are healthy are more promising. Studies show that a counseling style based on gradual change developed to reduce alcohol-related harm is useful in increasing exercise and other health behaviors as well. The application of harm reduction approaches to improving people's engagement in environmental change is newer, but it is an active area of research. For most of the things that we seek to change in private or public life, smaller, intermediate steps are often necessary before larger transformation becomes possible.[7]

"What [these] people are doing is a courageous thing and I believe in what they're doing," Joseph testified.[8]

UNLIKE THE OTHER DEFENDANTS, RICHARD ELOVICH SAT WITH ACT UP's three attorneys at a small, crowded table meant for two people, not four. That's because he was also acting in his own defense. He had sharp analytical skills—indeed, he later got a PhD in medical sociology from Columbia. Elovich was a performer as well. In the evenings while the trial took place, he starred in a semi-autobiographical one-man show at P.S. 122 in the East Village.

Elovich was also the person who had talked Joseph into testifying for ACT UP. They had gotten stranded together at the Atlanta airport; a hurricane had made a turn toward Georgia while they were attending a meeting at the U.S. Centers for Disease Control. With not much else to do to kill time, they'd begun a tentative but civil conversation.

Elovich listened sympathetically as Joseph expressed his anger about how ACT UP had treated him over the years. Although Elovich offered no apology, they began to connect, on a simple human level. That allowed him to ask—and Joseph to agree—to testify. Throughout the trial, most of the questioning was done by the other attorneys, with Elovich jumping in if he thought any crucial points had been omitted.

Among the experts who spoke, Yolanda Serrano was unusually open in her testimony. Typically, she kept her private life so private that even many of her friends had no idea about her personal connections to her activism. She was friendly and passionate about her cause but guarded about her own experience. Indeed, when she died of AIDS in 1993, just two years later, few had even known beforehand that she'd been sick. Fewer still were aware that she herself had a history of injecting drugs. Her obituary said that she'd died of cancer.

In court, however, while she did not come out about her own use, she spoke about her husband's injecting and the pain of losing him to AIDS. She noted that 80 percent of partners of injection drug users were not injectors themselves. Serrano also described ADAPT's bleach distribution and outreach work in shooting galleries—and why it was necessary, but not sufficient.

Another witness was Don Des Jarlais, who led research at the institute where Edith Springer worked and was fast becoming the world's expert on the science of needle exchange. His qualifications included being a research advisor to the programs that had begun operating out west, in Tacoma, Washington, and Portland, Oregon, in 1988 and 1989, respectively (see chapter nine). He noted that the U.S. was nearly alone in the developed world in rejecting needle exchange and described data from the U.K., the Netherlands, and Australia.

He emphasized that providing clean syringes didn't lead to new users starting to take drugs—nor did it increase or lengthen use by those who were already injecting. In fact, even the city's flawed and tiny pilot study had showed that it could serve as a pathway to treatment. There is "considerable" evidence suggesting that needle exchange participants are more likely to get treatment, Des Jarlais said.

Further crucial evidence came from New York state senator Velmanette Montgomery, a Black woman who defied the political consensus, despite the possibility that doing so would hurt her re-election chances. Representing the hard-hit areas of Bedford-Stuyvesant and Fort Greene in Brooklyn, she was nearly alone among politicians at the time in her support for needle exchange. Montgomery had introduced legislation to legalize it—but she said that despite the data that supported the policy, politically there was no way to pass it any time soon.

Some of the most moving testimony came from the defendants themselves. The sixty-seven-year-old nurse who'd joined ACT UP the day she got arrested with them, Cynthia Cochran, said it was "an abomination" that the medical profession itself hadn't acted urgently on this issue. With her silver and black hair in a bun, she wore oversize glasses, along with a snappy orange necktie that complemented her gray suit. Her voice conveyed her outrage. As she cared for late-stage AIDS patients, she said that she felt, "There was something almost indecent about taking wages when you're only keeping people alive with no prospect of getting them well."

That was why, when she heard about ACT UP's planned action, she'd been compelled to join in. "It was a wretchedly small contingent from medicine," she said of herself, but she'd wanted to show support as much as she could.

One of the key legal issues in the trial would be whether the defendants were primarily deliberately trying to get arrested—or if they had really planned on at least attempting to get needles to people who needed them. It was okay if there was some element of civil disobedience—but for the necessity defense to succeed, that couldn't have been the activists' only purpose on that day. Cochran hoped to provide ammunition for this part of their argument.

She told the court that she had personally seen people who wanted clean needles, just outside of the crowd of media, demonstrators, and police. They were hanging back where they could blend into the neighborhood and be less conspicuous. "The addicts I saw were indicating they wanted what I could get to them," she said, describing how she'd thrown bleach kits to those she could see raising their hands during the frenzied moment when the media had separated her from the rest of the activists. Because she was tall, she could see over the heads of most of the crowd. From where I stood, I saw what must have been some of the same people running away with bleach kits as the table and the activists were being taken away.

Jon Parker's testimony was also critical. Wearing a white oxford shirt, his blond hair feathered back with his long braid hidden behind him, he spoke so quietly at first that the judge had to ask him to speak up. Soon he was telling the court about own history with drugs and the criminal justice system. He described his path from "jail to Yale," as he later titled a memoir. In his broad Boston accent, he discussed founding the National AIDS Brigade and how Serrano had introduced him to ACT UP.

She had also helped him identify the decrepit hotel in Williamsburg where he frequently dispensed syringes, he said. The defense attorneys asked about his work there. "These people are very appreciative of our help," he explained. "They all seemed shocked to see people who actually care about them doing something to help them." He said that almost all of the needles he distributed were returned, noting that residents would keep them in bottles in their rooms, which meant they could be disposed of safely by the activists, rather than discarded on the street.

"What do you think you're accomplishing by distributing or exchanging needles with people?" the defense asked.

"We're allowing people the means to stay AIDS-free," said Parker. "I mean, otherwise most [of these] individuals [are] in a situation where they might feel the need to share a needle. I don't know how to explain it but . . . the most important [thing] is that we instill hope in people. We show them that someone cares. We allow them to maybe see a chance for their own rehabilitation."

The lawyer asked how exchanging needles could do that.

"When I was a drug addict, I thought I had to completely change," Parker replied. "There's two worlds: the drug addict world and the straight world. I thought to be in the straight world, I had to change. I had to go to school, get a job, get off drugs. When we do needle exchange, when we allow an active addict to exchange a needle, right then, he realizes that he's doing something for himself.

"That's very, very important," he stressed. "That takes the cynicism away [about their ability to change]. That's really—it's like the first step in the treatment, allowing, empowering the addict to realize he can make a difference in his own life. That's what we do the most. We instill this hope."

He added, "When they can make even a small difference in their life—even if it is just exchanging one needle—right then they know . . . [that] they are doing something for the good of themselves and that's very, very powerful. It shows them that they can keep going on and make other changes." In just a few sentences, he'd explained some of the key principles of harm reduction and how it helped small changes lead to bigger ones.

Parker was also questioned about why he didn't simply hand out bleach. "As a public health student," he insisted, "I was taught that any time you have an epidemic, you use every way possible. To use malaria as an example, when they had a malaria epidemic, they gave insecticides, they drained swamps, they gave mosquito netting. You have to use every weapon possible. Bleach is a weapon. I think needles are more powerful."

He added, "We gave this question some serious thought," noting that if you give bleach without clean needles, sharing will still occur. "That would reinforce the negative behavior. We want addicts to stop sharing needles," he said.

Kathryn Otter, the transwoman who was in recovery and had worked as a counselor, reiterated Parker's message. She had long, straight, light brown hair with bangs and a youthful look that made her seem, at twenty-four, like a teen with a bad attitude—an impression that was only bolstered by the black t-shirt that she wore and her tattoos. But she spoke earnestly.

"One of the things I did so often in my work as a counselor was education," she said, explaining that she was able to do similar teaching about AIDS when exchanging needles. She'd been moved to act because she'd seen the disease kill. "I've watched people for years die in [the twelve-step group Narcotics Anonymous] and that sickens me," she said. "There was a lot of discussion by people in NA of 'things I wish I would have known [while using].' And that's the thing that just got to me—that the knowledge wasn't out there."

Otter also provided one of the lighter moments in the trial, when she was asked about why she knew the area around Essex and Delancey so well. She and the judge, who is an Orthodox Jewish woman, soon bonded over having gone bargain shopping on nearby Orchard Street. Once settled primarily by Jewish immigrants, the corner where the arrest had taken place was in a part of the Lower East Side that was for known for deals in the rag trade long before it became known for its drug deals.

The trial's most important moments, however, probably came during the testimony of the prosecution's sole witness, Dr. Larry Brown. He would be the last witness to appear before both sides gave their closing arguments. The only evidence that the prosecution had presented in the trial thus far was a reiteration of the fact that the defendants had been arrested with needles; their opening statement had taken an entire thirty-two seconds.[9] And so the state's case relied almost entirely on Brown's ability to debunk the defense's science.

NUMEROUS EXPERTS FROM AROUND THE WORLD HAD BEEN EAGER TO TESTIFY in favor of the Needle Eight: the judge had been sent more than two dozen letters of support from needle exchange researchers and other experts in eight cities in five countries, including one from Amsterdam's Junkiebond. But the prosecution did not seem to have had this luxury of choice.

The most prestigious expert that they could have called was probably the city's new health commissioner, Woodrow Myers. He had led Mayor Dinkins's charge to shut the pilot program. But the commissioner did not appear—even though he'd said in an interview with CBS News Radio that he saw fighting drug use as "a higher goal than preventing AIDS"[10] and was vociferous in his opposition to needle exchange. An African American superstar scholar, he'd previously been the health commissioner for the state of Indiana and had graduated from Stanford at nineteen and Harvard Medical School at twenty-three.

A close second choice would have been Dr. Beny Primm, who had co-founded one of the largest methadone treatment providers in the city and was a respected expert on addiction. Like Larry Brown, who was actually one of his top employees, Primm was a member of the Black Leadership Commission on AIDS (BLCA). The group was basically a who's who of Black politicians and other power elite in New York City. Mayor Dinkins himself had been a member before taking office. It was one of the biggest forces acting against needle exchange in the state.

In fact, when Joseph had proposed the pilot program, the greatest opposition to it had come from these Black leaders, often echoed by addiction treatment providers, church groups, and law enforcement. Their attacks had only continued and were an important backdrop to the trial. For example, Mayor Koch's police commissioner from 1983 to 1989 had responded to a question from the *New York Times* about the needle exchange this way: "As a black person we have a particular sensitivity to doctors conducting experiments, and they too frequently seem to be conducted against blacks."[11]

His language was meant to elicit memories of the hideous Tuskegee syphilis experiment, in which doctors had left the debilitating disease untreated to study its progression in Black men—even when effective treatment became available. This "research" had been carried out and funded by the U.S. government from 1932 through 1972, when its unethical practices were revealed.[12] Within the Black community, Tuskegee remains an open wound, an ongoing emblem of medical abuse and neglect.

And indeed, many Black leaders and clergy in the 1980s and nineties made the comparison between needle exchange and Tuskegee explicitly. This unfortunately dovetailed with widely circulating conspiracy theories, which suggested that AIDS had been deliberately unleashed to kill African Americans. It sparked rumors that the needles the government planned to hand out would be tainted with HIV—to spread it, not prevent it. A 1990 poll of Black churchgoers in several cities found that two-thirds said they thought that it was possible that the government was deliberately spreading HIV as a form of genocide.[13]

During the fight over the needle exchange pilot, Harlem's city councilman had called needle exchange itself "genocide," adding that Joseph "should be arrested for murder and drug distribution"[14] for his part in sponsoring it when he was health commissioner. The pastor of Harlem's Abyssinian Baptist Church said simply, "I am not in favor of cooperating with evil."[15]

These positions were deeply held and genuine. They were based in a lengthy and horrific history of oppression and of underfunding of health care, which meant that addiction treatment was only available to one in ten people who needed it in New York. But, as in ACT UP's previous, failed necessity defense case, these were moral and political arguments, not medical or scientific evidence.

Any prosecution expert called for this case would be in the difficult position of having to argue against syringe exchange without being able to provide an alternative emergency action to take. That's because no one—not even the most ardent backers of treatment—could realistically say that it could be scaled up quickly enough. Nor could they honestly argue that relapse was rare. There was also no scientific evidence that needle exchange caused harm—all of the existing data showed the opposite. These stark facts may have deterred other experts. Brown, however, appeared undaunted.

As with all experts, Brown's testimony began with a recitation of his qualifications. He spoke proudly of his medical degree from New York University, his residency in internal medicine at Harlem Hospital, and of receiving his master's degree in public health from Columbia. He waxed on about his scientific publications but was eventually cut off by the judge when he digressed to say that he was "terribly uncomfortable" with discussing the scientific issues related to needle exchange in a court of law. His bearing seemed pompous: the impression he gave was that having to discuss science with mere lawyers and a judge was beneath him.

A new assistant district attorney appeared in court that day to question Brown. He was a confident looking man with brown hair and glasses. The defense was, in one sense, heartened to see that someone of higher status had been assigned to replace the previous prosecutor, whom they had jokingly termed a "baby DA" because of his inexperience. The move could imply that the leadership in the office was worried and had decided to bring in a bigger gun. But that had a downside, too: a more seasoned lawyer might present a stronger case. The ADA began the meat of his questioning by asking for Brown's position on syringe distribution.

Brown replied, "When that issue is broached, I find it difficult to say in one or two sentences. To me, the answer is not entirely that clear. What I mean is that, when one considers any intervention and its usefulness to society, you want to consider the issue of safety as well as efficacy and you want to investigate in well-designed protocols or studies." Then he claimed that all of the dozens of currently existing studies were irrevocably flawed.

He said, "While there is suggestive evidence that there is no increase in drug use, we need to recognize that that in and of itself does not prove safety. It certainly does not prove efficacy." He also testified that he believed that there were too many differences between American and European drug users to make the British and Dutch data relevant and that, in any event, the right questions weren't being asked. He claimed that it might not ever be possible to design a study that would provide acceptable evidence because the research would invariably have to rely on the unreliable accounts of addicts describing changes in their injecting behavior.

But under further questioning, Brown admitted that HIV among IV drug users in New York was widespread. He agreed that they were the largest group of people currently infected, as well as the population most likely to spread the virus to heterosexuals who didn't take drugs. He said, "If we had to have a program that would prove the efficacy [of needle exchange], we would need to get something that's close to a gold standard."

Then the prosecutor asked one of the most important questions of the trial. "How would you respond to the view that needle exchange is necessary because HIV is so very life threatening?"

Brown reacted with a deep, audible sigh. "That is similar to a lot of the ways that society responds—with a Band-Aid approach. If there was really some concern about chemical dependency, we then would not use these Band-Aid approaches and we would deal with the root causes: the poverty, the lack of employment, the problems with education."

He continued, "HIV, as bad as it is, at some point or another is going to come under control. We're going to unfortunately lose a lot of people and I regret that seriously, but HIV represents for people of color only the seventh horse of the apocalypse . . . To me, giving this Band-Aid approach to this problem is again repeating the same problem we have with respect to health care in this country . . . Needle exchange programs are an incremental and insufficient response, in my mind, to a very serious problem."

As Brown appeared to condone just letting AIDS kill people while awaiting a gold standard approach to prevention, the needle exchange supporters in the courtroom seemed to have a hard time restraining their rage. I myself had to bite my tongue. I could also see frustration and fury in Richard Elovich's eyes as he sat with the attorneys, desperate for his turn to respond.

Fortunately, he didn't have much longer to wait. The defense declined to cross-examine Brown, having determined that the prosecution had pretty much already demonstrated his inability to refute their arguments with data. Both sides rested. It was time for each side to make its best case in closing arguments.

ELOVICH BEGAN HIS CLOSING BY TALKING ABOUT NUMBERS: THE **100,000** deaths from AIDS that had occurred so far in the U.S., the 30,000 deaths in New York city alone, and the fact that half of the 500,000 people in America known to inject drugs lived in the state.

He said, "In the ten years that the AIDS epidemic has raged, while all of these people have died, while all of these people are being infected, we have come to distinguish between authorities and people who speak authoritatively through their own direct experience." The same thing, he argued, needed to be done with the evidence that had been presented at the trial.

"We have to make a distinction between a figure of authority, an expert like Dr. Brown who will say to us that, 'People will die, that's unfortunate, I deeply regret it,' and people who are, like myself, saying, 'Dr. Brown, that isn't enough.'"

Elovich went on to describe how detached experts who want to see perfect evidence and 100 percent proof before moving forward are different from those who are personally affected by AIDS, who "are seeing the body count, are seeing the people closed out of treatment." He noted that no one had disputed the fact that there are 250,000 injection drug users in New York state and only 40,000 existing treatment slots. He said that the health of this group should be given the same consideration as everyone else's.

"The lives of drug users are not expendable. The lives of their sexual partners and their children are not expendable," he said, practically shouting. The personal passion he felt about the humanity of people with AIDS and people who take drugs was clear in his intensity.

"I was in a rage when I left this courtroom yesterday," he went on, quite obviously still angry. Again, he assailed Brown's claim to "regret" the ongoing deaths. He thundered, "That is not enough." He mentioned sitting on a committee with Dr. Brown that had ultimately, after great effort, succeeded in getting the city to add a whole 600 new treatment slots. This was the first expansion of any size in many years. It didn't begin to meet the need.

Next, he talked about his personal experience. "I know how many times I went through relapses . . . you go through relapse over and over again," he said, indicating that even easily available treatment for all wouldn't be enough to stop AIDS.

Then he picked up a needle, displaying it to the judge. "This needle is not meant to be a cure for the AIDS crisis," he said. "This needle is not meant to be a cure for drug addiction. But I know that when I hand out this needle, when I explain to an addict to clean the needle, to keep this needle as his or her own—when we explain this, what we're doing is we're getting beyond the several dozen of us who are out in the street. We're actually changing drug etiquette.

"People are passing it on so that the next time they're in a shooting gallery, when someone hands someone a dirty needle, they think about it, and that's how behaviors are changed."

He concluded that, based on his own experience with addiction and his own experience exchanging thousands of needles with hundreds of people, "I can stand before this court today and say, 'I know when I go out doing the needle exchange, I know that I've saved a life.'"

After Elovich, another ACT UP defense attorney, Mike Spiegel, made more technical, legal arguments. He focused on how the testimony given had proved that the activists' actions were legally justified and not criminal. "The section of the law known as the justification or the necessity defense has been called the safety valve of the law precisely because it's the opportunity for the law to understand and conform itself to the situation people face in the real world," he explained.

He carefully went over the elements required to support a necessity defense, providing examples of situations in which it would apply. One was a case involving a mountain climber charged with burglary for break-ing into an empty cabin, seeking shelter and supplies to save an injured partner. Another was the case of a pharmacist who illegally provided a drug without a prescription to someone who would have died if he didn't get the medication right away.

To win a necessity defense case, the defendants needed to reason-ably believe that what they did was necessary, the lawyer noted. They also needed to show that the harm they were trying to avoid was imminent and could not be prevented in any other way. Finally, they had to have genuinely tried to reduce that harm—and not just conducted a political protest. He showed how it was clear from the testimony that all of these criteria had been met.

Echoing Joseph, the former city health commissioner, he compared the activists to John Snow, noting that AIDS was as terrifying and mys-terious to people now as cholera had been in London in the nineteenth century. Back then, he said, some folks were just as angry about Snow's removal of the Broad Street pump handle as others were about needle ex-change in our time. "We're still talking about John Snow a century later," he said. "We owe these people that same debt of gratitude that history has conferred on John Snow."

The final defense attorney to speak was Jill Harris. A lesbian activist who worked as a public defender for Legal Aid, she wore a gray jacket with a skirt that brushed her ankles. Her hair was short; her manner brisk. She continued the attack on Brown, calling his testimony "chilling" and contrasting his perspective with that of the activists.

"Dr. Brown said that he believes that needle exchange is a Band-Aid solution to a larger problem—and none of these defendants would dis-agree," she conceded. But the difference between him and the defendants is that he seems to be "very comfortable doing very little to help or letting very little be done."

As Harris described it, Brown was content to wait for the government to respond to the underlying causes of addiction, like poverty, unemploy-ment, and lack of education and health care. He was content to wait for a "gold standard" for HIV prevention. She called this "a perfect example of what Dr. Joseph called the best being the enemy of the good." Since we can't have the best, we won't try to take what we can get, but instead do nothing.

Harris argued that this was a "profoundly cynical" position. "Dr. Brown must know, as we all know, what the likelihood in reality of our government really addressing the underlying causes of drug addiction in this society," she said, explaining that that likelihood is zero—the same probability of the city suddenly providing treatment on demand to everyone who needs it. "It's just not going to happen and Dr. Brown knows that," she insisted.

Building up steam, she added that she guessed that his strategy was to just wait while people die until the government notices. "The bodies having been piling up for some time," she said, "and the government response has been one of inaction, denial, and of really murderous neglect. People are literally dying in the streets of New York City and Dr. Brown says that what we need and what we should strive for is the gold standard."

The defendants, in contrast, she argued, take action. "They respond. They're activists. They do what's necessary to save lives." She described their actions as hopeful, rather than cynical—trying to save lives, rather than simply waiting for AIDS to go away.

Next, she painted a picture of their work, saying that she wished the judge could watch them on the street, even as she knew that was impossible for legal reasons. "You'd see instantly what these defendants' presence means to those addicts," she told the court, describing how hope was visible in their mundane interactions and change could be seen as people began returning needles and asking about other ways to help themselves.

And as she spoke, I couldn't help but think about one woman I'd seen at the needle exchange during an early visit—and then again, several months later. I hadn't recognized her the second time, so completely had she been transformed by starting recovery.

"Your honor," Harris concluded, "these activists don't need studies to tell them that what they do saves lives—even you as you heard from the stand that the evidence does point in that direction. They don't need studies to tell them that. They know, just like Richard Elovich knows, that what they do saves lives.

"And, your honor, Judge Drager, you know it, too."

IN CONTRAST TO THE DRAMA OF THE DEFENSE'S CLOSING, THE PROSECUTION'S arguments were primarily about the technicalities of the law. While this might not have been effective with a jury, it was more likely to move a judge. The ADA argued that the defense had not met the burden needed to prove that the defendants' actions had been necessary. Their attempt at exchanging needles on the day of their arrest was merely "political," he said.

"Your honor," he continued, "the defense fails for four separate reasons in this case. First, the harm that the defendants sought to avert is speculative. Second, the defendants invited arrest. Third, the defendants had legal alternatives, and fourth, the defense were trying to change a statute."

He assailed the scientific evidence on needle exchange, saying, "None of the defendants can say with any certainty whether in fact a life would be saved by giving out a needle. They all hoped that harm would be avoided, but, your honor, the penal law is not about hoping."

He praised Brown's testimony, noting that the state's expert had said that "there is no evidence that needle exchange does any good. He also stated that the safety of needle exchange has not been shown and that, in fact, it could do harm."

The prosecutor also raised doubt about whether people who were actively addicted to drugs could ever behave rationally, citing testimony from defendant Gregg Bordowitz. "He testified that he became infected with the HIV virus because his addiction so clouded his judgment that he couldn't negotiate safe sex, couldn't use a condom. He had knowledge and the availability—yet his addiction caused his infection.

"This, your honor, is a well-educated founding member of ACT UP, whose addiction caused his infection," he said. "Ask yourself now how a down-and-out addict in a shooting gallery in a burned out building in New York City is going to act in the throes of addiction in light of Mr. Bordowitz's testimony. His testimony shows that addicts can't rely on common sense."

He concluded that ACT UP's actions were driven by moral and political concerns, not a genuine emergency. "The defendants are asking you to declare the statute void—unlike the mountain climber turned burglar who never asks for the burglary statute to be eliminated," he said. He concluded by saying that in a democracy, "elected officials make the ultimate decisions on health care policy. Throughout this trial, your honor, you have heard considerable testimony that ACT UP is a democracy. Let me just close, your honor, by stating the obvious, that so is New York state."

It would be nearly two months before Judge Drager would release her decision.

WHEN THE COURT ANNOUNCED THAT THE VERDICT IN THE NEEDLE EIGHT CASE would be read on June 25, the defendants and their supporters planned to show up in force. That day, the small courtroom was overflowing as Drager prepared to speak. All of the defendants were there with their lawyers, of course—as were many of their key supporters from within ACT UP, especially those who volunteered at the needle exchanges.

I sat as close to the front of the room as I could. Reporters from the *New York Times*, *Newsday*, the *Daily News*, and other media had also turned out. The activists were anxious—at least some had prepared for the possibility that they might be immediately jailed. A few had made contingency plans for pet sitting and other similar needs. Defendant Deb Levine was so nervous that she vomited more than once in the ladies' room. Monica Pearl had her parents and her sister accompany her to offer moral support.

However, as the judge began reading the verdict, excitement about the possibility of acquittal began to build. Drager described the arguments made by both sides. Then she went through, point by point, how the evidence that was presented satisfied the legal criteria required to support the necessity defense.

She said, "This court finds it reasonable for the defendants to believe their actions necessary as an emergency measure to avert an imminent public injury. Without doubt, AIDS has created an imminent crisis in New York City. There is no dispute that use of clean needles by addicts prevents the spread of HIV infection."

Nervously, the defendants began to look at one another and their lawyers. Had they won? Everyone was listening for a disappointing "But . . ." that could dash their hopes. And then, seeming to be headed toward such a destination, Drager began to describe Larry Brown's testimony about needle exchange being a mere "Band-Aid." Anxiety began to rise. I was so tense that my nails were digging into my skin as I tried to keep my hands still.

The judge said, "There is much validity to Dr. Brown's contentions." That sentence made hearts pound, including mine. Then, however, she continued, "[T]he issue before this court is not to choose between the different policy options offered by the witnesses, nor is it necessary for the defendants' efforts to be proven successful."

Our hopes began to soar again, as she laid out her reasoning. "Rather, the court must find whether it was reasonable for the defendants, relying on competent medical evidence, to engage in the conduct at issue. While the defendants' actions alone would not end the epidemic, it is reasonable to believe that their actions served to avert further risks of infection for some individuals. The court is satisfied that the nature of the crisis facing this city, coupled with the medical evidence offered, warranted defendants' action."

At that, smiles and gestures of joy and relief began to be seen among the activists, though they worked hard to contain themselves to avoid being reprimanded for improper behavior. Drager began her conclusion with a flourish that explicitly supported harm reduction.

She said, "This court is also satisfied that the harm the defendants sought to avoid was greater than the harm in violating the statute. Hundreds of thousands of lives are at stake in the AIDS epidemic. The crime of possessing a hypodermic needle was enacted as a weapon in the war on drugs. Although law enforcement officials believe the statute essential in this fight, available evidence suggests it has had limited success."

She followed this grave understatement with explicit evidence. "As the testimony revealed, only eleven states have statutes similar to New York's law," she noted. "Despite these statutes, these states—and New York in particular—have among the highest rates of addiction and there are still plenty of dirty needles available."

After citing a few cases that supported her decision—and qualifying that her ruling was not "binding on any other court"—she said that ultimately, other branches of government would have to decide whether to authorize syringe exchange.

"That having been said, for the reasons set forth in this decision, with respect to one count of criminally possessing a hypodermic needle, the court finds each of the defendants not guilty."

Now, loud cheers, clapping, hugs, and general euphoria broke out among the activists. They had done it! They had proven in a court of law that needle exchange was a medical necessity during the AIDS crisis. While there was certainly far more work to be done, contrary to the judge's claims that she was not setting a precedent, the case paved the way for the activists to continue their work in less of a legal gray area. And it also advanced the case for needle exchange and ultimately all syringe possession and sales without a prescription to be legalized in the state.

It was a stunning victory.

seven

Exposing Racism in the Drug War

AFTER THE VERDICT, THE ACT UP DEFENDANTS CONTINUED TO DO NEEDLE exchange and expand their underground harm reduction programs as much as they could. By the summer of 1991, they had regular sites in the South Bronx, the Lower East Side, and Brooklyn, which operated at least a few days a week. Collectively, they were distributing and receiving back around 8,000 syringes a month.[1]

But conflicts with politicians, and especially the Black establishment around Mayor Dinkins, continued to be a significant challenge, particularly for the few Black activists who openly favored harm reduction. If needle exchange were ever to reach the scale needed to truly fight the virus, this would have to change.

The issue was especially acute for ACT UP's Dan Williams, as he tried to win support for—or at least reduce opposition to—these programs from key community leaders. As he described it, "My involvement in the struggle to empower [drug users] is based on the conflicting experiences I have as a gay African-American male." This conflict, he felt, metaphorically split him in two.

"I am no good as half a person," he said. "I could not accept my identity as a gay man if my African-American identity could not be represented. The opposite is also true, but the existence of most persons of color is greatly threatened by inaction and lack of concern within, and outside, communities of color."[2] Experiencing this slow response to AIDS was deeply painful to him because it seemed to reflect how little his own community valued people like him.

He was particularly upset by the initial reaction to HIV from Black and Latino groups. "I expected an outcry from communities of color in the beginning of the crisis," he said, "but there wasn't any. I wondered why. The answer is both simple and complex. People of color didn't need another stigma. So, many of us denied it was happening until we were at the center of an epidemic." That denial, unfortunately, allowed the virus to spread. And the judgmental position taken by much of the leadership left people of color who were gay or injected drugs stranded and isolated.

Williams was all too familiar with being judged and rejected based on parts of himself that are essential to who he is. Raised in Beaufort, South Carolina, a tiny community made up of around 130 small islands off the coast, he knew he was somehow different almost as soon as he understood the concept of being unusual. "I never really fit into anything," he said. "I basically asked a lot of questions that people never wanted to answer. I was very inquisitive."[3]

Beaufort is best known as the location of Parris Island, home of the Marine Corps's demanding boot camp. Both of Williams's parents served in the military, but they were also deeply rooted in rural South Carolina. As a young child, he actually knew his great-great-great grandmother, who had survived slavery before Emancipation. When he was in grade school, his school was integrated for the first time. It happened without violence or protests. But as a bookish boy who, he said, spent an "inordinate" time reading, he gravitated toward kids with similar interests, many of whom were white. This caused friction—as did his growing awareness of his attraction to men.

After a stint in the Navy and periods spent in New Orleans and Italy, he moved to New York to attend Parsons School of Design to study graphic design. Then, he learned that his lover in Italy, whom he had considered a soul mate, was dying of AIDS. He'd already begun to hear talk about the disease, and now he was terrified.

He joined ACT UP in 1987. Initially, he was involved in Majority Action, the committee that focused on AIDS in minority communities. It was so named because people of color had become the majority of those with AIDS in New York. But the moniker often seemed ironic, given the overall whiteness of ACT UP. When Jon Parker showed up to ask the activists to do needle exchange with him, Williams was intrigued—despite the fact that he had no personal connection to drug injecting.

"It's the whole thing about a group of people who are totally outside—talk about being ostracized!" he said. He was especially compelled by the fact that even trying to save the lives of injection drug users was essentially criminalized. "You're trying to help somebody—and somebody wants to arrest you for it. It just played totally with me. And so, I was, like—I just did it," he said.[4]

Williams wore his hair closely shaved, almost military style, often with large, nerdy glasses. He became part of the needle exchange's supply chain. His neat appearance made it easier for him to buy syringes from states where they were legally available over the counter: he looked more like a dutiful grandson picking up diabetic supplies than someone who had drug-related intent. He made dozens of runs to get thousands of needles.[5]

But his passion for syringe exchange put him at odds with groups like the Black Leadership Commission on AIDS, which had made fighting against it a central cause. The battle in the Black community over AIDS and related to drug policy more generally was crucial to the development of harm reduction, in part because of the way it exposed an especially insidious aspect of racism. Essentially, the drug war turned out to be one of the most important ways through which much of the Black middle class and most leading Black politicians had become convinced to back the tough policies that produced mass incarceration.

This support was achieved in part by exploiting what historian Evelyn Brooks Higginbotham first labeled "respectability politics," which has been a major force in the African American response to both AIDS and drugs. Brittney Cooper, associate professor of women's studies at Rutgers University, defines respectability politics succinctly in one of her essays as the belief that "If Black people would just 'act right' and 'do right,' we would be all right."[6] The flip side of this, sadly, is that people who don't "act right"—like those who inject drugs—are viewed as drags on the community and are deemed unworthy of support.

As many have pointed out, this idea has long been used to divide Black people. In her landmark 2010 book *The New Jim Crow: Mass Incarceration in the Age of Colorblindness*, Michelle Alexander described it this way: "The criminalization and demonization of black men has turned the black community against itself, unraveling community and family relationships, decimating networks of mutual support and intensifying the shame and self-hatred experienced by the current pariah class."[7]

The drug war framed drug users and dealers as an enemy to be fought—not as fellow community members with a problem. Thus, locking them up seemed to be the answer. Indeed Yale law professor James Forman has argued that Black support for the drug war was not so much "respectability politics" as it was "responsibility politics"—leaders who supported the crackdown felt that there was no other alternative to save their communities.

It must be noted, too, that there was always also resistance to "respectability" politics within the Black community: for example, civil rights leader Ella Baker pushed for including those who were not seen as respectable like "drunks" and "prostitutes" in activist concerns. In 1986—when support for the drug war was nearly universal—the great Black writer James Baldwin said, "If you want to get to the heart of the dope problem, legalize it," arguing that otherwise drug laws would simply be used to oppress the poor. And sociologist Troy Duster was among the earliest to point out how ideas about who uses drugs—not pharmacology—shape our legal response to them.[8]

But, tragically, American drug policy has always been more a tool of white supremacy than an effective way of managing problems with substances. This is clear from the explicitly racist origins of the laws against cocaine, opium, marijuana, and even the passage of alcohol Prohibition. (See chapter four and, for more on Alexander's influence on bringing this racism to public attention, chapter nineteen.)

The drug war's hidden purpose is also demonstrated by the government's willingness to spend nearly endless amounts of money over many decades on policies that produce few, if any, positive results. Since Nixon first declared war on drugs in 1971, the federal drug control budget alone went from $100 million annually to over $15 billion per year in 2010, thirty-one times higher when adjusted for inflation. Total spending is well over a trillion dollars since the policy was initiated.[9] And funding increases have continued regardless of cuts in other areas—and in spite of worsening addiction, incarceration, and death rates. A policy this expensive and this disastrous on its own terms must be driven, at least in part, by something other than what it claims to be doing.

This means that an important part of the mission of harm reduction is to reveal the racist origins and intent of the drug war—and to show how the damage done by criminalization far outweighs any claimed benefits. Knowing how "respectability" has been used against Black people helps explain why a policy as clearly unsuccessful as the war on drugs has been is able to continue, regardless of its complete inability to solve the problem it purports to address.

For one, politicians have long used the drug war to seek the support of white racists. In the seventies, Nixon's infamous (and effective) "Southern strategy" to win white voters used code words like "tough on drugs" and "tough on crime" to imply that Republicans would be tough on Black people. Top Nixon aide H. R. Haldeman recalled that the president himself "emphasized that you have to face the fact that the whole problem is really the blacks. The key is to devise a system that recognizes this without appearing to."[10]

Sadly, this strategy became even more successful in the eighties and nineties. Ironically, that's because it worked for both parties. Republicans continued to use the drug war as a signal to white racists. But Democrats—including many Black politicians like New York representative Charles Rangel and 1988 Democratic presidential candidate Jesse Jackson—used it to show that they, too, were concerned about drugs and crime.

At that time, treatment was thought to be largely ineffective, and besides, it was too "soft." Any opposition to even the most draconian measures was framed as treason in the drug war—in other words, as being "pro-drug." Many well-intentioned people of all races bought in because they didn't see any other way to address the problem. Before long, this resulted in a herd-like consensus in both parties and the mainstream press, which generally ignored dissenting ideas about drugs. This led each party to aggressively try to outdo the other with ever more extreme sentences and sanctions.

The Anti-Drug Abuse Acts of 1986 and 1988 are some of the cardinal examples. Foundational to the modern drug war, these laws created federal mandatory minimums for crack. They made penalties 100 times greater for sale or even possession of this form of cocaine, based on the quantity of drug that was involved. In practice, this meant that the legislation targeted Black people, who were more likely than whites to use their cocaine in the form of crack, which is less expensive.

A mere five grams of the stuff—which a user could readily consume during a binge with a friend or lover—meant a mandatory five-year sentence as a trafficker, regardless of whether the person actually sold the drug. By 1995, some 80 percent of those serving federal time for federal crack offenses were African American.[11] And states joined in eagerly, creating or placing more emphasis on enforcing longer and harsher sentences for drug crimes than for rape or even murder.

In addition to driving mass incarceration, the legislation piled on all sorts of additional penalties. It banned people convicted of drug crimes from getting student loans. It cut them off from many welfare benefits and food stamps. It required eviction, and later laws permanently prohibited the return of anyone to public housing if they had previously used or sold drugs or even simply failed to prevent drug activity in their home.[12] This often meant that parents could not visit their own children, even if no one had taken illegal drugs for years. It also led to homelessness for many formerly incarcerated people. Rapists and murderers could sometimes be forgiven—but not people who used or sold drugs.

These laws didn't just criminalize and stigmatize drug users: they created overwhelming obstacles to recovery at every turn by reducing opportunities for employment, education, and housing. Since the Reagan era, literally tens of thousands of different restrictions barring people convicted of various drug crimes from everything from voting to becoming a lawyer have been added.[13]

The 1988 Anti-Drug Abuse Act passed the House 346 to 11 in November of that year. It's important to recognize that of those few who stood against it, six were members of the Congressional Black Caucus, who were already seeing the damage that such laws can do.[14] Another notable dissent came from Kurt Schmoke, the first Black mayor of Baltimore, who had shocked the U.S. Conference of Mayors earlier that year by going even further and coming out in favor of decriminalizing drug possession. Within the clergy, the minister of San Francisco's GLIDE Memorial Church, which welcomed people who used crack and helped them move toward change, told the Bush administration that he couldn't support its drug war. "You are interested in a policy of enforcement," said Rev. Cecil Williams. "We are interested in a public health policy that puts priority on recovery."[15] (GLIDE would later adopt harm reduction, including offering a syringe exchange program.)

As these drug policy dissidents could already see, our overwhelmingly punitive approach had resulted—at least in part, by design—in creating a stereotype of the "drug user" as an immoral Black person, heedlessly seeking selfish pleasure. (This is why you often hear white people with addiction saying, "I'm not your typical addict." The unspoken and racist assumption is that the typical addict is Black—or worse, that addiction is typical for Black people.)

Michelle Alexander put it this way: "Drug crime in this country is understood to be black and brown and it is because drug crime is racially defined in the public consciousness that the electorate has not cared much what happens to drug criminals."[16] This lack of empathy across racial boundaries is what makes American drug policy toxic to its core.

Our indifference to Black humanity is a critical aspect of what allows politicians and the media, deliberately or otherwise, to use ideas about drugs to dehumanize people who take them. It is also part of how America has come to accept the idea that taking drugs makes someone unworthy of life—let alone care and respect. Consequently, the overlap between stereotypes of people with addiction and racist stereotypes of Black people has been devastating for the African American community—and most of all, for Black people who use drugs.

This noxious mixture also created a level of stigma that is so blinding that few Americans ever thought to question why stopping people from taking certain substances was more important than protecting them from AIDS—even when that meant putting their children and partners at risk as well. This same stigma led directly to the deaths of thousands of drug users, mainly Black and Latino, as syringe exchange was delayed over and over again across the country by endless local debates about whether it "sent the wrong message."

As Cathy J. Cohen, now professor of political science at the University of Chicago, describes it, "In the outcry over needle exchange in New York City, black officials seemed to engage in a calculus of human worth, where the lives of 'innocent children' and 'regular law abiding community folk' were designated as more important and more worth saving than the lives of black injection drug users."[17] Her book, which is titled *The Boundaries of Blackness*, shows how respectability politics left Black drug users outside of the borders that encompass those who deserve help. Such people, she wrote, "were perceived as a disgrace to 'the community' and thus not worth the expense of the limited political capital controlled by black elites."[18]

The key idea here is that the existence of Black users can be used to justify white racism—and therefore, they must be expelled from both ordinary human concern and from Blackness itself. As fear of AIDS grew, a sign appeared on the lampposts of Harlem, saying, "When will all the junkies die so all the rest of us can go on living?"

Researchers conducted a study that took a closer look at the response to AIDS in injecting drug users by New York's Black communities at this time. "[M]iddle class black interviewees saw the drug issue as a reflection of an inadequacy of the black community to confront 'improper' behavior by community members, allowing conduct sure to increase the stigma and racism blacks experience," they noted.[19]

Or as Harlon Dalton, a Yale law professor, put it, "We as a community have a complex relationship with illicit drugs, a relationship that often paralyzes us. On the one hand, blacks are scared to even admit the dimensions of the problem for fear that we will all be treated as junkies and our culture viewed as pathological. On the other, we desperately want to find solutions." He noted that the rest of the community despises Black people with addiction "because they hurt us and because they are us. They are a constant reminder of how close we all are to the edge. And 'they' are 'us' literally as well as figuratively; they are our sons and daughters, our sisters and brothers."[20]

Worse, all of this stigma, racism, and dehumanization was exacerbated by the intensity and high visibility of crack cocaine use and sales in New York's poorest neighborhoods during the peak years of AIDS. Ronald Reagan and George W. Bush's "crackdown on crack" was the Southern strategy on steroids: not only could Republicans use the rise of this drug to demonize Black people and fill the media with images of their alleged depravity, it could also deflect attention away from the cuts in services and high levels of unemployment that might otherwise be blamed for the already elevated and still rising crime rates in cities. Only about 3 percent of the American population in the highest risk age group for use—white or Black—had ever tried crack when the hysteria about it was at its peak. Nonetheless, the media during this time was absolutely flooded with scare stories about the new "instantly addictive" drug that was surely headed to the suburbs from the ghettos.[21]

As a rare dissenting op-ed, published in the *New York Times* in 1986 and written by a lawyer, put it, "If we blame crime on crack, our politicians are off the hook. Forgotten are the failed schools, the malign welfare programs, the desolate neighborhoods, the wasted years. Only crack is to blame. One is tempted to think that if crack did not exist, someone, somewhere would have received a federal grant to develop it."[22]

During a period when the majority of Americans got their news from the three major TV networks' nightly shows—each only a half hour long—crack received a lopsidedly outsized degree of attention. In July 1986 alone, there were at least thirty segments focused on crack. In a print sector dominated by two major newsmagazines, *Time* and *Newsweek* called the rise of the drug the most important news of that year, with *Newsweek* saying that it was bigger than Watergate or Vietnam.

Until the mid-nineties, the crack story was constantly highlighted by newspapers, magazines, local and national TV newscasts, and documentaries. Most of this coverage suggested users were hopelessly hooked; almost none of it focused on recovery, even though recovery was, in reality, common. And little reporting suggested any remedy other than law enforcement. Crack users and dealers who were shown were almost always Black, despite the fact that whites often turned the powder cocaine they bought into smokable freebase, which is pharmacologically identical.

By September of 1989, two-thirds of Americans said that crack and other illegal drugs were the worst problem facing the country, despite an unemployment rate of 5.4 percent and an economy heading into a recession.[23] That year, a *Time* magazine columnist claimed that children born to mothers who used crack during pregnancy were doomed to be criminals and/or intellectually disabled. He wrote, "A cohort of babies is now being born whose future is closed to them from day one. Theirs will be a life of certain suffering, of probable deviance, of permanent inferiority. At best, a menial life of severe deprivation. And all of this is biologically determined from birth."[24]

Nearly all of these babies supposedly facing "lives of permanent inferiority" were, at least in the minds of white readers, Black. And their mothers faced the most extreme stigma of all: they were seen as so devoted to their own selfishness that they were willing to destroy their children. However, scientific evidence did not then and does not now support these claims: most cocaine-exposed children showed little effect beyond that of poverty, and the only common psychoactive drug linked to specific and irreversible damage to infants in the womb is alcohol. Most mothers of drug-exposed children, moreover, have histories of childhood and adult trauma so severe that it is difficult to even read about, never mind experience. Rather than exploring this, however, the media portrayed them as monsters.

In this context, it is hardly surprising that Black leaders wanted to distance themselves from people who use drugs and that many feared strategies like needle exchange that might make them seem "soft." Sadly, the AIDS years coincided with the crack epidemic and the drug war hysteria around it almost completely.

As a result, activists like Williams were constantly having to justify their support of needle exchange to other Black people. One Black harm reductionist from the West Coast told me about an incident she experienced at a community meeting. A member of the audience, also Black, accused her to her face of perpetrating a new version of the Tuskegee syphilis experiment by supporting syringe exchange. "That was extraordinarily painful, in a very visceral way . . . to be accused of this horrible betrayal of my own people," she said.[25]

At the same time, of course, Black harm reductionists also faced racism in mainly white activist groups like ACT UP. It made for lonely work. "For me, I don't say that things in ACT UP were 'racist,'" Williams said. "I think it was internalized racism that people sort of do, and they have no clue that they're doing it." Later, the lens of harm reduction would be used to shed new light on issues like racist policing, police violence, incarceration, restorative justice, and many other aspects of criminal prosecution reform. It would be adopted by Black Lives Matter activists, who would bring the idea to a new mass movement. But during the AIDS crisis, for the most part, activism around HIV and drug use was quite separate from Black-led activism on civil rights.

For his part, Williams described how he was frequently at odds with both white gay men and Black activists. "[You're] just ostracized every damn place," he said. "You're ostracized in the black community, because you're hanging out with gay people and the AIDS thing . . . [And] the white people never liked you in the first place. You're nobody. You're way down there."[26]

Fortunately, however, he soon found an ally in another African American member of ACT UP, who would also become critical to the rise of harm reduction.

eight

Housing Works

I N 1989, KEITH CYLAR, A BLACK, GAY SOCIAL WORKER FROM VIRGINIA, attended his first ACT UP meeting. Slim and muscular, with long dread-locks, he turned heads pretty much everywhere. Once he began engaging in activism, he was frequently highlighted in photos of demonstrations and other actions.

Around a year earlier, his partner had died of AIDS just four days after being diagnosed. At the time, Cylar was in New York to pursue his master's degree in social work at Columbia. After losing his lover and testing positive himself, he visited the Lesbian, Gay, Bisexual and Trans-gender Community Center on 13th Street in the Village to try to figure out what to do. He came upon a table filled with ACT UP pamphlets and handouts, which had been placed outside the irregularly shaped room where the group then met. But the real attraction was all of the men in black leather.

"It was the lit[erature] that made me stop. It was the black leather jackets that pulled me into the room," he said.[1] For a few weeks, as he describes it, he stood at the back of meetings, just listening and occasion-ally mumbling "Get the fuck out of here" in response to what he saw as clueless remarks from the speakers. Dan Williams began to stand nearby when he saw him at these Monday night meetings.

They started to connect, at first just nodding at each other when they agreed something was absurd. But soon they began to talk, and Williams invited him to join Majority Action. "I was kind of sweet on him," Williams admitted, noting ruefully that the romantic interest was not mutual. Nonetheless, they began to work together.

Cylar himself used drugs like cocaine, but he didn't get involved directly with needle exchange. Instead, he threw himself into many different groups and actions, including working with Williams to attempt to find some common ground with groups like the Black Leadership Commission on AIDS.

"The first time we went there, we went there very, very confrontational," said Williams, "and then, we got accused of being [sent] by the white boys. And that was painful, because, it was, like, 'No, you can't do anything on your own, you have to be directed.'"[2] Eventually, however, they began to forge some connections, laying the groundwork for the organization to eventually start to reconsider some of its positions.

Cylar's biggest contribution to harm reduction, however, started with his work on ACT UP's Housing Committee, which rapidly morphed into a separate nonprofit organization. Known as Housing Works, it pioneered housing for people with AIDS who used drugs. In other words, Cylar brought the concept of harm reduction to housing.

By 1996, Housing Works would become the largest provider of housing for people with HIV in New York—and by 2004, it had annual revenue of $26 million, much of which came from a network of high-end thrift shops, a bookstore, and a catering company. All of these organizations employ Housing Works residents—and the rest of the funding comes from government grants, Medicaid, and private donations.[3] The nonprofit has become a New York institution and remains highly successful. And it was co-founded and co-directed by a Black, gay, HIV-positive man who continued to use drugs and be open about that for nearly his entire career. Cylar's work was harm reduction in action.

Like many of ACT UP's subgroups, the Housing Committee had formed to address a pressing real-world problem. In the early nineties, New York's hospitals were overwhelmed by AIDS—and many of the people who had been infected via IV drug use were homeless or unstably housed. ACT UP began pushing for—and soon succeeded in winning—better treatment of opportunistic infections. But as this began to extend lives, patients had nowhere to go when they improved enough to be discharged. "I couldn't get people out of the hospital because they didn't have a place to live," Cylar said.[4]

Drug treatment centers and similarly abstinence-oriented residences were out. Not only were these institutions wary of having to deal with HIV, they were obviously not the place for people who had no intention of quitting drugs. But organizations that housed people with AIDS didn't want drug users, either: they were largely run by and designed for middle-class, white, gay men and were just as influenced by stereotypes and prejudice about drugs as everyone else. Similarly, the attitude of mainstream homelessness service providers had long been that people who won't stop taking drugs don't deserve a home. In fact, federal law on public housing projects specifically required expelling people who had criminal records related to drugs.

"Housing Works started when, after demonstrating, fighting and working in the AIDS community, the people that I cared the most about were the people least likely to get served," said Cylar. "And so, we decided we had to do it ourselves."[5]

Cylar and Charles King, who would become both his life partner and a co-founder of Housing Works, met cute in ACT UP. Outwardly it didn't look like a promising pairing. King is white and is the son of a fundamentalist right-wing preacher from Texas. He had become a minister himself, though admittedly one dedicated to antiracism. He'd left the ministry to go to law school. Like Cylar, King is striking. During his early days at ACT UP he had long, center-parted light brown hair, with a beard and mustache, which gave him the perhaps not unintended look of a rebel Jesus.

Their first few encounters were political or strategic arguments. Then someone at the Monday meeting called for volunteers to write a fact sheet and King raised his hand. The second hand to go up was Cylar's. He immediately told the floor that no further volunteers were needed. King recalled, "He comes over to me about five minutes later and says, 'I think we should go ahead and knock this out right away. You want to come over to my place and do it?'"[6]

"We walked over to his place, and I sit down on the couch and pull out my notepad . . . and the next thing you know he's kissing me and seduced me, and that was it. We were partners for life," King said.

HOUSING WORKS WAS FOUNDED AS A NONPROFIT ORGANIZATION BY CYLAR and King, along with two others, in 1990. They opened their first "scattered site" (that is, not all in the same building) housing for people with AIDS who used drugs in April of 1991. Initially, an anonymous benefactor funded the group, but they were soon able to get government money as well because they specifically wanted to house the people whom everyone else rejected. Before long, they were providing homes for dozens and then hundreds of people—eventually owning several buildings and having assets worth $27 million.[7]

No one had ever created a program like it before, so the founders had to think carefully. It was one thing to spout rhetoric about the importance of housing to the health of people who are HIV-positive and actively addicted, no matter how deeply that rhetoric was felt and believed. It was quite another to actually provide decent homes—especially since the majority of these folks also have serious mental illness that tends to make their lives even more chaotic. These were the homeless people that organizations designed specifically to serve homeless people couldn't handle.

Cylar was already determined that harm reduction should be the foundation for their work. He knew Edith Springer; he'd probably been to one of her trainings and may have even initially learned about the concept from her. And so Housing Works immediately turned to her to train its newly hired staff. This included familiarizing King with the basics of harm reduction. He was on board, at least intellectually, right away.

However, it was harder than expected to completely eradicate the standard rigid, infantilizing, and punitive approach. Even though Housing Works had been designed to give homes to people who use drugs, Springer found that many of the staff clung fiercely to the notion that their main goal was not housing, but abstinence. Maybe they could be okay with a bit of drug use early on or here and there, but they wanted to see progress toward quitting and wanted to expel those who didn't seem headed to total abstinence. She had to work hard to get them to think differently.

It would also take time and experience to develop policies that distinguished between genuine concerns about loud noise, disruptive behaviors, guests, and crime—and moralism about what health should look like for people with HIV, mental illness, and addictions. It would take even longer to develop and institute rules that were fair and flexible enough to cope with them.

"If you think about the fact that back then, having an AIDS diagnosis meant that you were going to die in six to nine months, can you give me one reason why I would not want to get high?" said Cylar. "For me as a social worker, it just made sense to say, 'Okay, get high. But how do we manage your life so you can live a little longer?'"

"Our bottom line, counter to all of the traditional drug treatment approaches was, if you can't keep people alive, you're never going to be able to help them into recovery," said King, acknowledging that abstinent recovery was initially still the goal. But as they worked with Springer and became more and more familiar with harm reduction, the program evolved over time to recognize that other outcomes like decreased or less chaotic use and improvements in health also counted and mattered.

The story of one of the first families to live in a Housing Works apartment shows how this played out in practice. This family included a husband, a wife, and two young children. The father died from AIDS almost immediately after they got their apartment. At the time, the mother, Laura (not her real name), who was also HIV-positive, was seriously addicted to crack. "She would binge pretty much every time she got money," King said. "And so, first of all, there's an issue with safety for her children, but also, she was running out of money because she spent it all."

To deal with her overspending, Housing Works helped Laura create a budget based on the public assistance payments she received. She would first use her money to pay for essentials for her kids and herself. But she also chose to set aside a certain amount for crack. Together, she and her counselor decided to have the program keep her money for her in a safe, with separate envelopes for each budget category. This would reduce temptation to break her budget and help her stay accountable, above all, to herself.

The intention was not to be punitive or rigidly controlling. But a key to successful harm reduction is finding structures that allow people to make better choices—not just setting them up to fail by either allowing no choice whatsoever or completely free choice without systems in place to help the person learn how to self-manage. Figuring out what works for particular individuals is often a process of trial and error, and it requires much more flexibility and creativity from staff than simply enforcing rules or teaching a set curriculum. This is critical to successfully housing people who use drugs.

These ideas would also be pertinent as harm reduction concepts began to be applied to other areas. For example, environmentalists began to realize that expecting people to make absolute behavior changes, like becoming 100 percent vegan, giving up cars and flying, and only purchasing new items when there is no alternative, was unrealistic and could actually cause backlash. But asking people to try one vegetarian day a week or experiment with cutting back on travel was more engaging—and could lead to greater change over time. Moreover, when small changes are adopted by large groups of people, they add up. Similarly, harm reduction approaches for overuse of cell phones and other technology have people make smaller changes first and try various technologies to limit use, rather than starting with complete abstinence. And during the 2020 COVID-19 pandemic, harm reduction concepts have been developed to allow for safer socializing—such as meeting outdoors and wearing masks.

Happily, not only did Laura's banking system at Housing Works help her manage her money, it also helped her with planning more generally. "That allowed us to have honest, open conversations to ensure that before she went on a run, she would take her children over to a relative to watch them," said King. Knowing that she was starting to behave more responsibly also allowed Laura to feel a bit better about her life. And that helped her begin to corral the crack use so that soon she was only using on weekends.

Laura had begun her budgeting process in the summer. That fall, she saw a beautiful red girls' coat in a thrift store window. She knew that her daughter needed one—and it was exactly the right size and not exorbitantly expensive. She talked to the counselor who was working with her. Together, they realized that she could afford the coat if she simply took two weekends off from crack. And so she did.

"What she learned from that was that she had the possibility of making a choice that she hadn't believed she could make," said King. This is exactly the same process seen with needle exchange: a successful small change sparks hope that much bigger change could be possible. Consequently, during the rest of that winter, whenever there was something she really wanted to buy for her kids or herself, Laura would cut her crack budget accordingly. By that spring, King says, "She just decided, 'I'm tired of wasting my money on crack.'" And without any further assistance, she quit, eventually going back to school and becoming a staff member.

Not all of Housing Works's clients have such a straightforward path or such an overwhelmingly positive outcome, of course. But over time, as the agency grew, King and Cylar could see clear patterns of change. At any given time, about a third of the clients living in the apartments that Housing Works now owns or manages are stable and drug-free, or pretty close to it. About a third are in a phase similar to what Laura experienced at first, where they can, for the most part, manage their drug use so that it doesn't completely dominate their lives, and they are reducing their exposure to negative consequences over time. And the final third are still using heavily, with little evidence of any change.

This last group, of course, is certainly better off being housed and having help managing their HIV and psychiatric medications. However, many still engage in disturbing behavior driven by their desire for relief and oblivion—and certain things cannot be tolerated within Housing Works and do result in expulsion. The most obvious of these is violence, which clearly harms the community. Overt racism is considered to be violence as well. So, for example, a man who ignored repeated warnings about racist language and then graffitied a racist manifesto on a publicly visible building wall was evicted. Generally, though, the idea is to do as much as possible to keep people housed and find creative solutions to ensure that potentially antisocial behavior doesn't harm others.

Indeed, the person whom King calls Housing Works' "prototypical" client, a man named Sterling Smith, was evicted from nearly every apartment the group managed that he had occupied. That was quite a few. One time, he was thrown out for running a brothel in his apartment; in another instance, the problem was drug dealing. While high, Smith could be extremely volatile, and this, too, resulted in trouble. During the last ten years of his life, however, he managed to control his use and his behavior enough that he was able to keep his Housing Works apartment in Harlem. When he became terminally ill, he died at home, with King by his side.

Cylar explained why the process of improving health is often so difficult for people who live at Housing Works. "For many of our clients, the first step toward becoming whole is to forgive themselves for all of the scary and insane things that happened to them and they may have done to others," he said. Often—as in Smith's case—their reaction to people who try to help is initially resistance—and even, sometimes, trying to deliberately mislead workers because they distrust pretty much everyone.

"It requires the staff to develop a real sense of compassion, as the clients often become abusive, self-destructive, and angry," said Cylar, explaining that it's a pretty natural response from people who have grown up in a world that is often actively hostile, where people and institutions are frequently unreliable or outright cruel. Virtually everyone who ends up homeless, addicted, mentally ill, and HIV-positive has a long history of childhood trauma, typically compounded by the experience of racism and the extreme distress and social rejection that comes with living on the street or being incarcerated.

Ironically, however, while King could clearly see the value of harm reduction at work, in his personal and professional relationship with Cylar, he took a more absolutist stance toward drug use at first. He knew that fighting for the rights of active users to have decent housing and clean needles was the right thing to do. He had made it his life's work. But was it even possible to have a long-term, loving relationship with a person who was actively addicted? And could a harm reduction organization really accommodate an employee at the highest level if he continued to regularly and enthusiastically take drugs?

Keith Cylar and Charles King would soon show the world how.

IT WASN'T LONG AFTER KING AND CYLAR MOVED IN WITH EACH OTHER THAT King realized that his partner had a problem with cocaine. They had done coke together at parties, but King found that the drug gave him a hangover that lasted a few days. A Saturday night staying up snorting lines, for King, meant a lost Sunday and a fog that persisted long into Monday morning.

"It wasn't really my thing," he said, explaining, "I hate wasting time." And once he realized that Cylar was addicted, he stopped snorting cocaine himself in hopes of encouraging his lover to do the same.

At this point in 1990, when Housing Works was just getting off the ground, Cylar was employed as a social worker at a Harlem community organization.[8] The plan was for him to quit that job to become co-president of Housing Works when it officially opened. King realized his partner had a coke problem when Cylar went out one Saturday night and didn't return until Monday morning.

And, when he finally came home, Cylar didn't just expect King to forgive him, either. He wanted his lover to call his boss and lie, saying that he was too ill to come to work. Already furious, King refused. He insisted that, if Cylar wanted to start at Housing Works in April as planned, he must get help first. After some argument, he agreed. They found a traditional twelve-step residential program in Minnesota that specialized in treating gay men. Cylar attended and made a serious effort. During the month that Cylar was in treatment, King flew out to visit and participate in the family members' program that was part of the rehab.

But Cylar's abstinence only lasted about six months. Before long, he'd begun drinking alcohol, which, like all other substances except caffeine and nicotine, is considered a relapse in the twelve-step model, even if it isn't the person's preferred drug. Eventually, he also returned to cocaine. Now King didn't know what to do.

He was running an organization based on harm reduction, which accepted the idea that many people can manage drug use and reduce its risks without abstinence. He believed that to be true. And yet here he was insisting that his partner and colleague could not remain employed at Housing Works unless he was abstinent. He struggled with himself and with Cylar.

"We had made a commitment early on that our staff would reflect who we serve," King said. And at the time, Cylar was the only one of the group's core leadership who was HIV-positive and Black—not to mention his drug use status. Should the group go as far as to have an active drug user—who was absolutely representative of the population they served—as one of its chief executives? Or was that taking harm reduction too far?

King felt conflicted. Like many partners and parents of people with addiction, he wanted the best for his loved one, and that seemed to him to be abstinence in this case. On the other hand, there was clearly value to Housing Works and its clients if its leadership modeled the kind of inclusivity it claimed it wanted to see for people who use drugs.

Also, since they were genuinely coequal in leadership, King couldn't just fire Cylar without the approval of the organization's board. The founders had deliberately created a strong board structure so that no single person had the power to take over—or let their personal problems take over—the entire organization. Unchecked power can cause problems in any institution, of course. But it is especially dangerous for organizations that deal with addiction and other mental health issues. For harm reduction specifically, having a clear and balanced management structure that doesn't rely solely on one person is essential.

Most of the time, King realized, Cylar's work was unaffected by his drug use. He brought a unique perspective to the organization—not just because of his race and HIV status and drug experience, but also because of his deep intelligence and understanding of harm reduction. The result was that, despite arguments, Cylar began and continued his full-time job at Housing Works as planned.

And, over time, King and Cylar developed ways to adapt the position to avoid problems related to Cylar's addiction—using many of the same methods by which a job would be adapted for any other kind of disability. The structure and systems devised by Housing Works and Cylar remain a model for coping with addiction-related disability.

"It came down to 'What is the value added, and is the value added worth the extra price?' And when you framed it with that kind of equation, there was no question," said King. Conflicts over particular issues—especially around time and speaking commitments that were made and not met—continued, but eventually work-arounds like having a backup person, just in case, were created. There was nothing inherently wrong with having an understudy, King realized. The theatre community, for one, had developed that role for a reason.

King had tried for much of his life to fight racism and bias. But during his collaboration with Cylar, he also continued to have moments when he recognized that he retained deep prejudices about addiction. When Cylar didn't show up for a critical court deposition, the incident sparked one of these reckonings. This happened at a time when the organization was under great threat. They had publicly attacked New York's then-mayor, Rudy Giuliani, and were at risk of losing millions of dollars in funding as a result of his wrath. They'd even had to lay off staff and delay payroll. They needed to win the lawsuit for which Cylar was being deposed.

King and everyone else at Housing Works who knew what had happened were furious. Didn't Keith know how important this case was? Cylar and King argued angrily. "How could he, of all days to get high or be hung over [choose this one]?" King recalled asking. He ripped into his partner, telling him "in very unkind terms how angry I was and how much he had let the whole community down." Then Cylar explained that the reason he'd been unable to attend was not drugs but an anxiety attack. He wasn't off having fun getting high—he was at home, paralyzed by fear.

From living with Cylar, King knew immediately that this was true: he'd seen how badly his partner suffered from agoraphobia and other anxiety disorders and how much he struggled with them. If he hadn't been so close to Cylar, he'd never have even guessed that this could be the problem. "This guy always fronted as the most together guy in the world," King said. The black leather, the cool attitude, and the sheer charisma Cylar exuded successfully camouflaged his vulnerability.

"It was almost easier for him to acknowledge that he was using drugs than to acknowledge that he was having an anxiety attack," said King, explaining that he felt tremendously guilty once he realized this. He had unconsciously continued to buy into the stereotype that people with addiction are just selfish and don't care about how their actions affect others. It hadn't occurred to him to think about the relationship between Cylar's drug use and his mental illness—and why the pressure of the situation might overwhelm him.

From then on, backup plans and substitute speakers were easier for him to accept. "I think that's what you have to do, but because it's so stigmatized, it took this learning process, which was really unlearning stigma associated with somebody using drugs," King said. The drug use didn't cause Cylar's anxiety and dyslexia—both conditions had long preceded it. Drugs, King added, are "just the distraction that catches our eye."

Another incident also illustrated the importance of what Cylar brought to Housing Works as co-president. In 2000, he was arrested in Chelsea for illegal possession of anti-anxiety pills without a prescription. He was diverted into an education program, rather than jailed. For everyone involved, that was a relief, even though it was almost certainly a class he could have taught himself—and probably with more evidence-based information.

But it also posed a serious problem. There would almost certainly be Housing Works clients attending as well, who would be very likely to recognize him. King's first thought was to try to cover it up, to avoid embarrassment for Cylar and the organization. Perhaps they could devise a story about how he was auditing the class to see what these services were really like?

Cylar, however, had a better idea. He attended the class, and when people recognized him, he simply said, "Yep, I'm just like you." With that humility, he flipped a situation in which he could have been seen as a poor role model on its head. By attending openly, he modeled for clients how to handle the often humiliating consequences imposed on people who take drugs, which must be endured regardless of whether they make any sense, and which are almost always imposed more harshly against Black people. As a Black leader within harm reduction, he'd had plenty of experience with such circumstances.

HOUSING WORKS WAS LIKELY THE FIRST AMERICAN ORGANIZATION TO PUT into practice what became known as the "Housing First" philosophy in services for people who are unhoused. Like most of harm reduction, the idea sounds obvious if you aren't immersed in the abstinence-obsessed addiction treatment world. Essentially, Housing First recognizes that it is highly unlikely that someone living in an unstable setting or entirely without shelter will be able to quit alcohol or other drugs while still on the street.

Requiring them to give up their only coping strategy before they are considered "eligible" for housing is asking the impossible for most homeless people—especially given that many are simultaneously experiencing mental illness, racism, HIV, hunger, the stress of living outdoors, and the psychological catastrophe of frequently being treated as the lowest form of human life. Moreover, repeatedly "failing" and being ejected from housing programs with unrealistic requirements is demoralizing and often leads people to give up on seeking help.

Another pioneering example of Housing First in the HIV field was known as Stand Up Harlem. Founded in the early nineties by a Black, homeless, HIV-positive, former heroin user named Louis Jones, the group was able to wrest a Harlem brownstone away from drug dealers and turn it into a multimillion-dollar AIDS center, complete with holistic health care and delicious chef-cooked meals.[9] Stand Up—so-named because Jones was moved to stand up and fight AIDS at a friend's funeral—was unique in including both active and former drug users in a single community based on harm reduction. It also melded activism and service. Unfortunately, it didn't have a strong board and collapsed in the late nineties, after Jones himself lost control of his drug use. But happily, Housing Works was able to acquire its assets and hire Jones as he recovered and went on to further critical work in organizing drug users. Today, Charles King lives in its building along with some of Housing Works' clients. It is now known as Stand Up Harlem House.

Outside of the world of HIV and harm reduction, Housing First officially began in 1992, in a program led by a psychologist in New York City. By 1997, researchers had shown in a randomized trial that Housing First was able to keep 80 percent of participants housed for four years, which is far better than the rate for traditional high-barrier programs.[10] Adopted statewide in Utah, it cut chronic homelessness by an astonishing 91 percent between 2005 and 2015—after which, unfortunately, budget cuts reduced its effectiveness.[11] Nonetheless, by 2010, the idea had become a principle of federal housing policy—with cities that implemented it faithfully showing similar successes.[12] Unfortunately, the Trump administration opposed it and, aided by the coronavirus catastrophe, reversed much of the progress that was made.

At the same time, however, the COVID-19 pandemic has also led to new glimmers of light for harm reduction in housing. Some cities gave homeless people hotel rooms—and provided methadone, other medication treatment, and even alcohol in some cases in order to reduce harm from viral exposure if people left to buy substances. Early research shows that these policies were successful, like other Housing First strategies, when implemented with proper support. In addition, during the outbreak, a nationwide moratorium on evictions was declared—to attempt to prevent a new wave of homelessness. While imperfect, it, too, showed how focusing on reducing harm—regardless of people's drug use status—is a better strategy than letting harm take place and trying to pick up the pieces afterward.

All this rests on the groundbreaking work of Housing Works and others, illustrating the power of harm reduction to manage complex problems like long-term homelessness that were previously seen as hopeless. The contributions of people like Cylar, who had lived experience of both racism and addiction, were critical to its development.

nine

The Heiress and the Biker

S TEPHANIE COMER SEEMED LIKE AN UNLIKELY CANDIDATE TO BECOME HARM reduction's first and perhaps most important benefactor. Her old-school Republican father had founded the outdoorsy clothes retailer Lands' End, which presents the sailing and yachting life as a WASPy ideal. When he took the company public in 1986, the family became immensely wealthy almost overnight. Stephanie's life transformed. It almost certainly had never occurred to her parents that their windfall would wind up funding one of the most radical—and life-saving—movements in American drug policy. But they did not stand in the way when it did.

Over time, the Comer Family Foundation would give harm reduction some $14.5 million.[1] At first, even small grants of a few thousand dollars were crucial in sustaining a new movement that had previously had no regular source of financial support and no national organization. Stephanie Comer's advocacy and funds would change that.

"We did not grow up with any of this," Comer said, gesturing at the swank Chicago boardroom around her, which is decorated with valuable original maritime paintings of sailing ships upon raging seas, in many shades of blue. Now in her fifties, she appears to have none of the snobbery or entitlement that might come from the station in life she attained when she was still an English major at Vassar College. She's dressed casually, in a flounced blue shirt with subtle orange stripes. She has shoulder-length black hair tinged with silver, a wide smile, and warm brown eyes.

The story of how an empire built on nautical accessories and preppy clothes became the first big funder of harm reduction—which has a decidedly more countercultural set of meanings—rests mainly on chance. Almost immediately after selling the company, Comer's father set up the foundation. In 1991, Stephanie was asked to run it. Since she was feeling directionless in terms of her career at the time, "I sort of shrugged and said okay," she explained.[2]

She began with what she knew. In New York, where she had gone to college, AIDS had affected everyone in the art scene. "I think just coming of age during that time you were caught up in it. You couldn't help it and you were so angry that more wasn't being done," she said. And so she decided that fighting HIV would be a good use of the foundation's money. Then she began looking for a specific area within this broad cause to support.

By this time, Comer had moved to San Francisco to attend graduate school in photography—and the City by the Bay was just as devastated as the Big Apple. She started researching and talking to friends. On both coasts, gay men were the most visibly and audibly affected—but they were already mobilized, as she puts it.

Meanwhile, her mother, Francie, knew that Stephanie was seeking a way to have a major impact in HIV funding. For philanthropists, one of the best methods to ensure that you can make a real splash is to be the biggest—or at least the first—donor in an area. It's an entrepreneurial mindset, where the aura of size and originality are king. In high-profile fields like cancer research or museums, there's little real estate that hasn't already been named and claimed. But the Comers found a rare cause that was a completely different story.

On August 6, 1991, Francie saw a segment on PBS's *MacNeil/Lehrer NewsHour* that would change the course of harm reduction in America.[3] That random viewing of a public television segment would set in motion a series of connections that would create the most important national harm reduction group and help redefine what it means to have and recover from addiction.

Unlike many people who focus their charity on drug issues, the Comers had no personal or family experience with addiction. They came to harm reduction almost randomly, simply seeking to maximize their philan-thropic impact. This turned out to be beneficial: it meant that they hadn't absorbed the truisms of the treatment field and drug war that made so many people wary of or outright opposed to harm reduction. What seemed like a terrifying controversy to insiders and drug warriors—giving needles to addicts! Treating them humanely, rather than punishing them to deter others!—seemed like common sense from a public health perspective.

"I came to it without preconceived notions," Stephanie said. Both her mom and dad did, too. And this outsider view allowed them to see an op-portunity to save thousands of lives—rather than a source of potential bad publicity best avoided.

The broadcast that Frances Comer had seen spotlighted a man named Dave Purchase. Several months before New York City's health department began its ill-fated pilot program, Purchase had founded the first needle exchange in the United States that was embraced and supported by local government.

Purchase handed out his first needles in Tacoma, Washington, in Au-gust 1988 and had since become a major expert in the field. The segment in which he appeared was tied to the news that the National Commission on AIDS—a group created by Congress to seek best practices—had just endorsed needle exchange. Research that Purchase had helped conduct was among the data that had led the influential group to reach its positive conclusion.[4]

A motorcycle enthusiast who looked the part, Purchase had spent time on disability after a drunk driver slammed into his Harley and se-riously injured his leg in 1983. Before that, he'd been the director of a methadone program and had become concerned about the HIV risk his patients faced. Within a year or so of the accident, he'd worked his way from using a wheelchair to crutches. But then a building site exploded as he walked by, rebreaking his previously injured leg in three places.

Purchase didn't let this double misfortune stop him. Not being some-one who could just sit around—and still furious about the government's indifference to the spread of HIV in injectors—he decided to start a sy-ringe program. He'd heard about similar work being planned in Oregon and had read up on its European origins.

By that point, there already were sixty-three known HIV cases among Tacoma's 3,000 needle users—and he didn't want to see anyone else needlessly get infected. As he put it—and he became well known in harm reduction for his aphorisms—"A dead person can't two-step, let alone twelve-step."[5]

Fully prepared to be arrested, Purchase informed local officials—including the mayor, the police chief, and the director of the health department—about what he intended to do. His daughter whimsically put $500 in her freezer in case he needed to be bailed out.[6] Using money he'd received from a settlement related to his accident, Purchase bought dozens of needles.

Finally able to walk again with aid from a cane, he set up on the side of a downtown street that he knew to be frequented by injectors. No buildings exploded. He hauled out a folding chair and a tray table meant for TV dinners, on which he placed the works.

Unlike Jon Parker and ACT UP on the East Coast, Purchase rapidly won community and governmental support. The county health department immediately sent an outreach worker to help him and to start to conduct research. Even the police chief didn't want to arrest him. Recognizing that criminalization of needles spread the virus, he left the syringe exchange alone. Within five months, Purchase was a paid employee of the health department and had exchanged 13,000 needles.[7] That bail money would be left to chill in the fridge for many years.

Purchase had been featured on PBS that night to talk about his work and why he did it. And the more Stephanie and Francie Comer looked into the matter, the more excited they became about trying to fund him. As it turned out, his needle exchange work was not limited to Tacoma or even Washington state. Purchase had a sideline in helping people across the country start and then maintain their own programs.

By 1991, THE U.S. HAD MORE THAN A DOZEN EXCHANGES IN AT LEAST NINE states. In San Francisco, the group who worked with Maureen Gammon and Sheigla Murphy conducted their first underground needle exchange on the Day of the Dead in November 1988—seeing that as an auspicious time, both to save lives and commune with those who had already been lost. Portland, Oregon, officially opened a program in 1989.[8]

In New York, little more than a month after the verdict in the Needle Eight Trial in August of 1991, the *New York Times* ran a front-page story about a new study conducted by researchers at Yale. This research would help break through the wall of opposition in the leadership of the Black community.

As Dr. Larry Brown, the sole prosecution expert, had testified during that trial, opponents saw most previous syringe exchange data as worthless because of what they believed to be a fundamental flaw. That is, the research was almost entirely based on self-reports from people who inject drugs about whether or not they continued to share needles. And obviously, given the well-known stereotype about junkies as liars, such studies couldn't be trusted.

But the new data—from one of the country's most prestigious universities—couldn't be dismissed so easily. A Yale professor of public health, engineering, and management had devised a clever way to let the needles speak for themselves.[9] By studying microscopic amounts of blood left inside returned syringes, researchers could find remnants of the HIV virus if they were present—regardless of whether the needle had been bleached and the HIV had been inactivated.

Using this method, along with statistical modeling techniques, he and his colleagues were able to show that eight months after a new needle exchange began in New Haven, the amount of HIV circulating in needles fell by 33 percent. In other words, needle exchange reduced the odds that a syringe on the street would have HIV in it by removing contaminated needles from the supply and increasing the number of clean ones. This data was hard to reject. On top of the existing studies showing that places with better syringe access had lower HIV rates and vice versa, it was pretty definitive.

However, perhaps at least as important as the research itself was the support offered for needle exchange by New Haven's Black mayor, John C. Daniels. Like New York's Mayor Dinkins, Daniels had originally been strongly opposed. "This program is not a solution to AIDS or to drug addiction," he told the *Times*, when the study was released. He stressed that, "It is one more Band-Aid, but it is a Band-Aid we cannot afford to do without."[10]

And indeed, by November 1991, Dinkins would agree to let the American Foundation for AIDS Research (AmFAR), which had been co-founded by legendary actor Elizabeth Taylor, fund legal needle exchanges at five sites in the city. Harlem's Rev. Calvin Butts, who had previously denounced the programs, also changed his view, saying, "We must keep these people alive if we are to deal with their other problems."

Activists had originally founded all of the programs that AmFAR supported. Three had their roots in ACT UP; two were created and run by needle exchange committee members in the Lower East Side and the Bronx. Another was located at Housing Works in Manhattan, which Keith Cylar and Charles King ran. The fourth, located in both the Bronx and Harlem, was operated by Yolanda Serrano and ADAPT. The last program, also in the Bronx, was founded and is still run by Joyce Rivera, another long-time harm reduction advocate.

Most of these were shoestring organizations. Outside of the few places like New York and New Haven that had sanctioned it, many were still operating illegally or quasi-legally. Their budgets depended mainly on small individual donations, community events on the scale of bake sales, and, often, their founder's ability to live without a salary or on near poverty wages. Ironically, in part because of his accident, Purchase and his Point Defiance AIDS Project in Tacoma had more funding than most.

But raising money remained a huge problem, limiting how many people could be reached. Federal funding had literally been banned in 1988, courtesy of legislation sponsored by the racist and homophobic North Carolina senator, Jesse Helms. His justification? Needle exchange "undercut the credibility of society's message that drug use is illegal and morally wrong," he claimed.[11] (Helms's attacks on gay people and AIDS funding in general were so vile that ACT UP once placed a giant condom on the roof of his house in protest.)

While plenty of wealthy gay men funded major AIDS work, people who used drugs had no organized community at all to turn to for support. The few known rich IV drug users—rock stars, mainly—wanted nothing to do with syringe exchange, even if they had made millions selling songs that extolled injecting, as Lou Reed and Eric Clapton had. (A notable exception was the Grateful Dead, who supported needle exchanges on both coasts, albeit relatively quietly.)

The Drug Policy Foundation (DPF), founded in 1986, was basically the only significant sympathetic political group at the time—and it did give needle exchange some crucial early political and financial support.[12] But it didn't have much money and, like ACT UP, tended to avoid backing initiatives that provided day-to-day services, preferring to fund actual political action. Moreover, DPF was small, with at most a few thousand supporters at that point; in 1991, the drug war remained wildly popular. Even marijuana legalization seemed far out. Only 17 percent of the public was in favor of it.[13] AmFAR had been the only major AIDS group to step up initially—but needle exchange was just a tiny portion of its portfolio.

The more the Comers learned about the situation, the more they realized that this was exactly the kind of cause in which their money could really matter. Needle exchange certainly wasn't an area dominated by big, established donors or organizations; in fact, nearly all of them tended to flee, screaming, if anyone dared propose such a controversial idea. Ultimately, billionaire financier George Soros would become the biggest philanthropist in harm reduction, but he did not begin his work in this area until 1994. Clearly, if there were to be enough exchanges to meet the need in the U.S., money would have to come from new sources.

Comer began to study up on AIDS and IV drug use, checking out San Francisco's Prevention Point. She started volunteering there, seeing how simple kindness without judgment could change so much. "Life is about stories, and you hear different stories and people feel comfortable to share—well, I think that just expands your heart," she said of the work. She then called Purchase to ask whether he might need additional money.

"I think everyone just thought I was crazy, to tell you the truth," she said, recalling her first conversations with Purchase and others whom she later contacted to offer significant donations. After all, it's not every day that the head of a foundation calls out of the blue and says she might solve your financial problems. Such experiences are rare for ordinary nonprofits—and even more so for needle exchanges, which are much more used to getting contacted by the police and receiving legal threats.

But Purchase was the kind of person who connected easily: he seemed to understand how to talk to anyone from homeless people who were injecting drugs to bikers to police commissioners, other bureaucrats, and, yes, potential donors. Those social ties had eased his way when he first started his needle exchange; for example, he had at least one close friend within the health department that ultimately hired him.

He and Stephanie clicked right away. Soon they were meeting in person regularly, talking for hours upon hours in various coffee shops in Seattle and San Francisco. Neither paid much attention to the quality or the specialty brews that were a subject of much snobbery in both cities. But over many cups, he began to teach her the theory and practice of harm reduction. They would have been an odd match: Stephanie, the heiress of a business that had begun as a catalog selling marine supplies and yachting outfits, and the biker dude who could be an extra from the TV show *Sons of Anarchy*.

Like Jon Parker back east, Purchase was a "Johnny Appleseed" of needle exchange, though he was better at community relations than his cross-country counterpart. Though Purchase looked like a guy who was ready to fight, it was Parker who had actually been punched in the face by a minister, angered by activists doing needle exchange in his neighborhood. In contrast, Purchase got community buy-in right when he started.

He also gave ongoing, practical advice and support to those who wanted to establish new and ongoing programs in their communities. Aside from the earliest groups on the East Coast, most of the exchanges around the U.S. had direct help from Purchase, right from the start. Much of this work was done via an organization called the North American Syringe Exchange Network, which he founded in 1989.[14]

Comer rapidly agreed to fund the group, which gave guidance, operational support, and sometimes a starter kit of needles and other necessary supplies to nascent exchanges. With this money Purchase and Comer helped seed new exchanges—and harm reduction—across the United States.

ten

Any Positive Change

I N August of 1993, a man named Dan Bigg was the recipient of one of Comer's life-altering cold calls. She left a message on his answering machine. The Chicago resident who ran that city's needle exchange heard a woman's voice saying, "My name is Stephanie Comer and I'd like to fund your work." Not surprisingly, he was suspicious. But he called her back, just in case.

He was promptly invited to a morning meeting with Stephanie and her mom. At the end of their discussion, the Comers told him to write up a wish list for funding. The next week, without delay, he received a check for $75,000.[1] In his work with Comer and through another initiative that he would simultaneously develop, Bigg would become responsible for several of the most crucial advances in the history of harm reduction.

Like so many others, he'd come to the movement via the goddess, Edith Springer. He'd attended a training or talk she gave in the late eighties or early nineties and instantly recognized that this was what he wanted to do. The son of a doctor and a nurse, Bigg had originally wanted to become a physician. But, feeling squeamish when faced with real patients in the hospital, he decided to be a psychologist instead.

While studying at the Chicago School of Professional Psychology, he began working at a methadone program. There, he learned about HIV as it began to spread among people who injected drugs. When his clients began telling him that they were being silenced if they tried to talk about the virus at twelve-step meetings, he helped found a support group where those discussions would be welcome.

Bigg lived up to his name in many ways: he was a large guy with a huge personality. Both goofy and persuasive, he had brown hair and puppy-dog eyes. "I used to say he could sell snake oil to a snake,"[2] his widow, Karen Bigg, joked, with affection. Like Dave Purchase, Bigg also had the skill of being able to connect with just about anyone, regardless of class, race, or status. A father of three, he loved dogs and all things canine. And like a puppy, he was also fundamentally gregarious.

Comer had reached out to Bigg because, in the early 1990s, he had co-founded Chicago's first needle exchange. The group had officially become a nonprofit in 1992. Critically, they chose a highly unusual name for a harm reduction program. They called themselves the Chicago Recovery Alliance (CRA). And rarely has an organization's name itself mattered so much.

The "recovery" label set CRA apart right from the beginning—in a way that would help shape the harm reduction movement and escalate its growth. Previously, harm reductionists had actively avoided using the "r-word" in conversation—let alone in organizational literature or nomenclature. Like most of the addictions world, they saw "recovery" as signifying only a path to overcoming addiction that involved complete abstinence and twelve-step groups. They didn't want to be perceived as having such a narrow view. In fact, some saw themselves as being in active opposition to it. Before CRA, harm reduction had ceded both the concept of recovery and that word for it to the abstinence field. One of Bigg's key contributions would be to change that.

CRA deliberately included "recovery" in its name for two reasons. For one, it sounded innocuous, so it was less likely to set off alarms among neighbors or others who might not like to be near a program associated with drug injection. More importantly, however, Bigg realized that harm reduction needed not just to redefine addiction, but to revolutionize recovery as well. Harm reductionists had already shown that active addiction wasn't the chaotic state of mindlessness so often depicted in story and stereotype. But it was Bigg and CRA who recognized that if addiction wasn't the zombiehood that abstinence-oriented people professed it to be, then recovery probably wasn't as clear-cut either.

Like the Liverpudlians, Bigg and CRA understood the importance of framing: using specific language to favorably set the terms of a debate. This has been critical in spreading the harm reduction message, especially with regard to recovery. If recovery is only abstinence, any harm reduction work that precedes it is erased and doesn't count as progress. And if only abstinence matters, harm reduction will always take a back seat. "'Recovery' in the name has been deliciously ironic for people," Bigg said, explaining, "We were taking the name back to what it really is and how it really applies to our species."[3]

But if recovery isn't just abstinence, what is it? Harm reductionists had long grappled with this issue, which manifested itself in a number of ways that caused serious problems. For example, abstinence supporters have stigmatized people on methadone and other medications for many decades as not truly being in recovery.

In fact, Narcotics Anonymous, the main twelve-step program for people with opioid problems, specifically states this idea in its literature. As one of their pamphlets describes it, "Our program approaches recovery from addiction through abstinence, cautioning against the substitution of one drug for another."[4] As a result, people who take medications such as methadone or buprenorphine—even exactly as prescribed—are viewed as being just as far from getting better as those who are injecting illegal drugs daily.

This means that if you treat your addiction with these medications— even if you comply perfectly with every other aspect of the program and are saintly and super-productive—you are not allowed to raise your hand and "share" at most NA meetings or count the days since you last used other drugs to set your recovery date. In NA's language, you are not considered "clean" with such substances in your body.

CRA recognized the dangers of such a circumscribed definition of recovery. As Edith Springer so often taught, this absolutist perspective keeps both counselors and clients frustrated, because making substantial and often difficult changes that people ordinarily value doesn't count as success. And it can do even more damage than that. Long-term use of buprenorphine or methadone is the only treatment proven to cut the death rate from heroin addiction by 50 percent or more. Telling people that they must stop taking potentially life-saving medications in order to be considered "clean" can—and has—led to loss of life.[5]

Even worse, the twelve-step concept of total abstinence is sometimes extended to include non-addictive psychiatric medications—although at least half of people with addiction have a pre-existing or co-existing mental illness. One harm reductionist tells the story of an AA friend who'd come out of a deep depression and gone back to work with the help of an antidepressant. When he shared his triumph at a meeting, an old-timer told him to "get off that crap" if he genuinely wanted to be sober.

"He did," she said. And then he killed himself. When his roommate shared word of the loss at the next meeting, he tried to rationalize it by saying that at least this man had died sober. "I will never forget that and how sickened I was—and still am—by those words," she said.[6] In other words, the old-timer—unfortunately, along with many others in the group—thought it was better to die than to recover with the help of medication. Being, acting, and feeling better didn't count.

CRA developed a more inclusive way to think about it. And they managed to do so succinctly, without getting bogged down in details or debates over which specific drugs are okay for recovering people and which aren't—or whether you lose all your "recovery time" and go back to day one if you use any proscribed substance, even once. They did so by simply removing—you could say undoing—drugs.

Around 1989, Bigg and some friends met up to hash out a new definition of recovery. They convened at a Swedish restaurant on the North Side of Chicago. With free pots of coffee and sweet rolls provided by the friendly owner, they sat down, fully expecting a difficult and probably interminable argument. There was no way around it but to start.

Immediately, however, John Szyler—an HIV-positive former IV drug user and a CRA co-founder—came out with a brilliant idea. Szyler was a close friend of Bigg's, who has described him as being "like a cross between Frank Sinatra and Jack Kerouac." And, in his typically chill manner, he instantly solved the problem.

Recovery, Szyler said, is "any positive change," with the qualifier that this must be defined by the person him- or herself. Everyone looked at one another. For a pregnant moment, no one spoke. Could it possibly be that simple?

"People wanted to say something critical or negative, but no one could," Bigg said. "It is a perfect working definition of harm reduction and recovery—it applies to all people [and] immediately removes the killer stigma and condemnation that comes with intoxication."[7] In essence, it's not about whether you are getting high—but whether you are getting better.

"In those three words was a revolution that we're still living to this day," Bigg added, saying, "It reclassifies all people based on whether you [or] I are making positive movements as we define [them] for ourselves."[8] It defines recovery by what you do, rather than basing it on what drugs you take.

Seeing recovery as any positive change also eliminates many extraneous debates. From this perspective, it doesn't matter what the precise definition of addiction is or whether one form of recovery is superior to another or whether medication use is acceptable. Instead, as Bigg said, "It becomes a matter of logistics and collaboration, cooperation, openness, willingness to accept another for what they believe. You know, some basic tenets of humanity. And [it] has guided us ever since."

"Any positive change" could be using a clean needle, it could be getting a job, it could be going back to school or trying a new antidepressant. It could even be abstinence. But what counts as progress toward getting better is determined by the people who are trying to improve their own lives—not counselors or cops.

No longer would recovery be ceded to self-help groups or "professionals"—or to anyone else but those individuals who were experiencing it themselves, in whatever way they chose to do so. Recovery can't be determined by testing someone's urine or blood or by quantifying how much or how often or when they use or abstain. It isn't even about drugs. Instead, recovery is about people, and what matters most to them, just as it is for those who are recovering from other mental or physical disorders. Quality of life is what's important—and that can only be determined by the person living it.

Although the "any positive change" definition spurred controversy—and even outrage from those whose recovery identity had been built on gaining status by having many consecutive days and years of abstinence—

ultimately even abstinence programs would recognize the need to get beyond their rigid view of the question.

For example, in 2006, a group of recovery advocates—including some who'd gotten better via pathways other than the twelve steps—convened at the Betty Ford Center. Their goal was to devise a more ecumenical definition of recovery that recognized that participating in AA or NA was not the only way. In this case, they did retain abstinence as a requirement for recovery as they defined it—but they also said that using methadone or buprenorphine as prescribed counted as abstinence, like other legitimate prescriptions—and contrary to NA's position![9]

Cheryl Hull, a former Black Panther, became one of CRA's first employees in 1994. At the time, she had two years abstinent from heroin—and at first, she was skeptical of harm reduction, even after she was hired. In NA, she had been taught to see handing out needles as "enabling" people to avoid quitting. But then she started to hear that many of her friends had HIV infections. Some were getting gravely ill. She realized that clean needles could have saved their lives. "I began to believe in my heart that in my job, I was doing something good," she said.

Growing up in the projects on the West Side of Chicago, Hull had lost her father at fourteen and then began drinking heavily. She started using heroin in her late teens after a stillbirth and botched IUD implantation left her unable to have more children. The pain that had led to her own addiction became part of her ability to be compassionate to others. At CRA, her job was to distribute clean needles and collect unsterile ones, working out of one of the group's silver vans, which would soon become iconic in Chicago. It was there that she began to see the philosophy of harm reduction and "any positive change" in action.

At first, some neighborhood residents would curse at her, believing she was selling drugs and not just providing clean needles. Initially, she'd curse right back at them. "I wasn't at the growth that I am now," she said, smiling. Soon, however, she was able to respond calmly. Often using her own early resistance as an example, she began to convince folks that needle exchange was necessary.

"'If a person dies from AIDS or a person dies from overdose or if a person dies from any blood-transmitted disease,' I said, 'how can they recover?'" Hull explained. Sometimes, she'd also disclose her own recovery path. "They come on this van, and they see me, and they know I used to be right there where they are, and they say 'How did you do it, Cheryl?' And I tell them. And they be like, 'Oh my God. Cheryl, would you help me?'" Before long, she'd see some of those same faces at meetings. Many told her later that she'd saved their lives, though she says she would prefer to credit God.

Hull was also quick to see how harm reduction could be applied outside of drug issues, such as in her own not-instant process of change when people who were angry about the presence of the van cursed at her. More recently, she says, "I've slowed down on my candy. But I love candy. And I had bought me some of this chocolate candy [that has] caramels in it, so instead of eating five of them, I've went down to three. So, that's harm reduction for me."

Others would soon pick up these ideas in many additional creative ways across disciplines. So, for example, like Hull, people who take a harm reduction approach to dieting may drop the idea of "forbidden foods" and instead work toward eating less of them or eating them less frequently. For anorexia, harm reduction can involve specific practices to avoid or reduce vitamin deficiencies or the use of other tactics to reduce the physical damage associated with starvation. Rather than expelling people who are not "compliant" with giving up their restricted diets, treating anorexia with harm reduction "meets them where they are." With any hard-to-change behavior, if there's room to use a gradual approach rather than requiring overnight transformation, there's room for harm reduction. And if there are ways to reduce damage associated with the activity even as it occurs, there is room for "any positive change" to open the door for further growth.

Of course, the specifics will vary depending on the problem at hand. For example, much of the severe brain damage that can occur with long-term alcoholism actually results from a thiamine deficiency, rather than from the alcohol itself. Supplementing this vitamin can reduce this particular harm. Medical knowledge allows this form of harm reduction, but it cannot be implemented without the perspective of heavy drinkers who have to be able to make this dietary change in the reality of their own lives if thiamine is actually to be protective.

Further afield, in business, you might see executives offering job sharing with reduced hours rather than layoffs or choosing the manufacturing process that is least harmful to the environment. Anywhere risks can be weighed in context—rather than taking an all-or-nothing approach—harm reduction ideas can be applied. Anywhere small steps can lead to bigger ones, the idea of "any positive change" can empower people to start the journey.

As CRA and harm reduction grew, their recovery definition would continue to change the way America sees addiction. It would also shape the fundamentals of harm reduction itself.

eleven

Refining Harm Reduction

ALTHOUGH THE COMER FAMILY FOUNDATION WAS BASED IN CHICAGO, initially Stephanie had remained in San Francisco where she'd attended graduate school. At some point in 1993, she invited Bigg to visit her there, along with George Clark, who ran San Francisco's needle exchange at the time. They convened at her apartment, where she had a spread of finger food left over from a recent event. "We were eating in her kitchen, standing up eating leftovers," Bigg said. Then Comer explained why she'd invited them.

"Gentlemen, I hope you can help me with this dilemma we have," she said. "We have an extra $300,000 and I hope you can help me spend it."[1]

Before long, the three had decided that half of the money should be used for continuing support of Dave Purchase's syringe exchange network, to help open more programs and to help keep existing ones running and well supplied. Comer's high-floor apartment had a balcony with a stunning view of San Francisco. They stepped out onto to it to consider what to do with the rest of the money.

"The three of us were looking out on the city," Comer said. Clark and Bigg started discussing the need to bring the leaders in the field together, which had never been done in the U.S. They suggested having a meeting. Comer said, "Great. I'll fund it." The goal of the gathering would be to consider creating a new organization to consolidate and then promote the key ideas of harm reduction—far beyond needle exchange.

Such a group was desperately needed if harm reduction was to spread further within America. Although the international harm reduction organization founded by the Liverpool folks had continued to hold large conferences and publish its journal, they were mainly reaching interested academics and others who already knew where to look for innovative drug-related information. Edith Springer was continuing to conduct her trainings—but there was no central place for Americans who were looking for new ideas to come together and strategize about harm reduction practice and policy. The lack of such a group was even more problematic because here, advocates and practitioners had a much bigger challenge with politicians and health authorities than did their Western European counterparts.

The United States was not only one of the harshest practitioners of the drug war internally—it was also its major booster internationally. If harm reduction was going to take hold, support had to be marshalled here in the belly of the beast and its ideas spread across the many disciplines and areas where they were needed.

Comer, Purchase, and Bigg began to consider how to create such an organization. And before long, they'd organized the first meeting of what would become known as the Harm Reduction Working Group (HRWG). At this event, the movement began to define and formalize the key ideas of American harm reduction—and start to try to figure out what else needed to be organized.

Starting on October 26, 1993, the first working group meeting was held in Santa Cruz, at an intimate, homey resort. Both Francie and Stephanie Comer—along with Bigg, Clark, and Purchase—attended as organizers. They had personally selected the invitees: a who's who of American harm reduction, a veritable Justice League of the superheroes in the movement.

The group came from across the country, with a variety of backgrounds. They were definitely not your typical professional meeting attendees. Everyone was dressed casually. Nearly all had actually been arrested at least once, and many risked it regularly. A good proportion were current or former drug injectors, with the track marks to prove it. Each was an outsider in his or her own way; all of them challenged conventional wisdom about drugs and addiction and, usually, many other dogmas as well.

Edith Springer herself was there, of course; she had personally converted or at least mentored many, if not most, of the others. With her hair in a full and elegant gray bob, she looked polished and confident. Seattle's needle exchange was represented by Imani Woods, an African American dynamo who had started at ADAPT in New York in the late eighties or early nineties.

Woods, who had recovered from an alcohol problem via twelve-step programs, had debated for years with Springer, at first seemingly intransigently opposed to anything other than abstinence. "I came to harm reduction kicking and screaming," she said, laughing.[2] Springer agreed, saying that Woods had given her the hardest time of anyone, ever. Her passionate nature, however, made her an enormously powerful advocate when she did come on board—and she was not afraid of a fight. She was devoted to bringing harm reduction ideas to the Black community—and beyond.

At nineteen, Heather Edney was the youngest in the group. With dark, wavy hair and a punk attitude, she ran a syringe program for youth in Santa Cruz—and she was there to ensure that young drug users had a loud voice. Los Angeles was represented by Renee Edgington, a member of ACT UP LA, who had founded that city's exchange. Its distinct style reflected her sensibility as a visual artist. For example, participants returned used syringes by depositing them in a Rube Goldberg–style machine. They'd load up the works, pull a lever with a big knob, and observe as the device loudly dumped the spikes into a bright red hazardous waste container.[3] Her straight hair glowed a supernatural strawberry blond, and she wore bright red lipstick and cat's-eye glasses.

Lisa Moore, a professor of public health at San Francisco State University, had worked with that city's syringe program. A Black woman and Buddhist who has three black cats, she brought an activist's heart—and a scholar's perspective—to the group. When she first started doing needle exchange, she said, "What broke my heart was how utterly grateful people would be—for so little. And it made me realize how horrifically they'd been treated." For her, she says, the spirit of harm reduction brought to mind the one line she had memorized from Shakespeare in junior high school: "As imagination bodies forth the form of things unknown, the poet's pen turns them to shapes and gives to airy nothing a local habitation and a name." Having a concrete way to describe harm reduction practices helped reveal their underlying logic—and Moore wanted to share and help define it.

John Paul Hammond, a Black queer Quaker who co-founded both the ACT UP chapter and the needle exchange in Philadelphia, brought North Philly to the table. Slim, he wore his brown dreadlocks almost to his waist. He summed up his AIDS work this way: "We shall overcome by any means necessary . . . the one part of the message is Dr. Martin Luther King Jr.'s, and the other part is Malcolm X's. Without Malcolm, there would have been no Dr. King, and vice versa. You need the people in coats and ties who work within the system, but you also need people like us in the streets."[4] He'd helped develop the first harm reduction measures for crack cocaine smokers.

Filling out the roster was George Kenney, an African American activist who worked within his community to get needle exchange established permanently in Boston—without the antagonism provoked by Jon Parker there. Also participating was Sara Kershnar, who had done most of the organizational work to make the meeting happen. Other than Springer, the only person from New York at the first meeting was Joyce Rivera, a Latina who'd founded St. Ann's Corner of Harm Reduction in the Bronx in 1990, one of the city's first five funded programs.

Rivera, whose father had been addicted to heroin and who had lost her brother to AIDS, had started as a researcher studying bleach distribution at the same institute where Springer began her harm reduction work. She had collaborated early on with ACT UP's Bronx needle exchange. "We were building the bones, the spine for a movement," Rivera said regarding the meeting.

For a group who had been brought together because of their shared ideas and goals, however, the event was quite contentious. Perhaps because everyone was so used to having to fight to be heard, they instinctively argued, even when among friends. There were clashes over almost everything, none of which anyone can remember now. As Moore put it, "When you put a bunch of people in a room who have been doing what they see as what must be done independently for years, they don't play well with others . . . all of the people were phenomenal, and everybody was a fucking pain in the ass."

It took time for these consummate outsiders to trust one another, time for them to realize that they truly were on the same side, and time for people to mark their places, reveal their multifaceted identities, and make themselves known. Nonetheless, it was immediately clear to everyone that an organization to promote harm reduction was desperately needed—and that they should continue to meet to try to form one, regardless of how fierce the debates might get. "We knew that what we embarked upon was important," said Rivera, "and we were quite up to the task."

Since the first order of business was to come up with a good, clear definition of harm reduction, this was also one of the first of many skirmishes. These days, no one can remember who advocated for what, but by the end of the meeting, they'd agreed on the following:

> Harm Reduction is a set of strategies and tactics which encourages users to reduce harm done to themselves and their communities by licit and illicit drug use. By allowing users access to the tools to become healthier, we recognize the competency of their efforts to protect themselves, their loved ones and their communities.

Over time, the definition would evolve, but this short statement evoked much of its essence. It implicitly highlighted the value of the lives of people who use drugs, explicitly stated that they are capable of changing, and stressed that there are specific tactics and strategies to help. It didn't say anything one way or the other about the role of abstinence; it didn't say that harm reduction must involve drug legalization, and it didn't represent the concept as being limited to a specific area of dealing with drug use, whether that be treatment, prevention, or government policy.

"I had a background in political theory and it was really helpful," said Rivera, describing how that perspective was useful in thinking critically about harm reduction. She—and pretty much everyone else who attended and discussed the meeting—noted the importance of the facilitator, who was hired to help manage the "strong personalities" of the attendees. "Some of the people had histories which were difficult and so sometimes some of that history came up," said Rivera.

Next, however, the group had to develop a unique mission for their organization. Comer and the other members were familiar with the group devoted to ending the drug war and reforming state, federal, and international law, which was the Drug Policy Foundation. Many of the working group's members had attended its conferences, often as speakers. In fact, one of that organization's co-founders would join the working group at its later meetings. They knew that their goals were aligned, but distinct.

"I wanted to see a strong movement in the United States that linked all of these exchanges together, that was or could be a political force to change policy [and promote] best practices," Comer said of what she envisioned. Needle exchange—and compassionate policies and practices like it—needed an advocacy group of their own.

Another critical goal for the new organization would be to fully formulate and promote the idea of harm reduction itself—so that it could be used to inform better treatment and policy across multiple levels and regions. This mission meant that people who used drugs themselves needed to be prominent within the movement—since its aim was ultimately to preserve and protect their lives.

At its core, harm reduction is a movement for the human rights of people who use drugs. However, those rights are impinged upon from every angle—by everything from racist laws and stereotypes that drive criminalization to stigmatizing, punitive, and incompetent "treatment." This meant that its ideas needed to be disseminated and understood across multiple disciplines and policy areas. And because of that same strong stigma, organizing users and having them lead harm reduction groups is extremely difficult.

As Tacoma's Dave Purchase described it, "Harm reduction is a current manifestation of the age-old struggle for the universal recognition of the inherent dignity in all life. This struggle is between those who see the infinite dignity in themselves and others—and those who, being unable to see it in themselves, suffer from an intense sense of inadequacy and must degrade, dehumanize and enslave others in order to elevate themselves."[5]

Consequently, the working group knew that the organization they created would have a huge educational task ahead of it. Harm reduction would have to be inherently poly- and trans-disciplinary, while constantly being sure to stay in touch with its highly vulnerable grass roots. It would also have to consider and balance many types of harm, which vary depending on context.

Take drug courts, for example. In a setting where the existing policy is to sentence everyone who gets convicted of a drug crime to a lengthy prison term, adding an option that allows at least some people to get treatment instead is likely to reduce harm. But, if it is politically possible to take prison out of the picture entirely, then it's the drug court that will be more harmful. That's because in drug courts, those whose treatment fails are sent to prison, often for longer terms than they would have served if they hadn't tried to seek help. Moreover, many drug courts ban the treatment that most reduces the risk of death: long-term medication with methadone or buprenorphine. In contrast, in the non-carceral model, the harm associated with prison and with judges making treatment decisions is removed entirely. And overall harm is reduced, because punitive policies within and surrounding treatment do not improve outcomes.

The fact that harm reduction is context-dependent means that determining what can be labeled as part of the movement will change over time and can be a subject of ongoing debate. At the same time, this difficulty and fluidity also gives it continual room for excitement, new ideas, and growth. The overdose crisis and the COVID-19 pandemic, for example, have now brought thousands of new people on board. Today, there are harm reduction policy makers and wonks, harm reduction nurses, harm reduction public health workers and epidemiologists, harm reduction doctors, social workers, psychologists, sociologists, counselors, outreach workers, therapists, and psychiatrists. That's just a short list of those in the professions within the realm of health and health policy, in professions that work directly with people who use drugs. There are now many others who call themselves harm reductionists—in areas far beyond drug policy. Harm reduction thinking is seen as useful in areas as diverse as corporate policymaking, public safety, climate change, restorative justice, antiracism activism, trauma treatment, education—basically, anywhere that risky or potentially damaging behavior needs to be addressed and must be understood in context in order to be effectively changed without unintended consequences.

Harm reduction can be applied to approaches like mask-wearing, physical distancing, or other measures to fight contagious viruses; it can guide changes in diet and exercise to improve health; it can make drinking less harmful and driving less dangerous. From the start, harm reduction measures have also been used to improve the lives and health of sex workers, beginning in the Netherlands and the U.K. and now expanding in Denmark, where a van provides a safer space for street workers to bring their customers. Sex workers themselves, from Liverpool onward, have been a crucial part of the movement, bringing harm reduction ideas related to both drug use and sex together and working in community with one another to promote policies like decriminalization and interim measures that reduce risks associated with violence and police.

These days, harm reduction ideas are also used by people with psychiatric disorders, who often have to balance the harms associated with psychiatric medication with the harms associated with particular illnesses. One group, known as the Icarus Project (now known as the Fireweed Collective), has created a harm reduction guide to stopping use of these medications for people who have found they are not benefiting. The guide helps people manage withdrawal symptoms and other issues that may arise, while not taking an all-or-nothing stance against or in favor of medication use itself. As the author puts it, "A 'harm reduction' approach means not being pro- or anti-medication, but supporting people where they are at to make their own decisions, balancing the risks and benefits involved."[6]

Harm reduction accepts that many human behaviors cause harm and that most people cannot or will not avoid all of them. It argues that if we can't be abstinent—from whatever potentially harmful behavior we may do—there are still ways to mitigate damage and that doing so can be a path to further change, rather than a replacement for it. It allows us many ways to become better citizens of this planet.

After a series of further meetings, the Harm Reduction Working Group decided to create a new and much larger organization, which they named the Harm Reduction Coalition. And as they grew, they tried to ensure that the many different aspects of the harm reduction agenda were being given appropriate weight and harmonizing with one another. This, too, would be an ongoing issue.

For one, it rapidly became clear that harm reduction had to be anti-racist and join in coalition with groups organized by and for people of color. These communities had independently developed many practices that can now be called harm reduction, although via different routes.

However, the national harm reduction movement in the U.S. was mainly led by white people at first, in part because there was still so much support for the drug war among the Black middle class and political leadership. The coalition had to try to manage the tensions that arose from this, which would remain another long-term challenge.

THE GROUP'S NEXT TASK WOULD BE TO EXPAND THE MOVEMENT, BEGINNING with a large national conference to introduce itself and connect those across the country who worked in organizations like syringe exchanges, were already interested in the idea, or had become curious about it through encountering people like Edith Springer. To start to make the changes they wanted to see, harm reduction would also have to reach several key professional groups outside of needle exchangers, particularly providers of addiction treatment and the researchers who studied it.

In addition, they would need to reach people within the criminal prosecution system, including law enforcement. Without at least some of these folks on board, it would be difficult to make real inroads in reducing drug and drug war–related harm. With this in mind, the working group began organizing the first American harm reduction conference, aiming to include as many people from these varied areas as possible. And while planning for the big meeting continued, Dan Bigg also began working on a new practice that would ultimately supercharge the movement.

twelve

Undoing Overdose

THE FIRST TIME DAN BIGG REVERSED AN OVERDOSE, THE VICTIM COULDN'T believe that she'd ever been unconscious—let alone that she'd nearly lost her life. The woman who had OD'd was a gorgeous blue-eyed blonde from a prominent, wealthy Chicago family, like something out of a made-for-TV movie plot. She was unconscious and unresponsive, her skin turning blue in the front seat of a car. Her boyfriend, a regular client of the needle exchange, had driven up to its offices and run in. He was a tough Polish working-class guy, panicking and clearly terrified.

A long-time heroin user, he knew that if a man like him took a "high-class" woman like her to the ER and she died, he'd be looking at murder charges. To make matters worse—and perhaps even more Lifetime movie–ready—the victim was just eighteen. Fortunately, in his terror, the boyfriend recalled hearing that they had something at the needle exchange that could reverse overdose. So he rushed to the South Side warehouse office of the Chicago Recovery Alliance. There, Bigg was eating pizza and joking with his colleagues. The man ran to the door, crying, "Please help." Bigg and a co-worker sprinted outside immediately.

But when they got to the car and saw the victim, Bigg was, at first, not hopeful. The woman looked as dead as anyone can look, as he described it. Immediately, he began their overdose response procedure. It started with checking to see if she'd react to painful stimulation, by rubbing his knuckles on her lips.

Since she did not respond, he prepared an injection of naloxone (brand name: Narcan), which is the antidote to opioid overdose. Although most overdoses actually consist of mixes of depressant drugs—like opioids, alcohol, and anti-anxiety medications like Xanax—if an opioid is in the cocktail, naloxone will usually be enough to revive the person. It will not do harm if used in error: other than blocking opioids, the drug is inert. So while it won't save people from pure cocaine overdoses or other conditions that might leave them unconscious, it won't make them worse, either.

As Bigg readied the shot, his colleague tried to take the woman's long-sleeved blouse off, to give them better access to her arm. Her designer garment had some kind of complex fastenings that neither could work out. So, not wanting to waste any more time, Bigg injected the drug right through the shirt.

Then he reclined the passenger seat where she was sitting and began rescue breathing. "I breathed for her maybe three or four times. Her color got better, very, very fast," Bigg said, referring to the fact that overdose victims turn blue or gray when their bodies stop getting sufficient oxygen. A healthier pink tone became visible.

But seeing that, and becoming confident that she would survive, the boyfriend freaked out. To him mouth-to-mouth suddenly seemed way too close to kissing. He took over and breathed for his girlfriend once. And then Sleeping Beauty awakened. A long, sighing breath emerged from her lips.

As she slowly returned to herself, the woman looked up at the scene around her. She was disoriented and confused. She could tell that her boyfriend had been crying, which itself was shocking. Everyone tried to explain to her that she had just overdosed—and been revived. But she couldn't or wouldn't believe it.

Trying to get through, Bigg pointed out the hole in her shirt sleeve, which had a spot of blood on it. She dismissed that—she was a drug injector, after all, it could have happened at any time. He suddenly thought to ask her what her mouth tasted like and if she had recently eaten mushroom pizza. Only then did she recognize the taste and see a slice of the pie that the CRA folks had been eating, but that she had no memory of. It was icky, albeit undeniable, evidence of what had just happened.

After she'd recovered a bit more, she asked Bigg to train her and her partner about how to use naloxone themselves, which he did. Afterward, the couple left with several vials of the drug, as well as the knowledge needed to use it.

Scenes like this overdose rescue, unfortunately, are now pretty commonplace. But before Dan Bigg took action, they were far more likely to be deadly. It was his activism and that of CRA that first made the overdose antidote available to laypeople. In fact, while he was helping organize the first national harm reduction conference, he was simultaneously working to liberate naloxone from the bureaucracy that kept it off the streets and out of the hands of those who needed it most.

Before Bigg decided to act, naloxone was only available in medical settings, like hospitals and ambulances. All of the news accounts we see today about overdose reversals by drug users, parents, police, and other nonmedical folks are a direct or indirect result of his activism. This work started as he mourned the loss of a close friend.

John Szyler, the man who'd come up with the definition of recovery as "any positive change," had died of an overdose in May 1996. After years of surviving HIV and being abstinent from opioids, he'd begun using again after a long-awaited romantic weekend went wrong. His girlfriend, who was also HIV-positive, had had to cancel their date—not because she wanted to do so, but because she was sick. Sadly, disappointment is one of the most difficult emotions for people in recovery to manage. Szyler, unfortunately, succumbed to his attempt to medicate it.

When Bigg learned about his friend's death, he was devastated. Not long afterward, he met up with his fellow activists, trying to grapple with what had happened. He said, "I thought, what positive change can we make in John's memory?" Szyler had helped Bigg devise a list of harm reduction tactics, which they had listed on a t-shirt that they were planning to sell at the upcoming conference. Bigg recalled that one of them was "Keep Narcan around."[1]

This suggestion had been included almost as a throwaway line—in part because, in reality, doing so would be nearly impossible for anyone who wasn't a doctor or EMT. At that time, it was essentially locked away, reserved for use by medical professionals.

Bigg and the harm reductionists he inspired would change that; their advocacy would ultimately save the lives of many thousands of people. To memorialize Szyler, he and his co-workers vowed to free naloxone from the medical system and make it available wherever possible. Opioid overdose deaths were preventable—people just needed the right tools to save lives, they thought.

There was already a great deal of evidence to support street naloxone distribution. Bigg knew—and research also showed—that most overdoses are witnessed by at least one person. And, typically, there is time to intervene: most opioid overdoses slow breathing over the course of minutes to hours, not instantly (although fentanyl and other synthetics can require faster action).

His first reversal showed that this was indeed the case. Initially, he had thought the young woman he saw in the car was already dead, but he had been able to revive her. The experience also demonstrated to him how fear of legal consequences delays help-seeking: the victim's partner had deliberately avoided taking her to the hospital due to exactly that concern. If Bigg, a layperson who was not part of the medical or criminal legal system, hadn't had naloxone on hand, the eighteen-year-old woman would likely have died.

Her response to his intervention also turned out to be typical. "I would say the number one reaction among people being revived is surprise. They just don't get it," Bigg said. He noted that frequently, as in this case, survivors are also moved to return the favor. "They're motivated to be protective of other people," he said. "They want to help others stay alive as they were helped—and they'll be the last one to use because they want to watch over people and they know what to do." He added, "The whole idea that drug users are not caring, are not helpful, is insane. And there's nothing that proves it more dramatically than overdose prevention."

Indeed, both the woman whom Bigg had saved and her boyfriend would later have several more brushes with death. They would each use naloxone to revive the other at least once. That, however, allowed them to survive their addictions and go on to live full lives afterward.[2]

Naloxone was not classified as a prescription-only drug because it is dangerous or produces a high. In fact, it does the opposite: it can cause severe and distressing withdrawal symptoms in people who are physically dependent on opioids. Instead, the medication was restricted due to bureaucratic inertia and prejudice, including the usual fears about "enabling" heroin use and "sending the wrong message" by making it less risky. Bigg's most important contribution to harm reduction would be to change that.

The drug was invented in 1960 by a researcher seeking medications for constipation, which is associated with long-term opioid use. But he found a far more useful substance, one that can save lives. The FDA approved naloxone in 1971. It works by rapidly displacing opioids from the receptors that they occupy in the brain, some of which are involved in creating "air hunger" or the drive that makes us breathe. Opioid overdose kills by stopping respiration. Naloxone restores it.[3]

After naloxone was introduced, hospitals immediately began using it to reduce oversedation or outright accidental overdose from opioids used in surgery or pain care. Soon, it was also given to street overdose victims who managed to make it to the emergency room—and some ambulances began to carry it in neighborhoods where overdose was common. But for many decades, it wasn't available, even by prescription, outside of those settings.

The idea of using it on the street wasn't completely unprecedented, however. As early as 1971, San Francisco's Haight Ashbury Free Clinic began to stock naloxone in case of overdose. The clinic's founder actually saved singer Janis Joplin once, before she'd released a single record. Soon some medics serving concert promoters and doctors who worked with rock stars began to keep it on hand to avoid losing irreplaceable and highly profitable opioid-addicted musicians. If you weren't rich and famous or didn't live near the Haight, however, you were out of luck.

Though opioid overdose was killing thousands of people by the 1990s, the antidote sat on hospital shelves and in the back of ambulances for years before anyone with the power to make change even thought to try to make it broadly available to those at risk. It would take the advent of harm reduction to free naloxone from America's prejudice and indifference toward the lives of people who use drugs.

Naloxone distribution was first proposed as a harm reduction technique in 1992. It was pitched by a British researcher and physician, who began publishing papers in medical journals, arguing for what he called "take home naloxone."[4] A voracious reader of research, Dan Bigg had read at least one of them.

In fact, even before Szyler died, Bigg had begun gathering information on how he might practically and logistically get naloxone onto the streets. Secretly, drug users in California and New Mexico who knew friendly paramedics would sometimes obtain it and distribute it when they could. But when Bigg learned of his friend's death, he said, "I thought, we got to do it, we can't just talk about it."[5] However, there were many barriers, not least of which was the prescription issue. At least as pressing was the fact that on the street, naloxone had an awful reputation.

BECAUSE MOST PEOPLE WHO HAVE OPIOID ADDICTION OVERDOSE AT LEAST ONCE during their drug use, many have had at least one nasty taste of naloxone. Since the drug displaces opioids from the brain receptors where they act, it can bring on withdrawal rapidly. One doctor described what she saw when naloxone was used in the hospital to treat overdose victims this way: "It left people screaming, puking, shitting . . . and they would go out, use, and die."[6]

Fortunately, such experiences aren't the automatic result of the medication. The devil is in the dosage and how it is administered. With a small amount given slowly, an overdose can be reversed gently, producing mild or even no withdrawal symptoms. With a high, rapidly infused bolus, however, the victim can wind up unsure which end to place over the toilet first, as they shake with chills and shiver in total dread.

In other words, the reason for the lifesaving antidote's terrible street rep isn't inherent to its pharmacology. Instead, it is yet another example of the casual cruelty that the medical system so often exhibits toward people who take drugs. The initially recommended dose range and way of administering naloxone was probably well-intended, designed to ensure that the overdose was well and truly reversed. But in clinical lore it rapidly became clear that there was an easy way and a hard way, and many chose to go hard. Some nurses and paramedics even boasted about such sadism, saying it was "tough love" to "teach them a lesson." Unfortunately, the message that was most likely to be received from such disrespectful treatment was instead "don't seek help."

Once assured that it was possible to dose naloxone in a way that isn't overwhelmingly uncomfortable, Bigg and his fellow activists went to work. By this point, they had learned that it was legal for doctors to prescribe naloxone in Illinois. Now what Bigg needed was at least one Chicago physician willing to take the risk of prescribing the medication "off label" for direct use by laypeople, not just professionals.

This doc also had to be willing to risk dealing with legal issues that arose from the fact that the drug might not be used on the person to whom it was prescribed. The people who needed it would typically be unconscious and unable to take it themselves. And legally, this made it unlike the vast majority of medications.

The closest analogy is the EpiPen, which is used to treat severe allergic reactions. Here, the drug is directly prescribed to at-risk patients—though the intent is for others to administer it if the person has an attack. With naloxone, however, the idea is for people at risk to have it to use to save each other or for family members to use if an addicted loved one ODs—regardless of whether that specific dose had been prescribed to them. This issue evoked fear in the conservative medical profession, already unfriendly to addiction issues. Rescuers also faced liability issues, which would eventually prompt state legislation to ensure that no one could get sued for using naloxone in an attempt to reverse an OD.

Nonetheless, Bigg managed to find not just one but two physicians willing to step up. Chicago doctors Shawn Delater and Sarz Maxwell were friends from medical school. Both agreed to write prescriptions for people who visited CRA's roving needle exchange vans or their offices. Maxwell, whom Bigg had sought out because she was known as a compassionate prescriber of methadone, would soon become known as "the mother of naloxone." She also had a personal history of addiction, to alcohol. When he broached the idea of street naloxone to her, she said she told him, "'What a great idea!' And he said, 'Do you want to do it?' I said, 'Absolutely!'"

Maxwell has a memorable way of describing the safety of the drug. "Naloxone is ridiculously safe . . . I always say that if you want to hurt yourself with naloxone, the only way to do it is to break the vial and slit your wrists with the shards . . . It's a hundred times safer than aspirin."[7] Indeed, as with marijuana, it's not physically possible to administer a lethal dose—something that cannot be said of water.

Before they started to distribute it widely, however, Bigg needed to be sure that a large enough number of CRA's clients would actually use naloxone if faced with an overdose—and would be able to learn to do so correctly. To find out, they interviewed folks about their experiences of overdose and asked whether they'd be interested in free access to an antidote.

Not surprisingly, most people said yes. And so the group developed a training program to teach rescue breathing and how to administer the drug. Even with access to naloxone, rescue breathing is required knowledge for anyone who might potentially be faced with an overdose. It is done while the naloxone is being prepared for injection, while waiting for it to take effect, and of course, if it isn't available immediately for any other reason. In situations of oxygen deprivation to the brain like overdose, as doctors put it, "time is brain." What this means is that the longer the brain goes without oxygen, the more likely it is to be damaged or die.

During its trainings, CRA always emphasized that a call to 911 should be the first action taken in event of an OD. However, they soon found out from their own interviews and other research that about two-thirds of people would be unwilling to call for fear of either being arrested or treated poorly by medical professionals, or both. At least, though, recommending 911 contact would help tame the fears expressed by some doctors and paramedics that offering naloxone would cause more death by making people think they could avoid medical care. (And research ultimately found that receiving additional medical attention after having an overdose reversed on the street isn't necessary to reduce mortality.)

CRA also knew that they'd have to overcome some resistance to utilizing the drug, despite the clear interest their clients showed in having it available. Because so many people had had a horrific personal experience, there was concern that they might hesitate for fear of putting their friends through that or because they were afraid of causing harm if they made a mistake.

To overcome this problem, CRA used two strategies. First, they emphasized that the dose they were providing was far lower than that typically used medically. The vials they distributed contained ten milliliters, which included ten doses of .4 milligrams each, along with enough clean needles to inject it with. This would make being revived a much gentler experience, even if more than one dose turned out to be necessary. Convincing drug users of the importance of dose was not hard: nearly all know only too well how much the amount they take matters.

Secondly, they directed potential rescuers to inject the drug into the victim's muscle, rather than intravenously. This had two benefits. The onset of action is slightly slower with intramuscular injection, further minimizing the risk of inducing severe withdrawal. Also, it is far faster to simply stick a needle into someone's butt or bicep than it is to try to find a vein, particularly with a victim who has likely already damaged the most accessible routes. Eventually naloxone would be made available in an intranasal form, which made experiencing reversal even kinder and spared rescuers from having to deal with needles and glass vials. At first, though, the only version available was injectable.

Although CRA began planning its program and distributing some naloxone informally in 1996, they didn't bring it to scale until 2001. By that point, the staff had all been trained in overdose reversal, and Bigg had been able to wrangle a regular, inexpensive supply directly from a manufacturer. It took a little while before the impact of their work became clear.

"We did it for some months until we started getting back reports," said Maxwell. "And these reports were so life fulfilling that I couldn't stand it anymore. I couldn't sleep at night. I wanted to drop this stuff from helicopters."

People were calling it a miracle drug—or for the more biblically inclined, the Lazarus drug. It genuinely did bring people back from the brink of death. Said Maxwell, "Pioneering naloxone distribution is still the single thing I'm most proud of in my career."

She added, "Those were heady days indeed, and I was flying all over the U.S. and Europe to talk about naloxone. I'd always bring a suitcase full of naloxone and sample 'patient chart' forms, and at the end of the talk I'd dump it all on a table and say, 'Help yourselves!' There was never a vial left."[8]

Meanwhile, Bigg himself was doing the same thing, though he carried his naloxone in a duffel bag. When drug policy reformers held a conference in Seattle in 1999 about overdose, he was featured, along with his sack of naloxone and his demand that others join him and start creating their own programs. As Dave Purchase had done with needle exchange, Bigg began spreading the word about naloxone and helping people set up their own distribution sites and trainings, typically within existing needle exchanges. Often, he'd supply them with their first doses of the drug.

BY 2002, CRA HAD DISTRIBUTED MORE THAN 550 VIALS OF NALOXONE, AND fifty-two people reported having successfully reversed an overdose with it. That is likely an underestimate: reports are not required, and some people may prefer not to report or just forget to mention it during the brief time they visit CRA to get clean needles and other supplies.

Moreover, as with prior harm reduction programs, none of the concerns raised by critics were realized. People didn't suddenly start using more drugs because they felt they were safer since they had naloxone, nor did children decide to take up injecting because overdose might be less of a worry. Although the media reported anecdotes about "naloxone parties"—where people supposedly took extra high doses of drugs, knowing they could be revived—these were always secondhand, friend of a friend, or law enforcement sourced stories. In reality, the experience of having an overdose reversed is so unpleasant that no one deliberately seeks it: these were new urban legends, as factually dubious as accounts of LSD being placed on stickers to be given to kids or Halloween candy being laced with poison and distributed to neighborhood trick-or-treaters. As one CRA client put it after being given naloxone, "It doesn't influence me to do more; it actually influences me to do less," explaining that this was because he wanted to be sure he was awake enough to help his friends if they needed it.[9]

In 2001, the year the program started in earnest, Chicago saw a 20 percent decrease in overdose deaths. This rate continued to decline by 10 percent in each of the two following years. Since there was no randomized trial, the research conducted on CRA's program cannot prove cause and effect, but it is certainly telling that the OD rate in the Windy City had quadrupled between 1996 and 2000, before significant naloxone distribution began, and began to fall thereafter—at least until the city later fell prey to one of the nation's first fentanyl outbreaks.[10] (Naloxone can reverse overdoses of fentanyl and related drugs—but because these opioids kill far more quickly, there is less time for people to act to save lives.)

Between 1996 and 2010, forty-seven other naloxone programs were started across America, adding up to 188 sites distributing the drug in fifteen states. Nearly all of their founders were directly inspired by, mentored by, and/or supplied by Bigg—more often than not all three. Collectively, during that period, these groups gave out some 53,000 vials of naloxone, and more than 10,000 overdose reversals were reported back to them.[11]

Perhaps even more remarkable is the experience of people who had saved a friend or relative. As Bigg once told me about the half dozen or so reversals he'd personally performed, there's nothing more empowering than saving a life.[12] Another harm reductionist put it this way: "It's a profoundly moving moment when somebody is that close. There's still a pulse, but they're no longer breathing. They're on their way out to whatever—to just nothingness or whatever else you think there might be—and to be the one who interrupts that and maybe put [them] on a different path is a really emotional thing."[13]

In other words, the "side effects" of distributing naloxone are not increased drug use or worsened addiction. Instead, this drug not only saves victims' lives, but can also improve the quality of life for the rescuers as well. Injection drug users have many reasons to feel worthless—self-hatred both predisposes people to addiction and is escalated by it, with stigma and criminalization making matters even worse. But there are few actions a person can take that are more universally acclaimed and morally elevated than saving a life.

And so, by empowering addicted people to save each other, naloxone often helps them save themselves. Research shows that, as with needle exchange, naloxone distribution decreases injecting and often serves as a pathway to treatment and recovery. As Maxwell put it, "They would say things like it made me feel worthy again. The people who performed reversals—their lives were transformed." Without the work of Dan Bigg and

CRA, however, none of those lives would have been saved. And, harm reduction's overall growth would likely have been far slower, if it had happened at all.

The advent of street naloxone was one of the most critical events in the history of harm reduction, for at least two reasons. For one, it's almost impossible to argue against access to a virtually harmless drug that can instantly revive someone on the brink of death. And secondly, when America later began to face an unprecedented rise in opioid overdose during the early twenty-first century, naloxone would be there to help sell harm reduction to the masses.

thirteen

Undoing Treatment

W HEN PATT DENNING WALKED INTO WALDEN HOUSE, THE BAY AREA
psychologist was horrified by what she saw. On the outside, the
widely respected San Francisco rehab didn't look much different from
other residential facilities for people who are down on their luck. But the
"treatment" she saw inside was unlike anything she'd been exposed to in
her PhD training—and unlike anything she'd seen in her therapy practice,
supervision, or continuing education classes.

It was the early 1990s—around the same time that Dan Bigg was getting the Chicago Recovery Alliance up and running and Stephanie Comer
and Dave Purchase were trying to figure out how best to spread the gospel
of harm reduction. In an otherwise ordinary hallway, Denning came upon
a bizarre scene.

Several adults were sitting on high stools with their faces to the wall,
backs outward. They were wearing what seemed to be some sort of dunce
caps. The people with the odd hats were completely silent. They didn't
talk among themselves. In fact, they barely moved. Those who walked by
pointedly ignored them. It was as though they were invisible to everyone
but her. And the longer her visit continued and the more she saw, the more
disturbed she became.

Denning's experience at Walden House would set her on the path
toward harm reduction. At the time, the movement itself had little connection to mainstream addiction treatment: it had started as a public
health response to AIDS, not as a trend in the rehab system. In fact, many

treatment providers saw harm reduction as the opposite of treatment—as something relegated to people who weren't prepared to stop using. Few even considered that its ideas could be integrated into recovery or counseling. Denning would be among the first to try to change that.

As a psychologist in San Francisco's Castro district during the AIDS years, she had spent much of her professional life trying to help gay men cope with the onslaught of illness and grief. A lesbian, she'd co-founded the first feminist counseling center in the U.S. in the seventies. Perhaps as a result, she has always seen therapy as being at least as political as it is personal.

"People often say to me, 'You know, Patt, you are a psychologist. You are a therapist. Why are you talking about all this politics?' I am talking about politics because you can't separate our drug policy from our criminal justice system and from our treatment."[1]

That perspective would make Denning—along with an alcohol researcher with whom she collaborated named G. Alan Marlatt—into critical ambassadors from the world of harm reduction into the world of addiction treatment. They would begin the process of bringing harm reduction off the streets and into counseling sessions and rehabs. Unfortunately, because addiction treatment and counseling themselves had developed outside mainstream medicine and psychology, the idea of "first do no harm" was shockingly absent from the most widely used programs and philosophies.

Denning had first decided to visit Walden House because she was curious about the treatments to which she'd been advised to refer addicted clients. In her PhD training, she'd been told that specialized knowledge beyond her degree was required to treat addiction—and that no one with the disorder could benefit from therapy without quitting drugs first. So she made referrals. But she wasn't impressed by the results she'd seen with clients she'd sent out—and some of what they told her about their experiences didn't sit right with her. Now she was beginning to understand why.

After she passed through the hall of dunces, Denning was allowed to sit in on a group. Around ten people were participating, including the leader. One by one, the members talked about what terrible people they were. None of them said positive things about themselves; what they described were only flaws and dishonest, hurtful, or predatory acts they'd engaged in while addicted. They seemed cowed and often had their heads down, looking at the floor. Almost any of them could have served at that moment as a stock photo illustration for the concept of shame and shamefulness.

But one woman, perhaps new to the program, resisted. When it was her turn, she said that she really hadn't done particularly bad things. Mostly, she said, she'd simply stumbled around drunk. Almost instantly, however, the group leader cut in. He insisted that she wasn't being honest and that she wouldn't be in treatment if she hadn't done wrong. The woman thought about it for a minute and then said that she thought that maybe she'd once missed work. Now, he pounced. "See, you've done bad things, why are you lying?" The viciousness of his response stunned Denning.

And then the rest of the group piled on, too, accusing their fellow patient of trying to manipulate them and saying that, because they had been there during their own addiction, she couldn't fool them with her cheap attempts at deceit. "You can't con a con" was the general sentiment. Nearly everyone in the circle joined in, continually escalating the attack. "It was a scene of humiliation and taunting," Denning said—and it ran counter to everything she knew about how to do therapy.

Later, she asked a staff member about the people with the weird hats in the hallway. They were being punished, she was told. "They broke a rule. 'Addicts have to be taught to be responsible.' That was one of their big mantras," Denning said. The counselors also advised her that "you can't take them at their word, because they're always scamming you." Denning was floored. The way these so-called professionals spoke about and acted toward the people they were supposed to be treating was offensive to her, both as a professional and just as a human being.[2]

Denning's shock didn't come from inexperience or lack of knowledge about mental health care. By that point in her life, she knew a great deal about what makes for good therapy and what is ethically acceptable and appropriate. After all, she had a PhD. And she was not just some early-career employee of a mental health center—but its director.

In her work in the Castro, she had become distressingly familiar with helping clients cope with the horrors of AIDS and the ocean of loss they faced. It hadn't surprised her that many had turned to alcohol or other drugs for relief. This was hardly an irrational response when literally half your friends were dead or dying—and you might be next.

But before her visit to Walden House, when clients developed outright addictions, she'd unthinkingly done as she was trained to do and referred them out for treatment. At first, when they came back with bizarre stories, she thought perhaps that particular person had happened to have an unusually bad experience. Or maybe they'd misinterpreted something. It wasn't that she didn't trust her clients or thought they were dishonest; quite the contrary. Instead, the practices she was hearing about sounded so damaging and frankly crazy that she found it hard to imagine that they were used at all. That was why she had decided to see for herself.

The first thing that had raised her antennae at the rehab she visited was the fact that she was immediately allowed to sit in on a therapy group. Typically, permission would have to be given by each of the therapy participants themselves first, not just obtained from the staff. But that was only one of many signs that addiction treatment had a completely different relationship with those who received help than was acceptable, let alone widely practiced, in psychotherapy.

Tactics that would be considered abuse in any other type of care—screaming at patients, humiliating them, cursing them out, dismissing any objection or complaint, expelling them from treatment for being symptomatic—appeared to be commonplace. "I'm like, 'No, they didn't say that to you.' 'No, they didn't do that.' What?" she said. To be sure that Walden House wasn't just some outlier, Denning also visited other facilities and even attended a number of twelve-step meetings.

Regardless of what kind of program she visited, however, Denning did not like what she saw. "I was just personally and professionally appalled," she said.[3] Like most psychologists, Denning had been taught to practice in a way that was respectful and client centered. Therapists were not supposed to order patients around or treat them like children. They were absolutely forbidden to misuse their power by humiliating and demeaning clients. Such tactics had proven to be counterproductive and could even be traumatic. In fact, research done as far back as the seventies on attack-therapy groups like the one she'd seen at Walden had found that it caused psychological damage that lasted at least six months in nearly

10 percent of participants.[4] Since then, hundreds, perhaps thousands, of papers had been written about the power dynamics of therapy and how careful clinicians must be with it in order to safely and ethically treat vulnerable patients.

Not surprisingly to Denning, the disrespectful and sometimes outright abusive treatment she saw also didn't seem to help many people. Few of those Denning referred to rehab came back better, and some were worse. A few just disappeared. Now she knew why.

AFTER HER VISIT TO WALDEN HOUSE, DENNING RETURNED TO HER OWN offices enraged. She would not allow another person facing AIDS to be referred to a program where he or she would be treated so disrespectfully. She told her staff, "I don't know what we're going to do, but we're not referring to these programs," she said. And in 1995, she met Edith Springer.

A friend of Denning urged, or more like commanded, her to attend a talk scheduled at San Francisco General Hospital. Yes, it was at eight a.m. or some other ungodly early morning hour, but she had to go. She had to meet this crazy social worker from New York who had absolutely transformative ideas about drugs and addiction.

Denning agreed, in part just to get her friend off her back. She figured that he had to be exaggerating. But he wasn't. Before listening to Springer, she'd had no idea what harm reduction was. Now she became immediately convinced of its value and why it had to be popularized. And she also had a name for the type of care she wanted to provide.

"It was astonishing," Denning said, "I laughed hysterically. I thought, 'I love this person.' And it was the first time I'd ever heard anybody talk about things that I was thinking about the attitudes that people have toward drug users." Denning and Springer also soon became close—though bicoastal—friends.

With Springer's encouragement, she continued to study the problem and develop better ways of working with drug users. "I started reading research that showed, 'Oh, we actually do know what *doesn't* work, which is confrontation. We're getting an idea of what *does* work, which is empathy, and cognitive behavioral interventions,'" she said.[5] Unfortunately, the practices that were the most common were those that were the most harmful and the least effective—like group confrontation and humiliation. Conversely, it was nearly impossible to find treatment that used the therapies that had good data behind them.

Drawing from this research, Denning would help create harm reduction psychotherapy. Born and raised in small town Steubenville, Ohio, she describes herself as a "child of the sixties," who had some of the best experiences of her life on drugs, "but luckily, none of the worst." Fascinated by the mind and the way drugs could affect it, she studied psychology and also did a postdoc in psychopharmacology, with her own experience keeping her wary about exaggerated claims.

Later, she would co-found the Center for Harm Reduction Therapy with her partner in both life and work, Jeanne Little, who is a social worker. It would take many years for harm reduction to firmly take hold in the addiction treatment world—and, even now, while growing, it is still a minority perspective. Denning and Little, however, have been critical to its spread. Together, they have trained thousands of people in harm reduction therapy, greatly magnifying the impact of what Springer first taught Denning.

PART OF THE REASON THAT HARM REDUCTION WAS INITIALLY SLOW TO INFIL-trate addiction care was that it developed separately and outside of traditional channels. Because the movement started as grassroots HIV prevention, the professional ties that harm reductionists had, if any, were initially to public health, sociology, and infectious disease researchers, not drug treatment or even social work. As a result, harm reduction was first framed as being in opposition to "real" addiction treatment—or at least it was seen as necessarily separate.

This meant that, initially, the movement had almost no impact where it would seem to matter most: in places supposedly designed to help with drug problems, like rehabs, counseling centers, and other addiction care. Even the rare treatment providers who didn't outright oppose harm reduction tended to see it as a second thought, at best a way to prepare people for abstinence while protecting them from AIDS—not an over-arching philosophy that should be in place wherever drug policy affects people who use drugs.

Consequently, many of the most harmful practices in the addiction field—which run contrary to what harm reduction and other empirical research demonstrates—remained unaddressed for many years. In order to understand just how revolutionary harm reduction is to addiction treatment, it's critical first to understand the problematic ideas at the root of most current care. In each of the three main types of treatment—the twelve-step/Minnesota Model, the therapeutic community model, and medication treatment—some core ideas and common practices are at odds with both research evidence and harm reduction. This is due in part to the fact that the addictions field developed after mainstream medicine gave up on treating the problem—and left it to laypeople to devise responses, which were then replicated without much evidence beyond anecdotes.

The first—and still most common—type of addiction treatment to become widespread in the U.S. is known as the twelve-step/Minnesota Model. Created in the 1940s in that state, the model is based on the idea that AA's twelve steps and complete abstinence from all psychoactive substances (other than caffeine, nicotine, and sugar) are the only route to real recovery. Originally developed as a month-long inpatient program aimed at inspiring lifelong twelve-step group membership, this approach is now also used in outpatient treatment and long-term residences called "sober homes." At least two-thirds of American rehabs require twelve-step participation, as recommended in this treatment philosophy.[6]

In Minnesota Model treatment, most of the treatment day is spent learning about twelve-step programs and being taught to see addiction as a chronic, progressive brain disease. In many centers, patients are told that the only alternative to lifelong meeting attendance is "jails, institutions, or death." Although the model has been updated with the addition of family therapy, psychiatric care for coexisting disorders including medication, and sparing use of addiction medications, the core idea remains that the path to recovery is surrendering to a higher power, taking moral inventory, making amends, and carrying the message of the steps to others. And any resistance to these ideas is seen as resisting recovery, rather than as a need for a different approach.

In contrast, Walden House and similar ninety-day or longer residential programs use what is known as a "therapeutic community" model. Incredibly, American therapeutic communities have their roots in a literal cult called Synanon, which was founded in 1958. Developed by an AA member who thought that the ideas used in the steps should be imposed forcefully, rather than voluntarily, Synanon became a Hollywood and media sensation after it claimed to have cured a man's heroin addiction. At the time, that was seen as impossible.

The fundamental idea of therapeutic communities is that people with addiction are so marred by "character defects"—a concept Synanon took from AA—that their personalities have to be completely broken down. This was originally accomplished in part by punishments like shunning, dunce caps, head shaving, forcing straight men to wear drag and women to dress as sex workers, and many other humiliating tactics. But the main tool was "attack therapy," which Denning had seen in a mild form. In many cases, these group attacks occurred in "marathon" groups that continued for hours or days, without bathroom or food breaks.

Although it now sounds hard to believe, once Synanon claimed to have a heroin cure, state health and justice officials from across the U.S. immediately began copying it, not waiting to study the outcomes. This resulted in the creation of programs like Walden, Phoenix House, Daytop, and Delancey Street, which dominated publicly funded treatment for addiction from the seventies through at least the early 2000s. Practices that would have been rejected as traumatic and abusive for other conditions were simply accepted for addiction—yet another indicator of stigma and criminalization.

Eventually, Synanon itself began proclaiming that it was a church, hoarding guns and forcing men to have vasectomies—even as juvenile justice systems around the country were mandating teens to participate in it or go to jail. In 1978, members placed a de-rattled rattlesnake in the mailbox of an attorney who had begun to win cases against it; the angry snake bit the lawyer, but fortunately, he survived. Soon, Synanon's leader was convicted of conspiracy to commit murder for that attack. But by then, its many descendants in both addiction treatment and treatment for "troubled teens" were well established, and hundreds live on.[7]

Today, most therapeutic communities—including Walden House and the others listed above—publicly disavow humiliating punishments and have tried to eliminate them. Many operate outpatient programs, which by nature are less intense. But this remains a work in progress: like fraternity initiations, confrontational therapy and harsh discipline are remarkably resilient in places where many of the employees are former clients who received punitive initiations themselves and still believe in them. For example, a 2012 study found that more than half of residential therapeutic communities still use tough confrontational therapy.[8]

Finally, the third form of treatment, which is aimed at opioid addiction, is medication treatment. This is the system of methadone clinics and doctors who prescribe buprenorphine—both of which are opioids themselves and strictly regulated. Talk therapy provided with these medications tends to be based on twelve-step approaches—despite the anti-medication ideology that is prevalent in many groups.

As Denning learned more about addiction treatment, she continued to be outraged by the lack of scientific justification for its practices and the harmful nature of so many of them. Nearly all of the programs she visited and read or heard about from attendees were utterly blind to ethical considerations around power. It was as if someone had read Michel Foucault's *Discipline and Punish: The Birth of the Prison* and decided to use the panopticon as a clinician's guide to the treatment milieu—or chose to copy the brutal tactics that appeared among the "guards" in the Stanford Prison Experiment as a model for therapy. Absolute power on the part of the treatment program and complete obedience by patients were simply assumed to be acceptable and appropriate—with little room for disagreement, rare or difficult access to any reliable form of complaint procedure, and no recognition of how frequently unchecked power leads to abuse and atrocities. The increasing rejection of paternalism seen in general medicine was almost nowhere to be found here.

While this was most extreme in therapeutic communities, it wasn't limited to them. In many medication and Minnesota Model/twelve-step programs, clients are frequently and repeatedly told to "shut up and listen." (One saying: "Take the cotton out of your ears and put it in your mouth.") Even programs with the most caring, gentle reputations—which would never allow anything as extreme as attack therapy—are still likely, even now, to have counselors who "joke" that every time their patients' lips move, they are lying.

Obviously, all of this conflicts with harm reduction ideas of "meeting people where they are" and following their lead as they set their own goals. The Minnesota Model and harm reduction clash not just because the former has only one acceptable goal for patients, but also because the twelve-step view of complete "powerlessness" during active addiction is falsified by the demonstrable progress toward health seen in programs like needle exchange. Confrontational therapeutic communities are clearly incompatible, too: breaking people down emotionally in order to rebuild their personalities cannot be reconciled with patient dignity and autonomy and has been shown to be harmful.

Even medication treatment, which is potentially philosophically harmonious with harm reduction, is often problematic in practice. For example, clients practicing harm reduction by, say, using marijuana instead of cocaine, can be expelled from medication treatment for opioid addiction, since they are not completely abstinent. Such a policy is clearly not compatible with harm reduction because it both imposes goals on patients—rather than meeting them where they are—and increases their risk of death.

None of this is to say that these approaches can't be modified to be more congruent and evidence-based, simply that they typically aren't. Many people within harm reduction have found twelve-step programs useful—including me. The real problem is claiming that one approach is the only way and contains the only truth about addiction—rather than, as one twelve-step slogan has it, telling people to "take what you like and leave the rest."

In light of this messy and frequently hostile treatment field, harm reductionists faced an enormous challenge. The vast majority of programs weren't going to change just because research showed that their practices were ineffective or harmful, despite the fact that this seems like the rational thing to do. It would take much more than that.

In fact, changing practice to fit evidence is slow, hard work—even among people who are educated specifically to do so, like doctors. But in a workforce where most people's training is based on teaching clients to recover the same way they themselves did, it's an order of magnitude more difficult. If you feel that your recovery depends on following a particular path, it's much easier to dismiss alternatives and blame clients for not following instructions—rather than learn new ideas, especially those that might threaten what you previously thought to be universal truths about addiction.

To make inroads, harm reductionists began by working outside of traditional treatment, in their own psychology, social work, or counseling practices. Slowly, through trainings, workshops, and conferences, they tried to reach others who worked in the field and make them feel comfortable enough to import harm reduction ideas into their own practice. Sometimes, their trainees would have conversion experiences like Springer herself did when she met Allan Parry—just as some folks with addiction do become fully abstinent the first time they try. But more often, there was a slow, circuitous process—in the same way that harm reduction itself works through small, gradual changes.

For example, in 2012, the pioneer Minnesota Model program Hazelden (now the Hazelden Betty Ford Foundation, after a 2014 merger) finally began allowing opioid addiction treatment with buprenorphine rather than requiring total abstinence. Its own figures had shown that many patients were dying of overdose immediately after leaving, through the same deadly process of loss of tolerance that triples overdose risk following abstinence during incarceration. While this program still tends to push abstinence after only short periods of medication use, the change shows that it is beginning to recognize the need to reduce harm.[9]

Meanwhile Denning helped develop a completely new model. In 1995, almost immediately after meeting Edith Springer, she began to do further research and start formalizing the ideas of harm reduction psychotherapy.

She also dove in politically, connecting with other key figures in the na-scent movement.

And simultaneously, the idea of harm reduction therapy for drug prob-lems was also sprouting on the East Coast. That year, Springer had co-founded a group called Mental Health Professionals in Harm Reduction, along with a New York psychologist named Andrew Tatarsky, who had been developing the practice as well. This group would help professionals integrate harm reduction into social work and psychology practice and training—and soon had hundreds of participants involved in its meetings and events.[10]

Because Denning had become so active so quickly, by the time the Harm Reduction Working Group started planning its first national confer-ence for 1996, she was prominent enough to be asked to speak at a ple-nary session. That conference would be where American harm reduction truly became a movement—among both activists and professionals.

fourteen

Come as You Are

WHEN G. ALAN MARLATT ARRIVED AT THE PARC OAKLAND HOTEL IN late September 1996, he had no luggage, thanks to an airline error. The University of Washington psychology professor and founder of its Addictive Behaviors Research Center had focused much of his previous work on alcohol. But he had become intrigued by the idea of harm reduction and had been invited to speak at the movement's inaugural conference. To him, undoing the distinction between alcohol and other drugs seemed like an obvious way to advance harm reduction. Indirectly, his missing baggage would inspire decades of work within the movement.

As he checked in, Marlatt realized that he would need a clean shirt. All of his clothing was in the bag that had been lost. Conveniently, Dan Bigg's Chicago Recovery Alliance had set up a table near the registration desk, selling the t-shirts they'd designed for the conference. On the front, they read "The Power of Any Positive Change!"—touting their new harm reduction definition of recovery. The professor decided to buy one and did not look at the back before immediately donning it.

Heading for his room, he got into an elevator, which was somewhat full. Within minutes, some executives who were standing behind him began whispering to each other and not too subtly pointing at him. In that t-shirt and jeans, Marlatt did not look like the highly accomplished scientist that he was. The suits' derisive tone suggested that they were not pleased—and perhaps were even shocked.

Curious about what had set them off, when he got to his room, he took off the shirt. For the first time, he read what was listed on the back. Some forty-four harm reduction tactics were included, ranging from utterly un-objectionable—like "build strong relationships," "choose not to use drugs," and "work for peace"—to the less so, such as "use a sterile syringe for each shot," "learn to inject yourself," and "enjoy your high in a safe place." It was the same shirt on which Szyler and Bigg had also included "keep Narcan around"—and which had helped spur Bigg to begin to distribute that antidote after his friend's death.

Marlatt later wrote, "No wonder the businessmen were talking be-hind my back!" On one hand, his experience with them was one of many illustrations of the stigma related to addiction that he constantly worked to fight. On the other, the slogans on the shirt were themselves a great introduction to many of the specific strategies of harm reduction. He used the incident and the list to introduce the first book on harm reduction for clinicians, which he published in 1998.

By the time he attended the 1996 conference, the bearded Canadian-born psychology professor had already become one of the most prominent alcohol researchers in the world. His work would be critical in bringing harm reduction into psychology and addiction treatment—and across the often-separated fields of alcohol and other drug research.

As Edith Springer and Patt Denning had done, Marlatt became an emissary of harm reduction in his field of expertise. This was especially important because psychology is one of two disciplines that dominate aca-demic research on addiction and its treatment, along with psychiatry. Hav-ing one of psychology's most respected researchers on board meant that harm reduction would develop a research base that could start to address the dangerous practices that Denning had seen and that I had personally experienced in treatment.

The conference itself would be the big debut for the Harm Reduc-tion Coalition, which had, by then, been formally established by the working group. A full 700 people attended the four-day event. Writ-ing later about his experience, Marlatt described the organizers' goal as "marking the national birth of a U.S. harm reduction movement."[1]

It certainly did that, giving participants a crash course in all of the key elements of the work.

Born in Vancouver in 1941, Marlatt had initially wanted to be a therapist but, in college, he found himself drawn to research instead. Like Springer and Denning, he inspired countless students. He was also a seeker, bringing the fruits of years of experience with Buddhist meditation and mindfulness to his science.

Marlatt's seminal work began in the 1970s. Like the later needle exchange data, his alcohol research threatened some core concepts of the twelve-step/Minnesota Model. Both sets of data show that people with addictions are not completely out of control, even while under the influence of their preferred substance. This is a very hard concept to study experimentally. But Marlatt developed an ingenious method to explore which factors really determine how much someone will drink at a given time.

The work was conducted in a lab he had turned into a realistic replica of a bar. The "BAR Lab"[2] had rows of wine and liquor bottles, a polished wooden surface to lean on, barstools, fellow drinkers, mellow lighting, and, of course, a bartender. Some of the participants in the study had been selected to take part because they had alcohol use disorders, but no desire to quit; others were social drinkers. In order to keep them from focusing on their drinking patterns and potentially trying to hide them to try to please the researchers or make themselves look good, they were told they were participating in a consumer taste test, not a study of drinking behavior.

In some parts of the experiment, the researchers-cum-bartenders served vodka tonics. In others, the participants got tonic alone. And, in some of the conditions, the drinkers were told they were getting booze—but received only tonic. In other iterations, of course, the opposite was true.

This apparently frivolous research was designed to answer a serious question. If even a sip of alcohol can cause alcoholics to lose control—as AA and the Minnesota Model frame the disorder—the genuine drinks should have prompted higher levels of drinking later in the session. But that's not what happened. These studies found that it was people's *belief* that they were getting booze that led to increased drinking—the actual content of the beverage didn't matter.

And this was even true for those with severe alcohol use disorder: whether they got tonic and were told it was vodka tonic or whether they actually got the real thing, what mattered was what they expected, not what they received.

Expectations about alcohol, rather than alcohol itself, drive escalation of drinking. And that means that chemically, addictive disorders cannot be linked solely to a simple interaction between the brain and the drug. Learning and culture matter, too. This also means that alcoholics are not automatically "powerless" from the time they take their first drink. This research, which has been replicated, is considered to be a major contribution to the field.[3] It added to a growing controversy in alcohol studies that paralleled the fight over needle exchange and other forms of harm reduction with other drugs.

Marlatt was a key figure in showing that harm reduction ideas—across substances—more accurately fit with how people behave in their everyday lives. In doing so, he helped unite harm reduction activists who focused on illegal drugs and researchers and activists who were critical of the overwhelming focus on abstinence in treatment for both alcohol and other drugs. This not only added new supporters to the harm reduction movement, but also slowly began to change treatment.

Marlatt first learned about harm reduction from colleagues and research papers describing what was going on in the U.K. and the Netherlands. He'd arranged to spend a sabbatical in Amsterdam and visited Liverpool as well, seeing for himself what the first harm reductionists were up to and discussing it with its originators in the eighties. When he got back to Seattle, he understood that "harm reduction" accurately described his own work, which was at that point focused on reducing college binge drinking.

The program he developed is known as BASICs and has now been adopted by some 2,500 universities—more than half of the universities in America. It isn't aimed primarily at reducing drinking frequency or quantity, but on cutting risky behavior and resulting damage. "I think I have a name for that now," he told one of his colleagues, after learning about the practice in Europe. "It's called harm reduction."[4]

AT THE OAKLAND CONVENTION CENTER IN 1996, THE FIRST NATIONAL CONference of the Harm Reduction Coalition opened with an enthusiastic call to action by Allan Clear, the group's new executive director. A British photographer who had immigrated to New York in the early eighties, he'd helped found ACT UP's illegal needle exchange on the Lower East Side—and had headed up that organization as it transitioned into a successful independent nonprofit. Initially a twelve-stepper, he'd come to the movement via his own recovery from alcoholism. He was excited by the big turnout.

"This is a historic meeting," he said. He described HRC's work, saying that its vision came from people who knew there was an alternative to the maltreatment that marked so much of American drug policy. The group's goal, he said, was to make harm reduction into national policy for drugs and drug users.

Clear described how isolating it could be to be one of a tiny number of people trying to fight against both AIDS and the drug war. Many attendees had not previously met more than one or two others who shared their views, except perhaps online. Simply being together in one place with hundreds of like-minded people was electric. One of the other organizers of the conference remarked that the team was simply amazed that they'd managed to bring off the event at all. They were astonished that so many people had shown up.[5]

Next to speak was Dave Purchase, the Tacoma needle exchange innovator and co-founder of the working group, which had made the conference and HRC itself possible. After riffing on how hard it could be to define harm reduction concisely, he went on to sum it up in a single sentence. "Harm reduction is against harm, neutral on the use of drugs per se, and in favor of any positive change as defined by the person making the change," he said.

Cautioning practitioners that they needed to be just as sure to be kind and nonjudgmental to themselves and each other as they aimed to be with

their clients, he emphasized the importance of pleasure. "[H]arm reduction—being logical, practical, right and effective—is more enjoyable than
following a path that leads nowhere and supporting 'laws' of behavior that
do not work. Harm reduction is fun, and fun is what I suggest you [have]
here."[6] From the fact that so few people can remember any specific details
of the conference, I am certain that many people followed this advice.

Edith Springer's subsequent talk covered many of her key themes,
exploring the difference between the all-or-nothing abstinence approach
and the more gradual view of change embodied in harm reduction. She
stressed that most current treatment fails to treat patients respectfully.
And she emphasized how dangerous this can be, noting that in clinical
training, therapists are taught never to try to break down people's defenses
before alternative coping skills are in place. When this is done—as it so
frequently is in rehabs and therapeutic communities—she noted, "we run
the risk of causing the person to decompensate and become worse off
than . . . he or she was before."[7]

Imani Woods—whom Springer had described as her most difficult
student ever—followed her mentor and teacher up to the podium. She
was all-in on harm reduction now, but that didn't mean she completely
disavowed her past.

"I'm here to represent all of us who believe in abstinence," she began
defiantly. "That's where I come from: abstinence. Years ago, when I would
come into a room and hear someone say 'harm reduction,' I said, 'You must
be crazy.'"

Proudly stating that she'd grown up in Bedford-Stuyvesant and citing
Malcolm X's guidance about how it is okay to admit that you have been
wrong, she described her previous self. "I was one of those dogmatic counselors, you know, 'I came up the hard way and so can you.'" When HIV
began devastating the Black community, however, she began to question
this approach. "What is more important? That people stay alive or that
people not use drugs?" she asked. "And then I heard Dave Purchase say,
'Dead junkies can't get clean.'"

At the same time, Woods began to examine the outcomes of her own
counseling work, recalling how she and her co-workers often told their
clients that fewer than one in ten of them would genuinely succeed at

quitting drugs. "I had to ask myself the simple question: what about the other ninety percent? What about the ninety percent for whom abstinence didn't work?"

She went on to explain how hard it was, specifically, for people of color to buy in to harm reduction. She noted the actual harmful effects of drugs like crack on families as well as issues of respectability and racist enforcement. She said, "Let's be realistic. It's a whole different ballgame when we're talking about black folks and Latin folks. Because the effects on the community are different . . . Our community, we see drugs as a barrier. It keeps us away from all that good stuff like family life, ambition, achievement and so on." White drug policy reform advocates, in their efforts to distance themselves from drug war scare tactics, had often minimized this.

Addressing white people specifically, she said, "I must tell you: y'all use most of the drugs. Y'all just don't go to jail . . . we're the ones who end up going to jail. When you go into the black community and talk about harm reduction, you got a whole other ball of wax to deal with. All people can tell you is, 'Reduce this! Reduce these police taking me to jail . . .'"

Woods ended her talk with a call for unity, noting that there would undoubtedly be many arguments and clashes along the way. "Everybody thinks they're right, including me," she said. "With all that, you know it's going to be a mess. But if we don't do it, nobody's gonna do it. Somebody's got to make the change."

Other movement stars like Dan Bigg and Joyce Rivera also spoke, and there were sessions related to medical marijuana, which had just been legalized in California and was an issue that could get people who hadn't really thought about drug policy to recognize how it did harm. Also, at least two high-ranking police officials, from Connecticut and California, spoke, advocating gentler policies like diversion to treatment rather than incarceration.[8] Later, the question of whether law enforcement could ever practice genuine harm reduction would cause conflict. But at first, the movement welcomed all comers and deliberately brought disparate and sometimes clashing views together. To make change, harm reductionists would at the very least have to know how to engage with the mainstream.

ALAN MARLATT'S TALK COVERED HIS OWN WORK WITH ALCOHOL—HIGHLIGHT-
ing the controversy over whether people with severe alcohol problems
can ever learn to moderate or "control" their drinking. This acrimoni-
ous debate neatly paralleled the fight for needle exchange for drug injectors. Just as traditional treatment providers had argued that drug injectors
couldn't improve their health without kicking drugs first, they also claimed
that no positive change could occur for those with alcoholism without
total abstinence. And by showing that alcohol behaves just like other
drugs, Marlatt helped dramatically expand the scope of the movement.
That's because, while less than 2 percent of Americans regularly inject
drugs, at least 70 percent of the population has had at least one drink in
the past year.[9]

Illustrating these parallels to expand the reach of harm reduction was
a deliberate strategy. Marlatt knew that "undoing" drugs was essential to
the mission: if alcohol isn't seen as the drug that it is, its many users can
easily dismiss "druggies" as some alien group whose experience is completely unlike their own. The spectrum of substance use must be seen
in its entirety, so that we can recognize that it is indeed universal, across
cultures and time.

Years later, Marlatt would tell his students explicitly that he saw alcohol harm reduction as a Trojan horse: a way to get people to take in the key
ideas of the movement without immediately raising their defenses about
their implications. He told one postdoc, "When I started doing this work,
I had a feeling that harm reduction was the right way forward, but I knew
people weren't ready to hear that message." And so he worked first on
more acceptable approaches. One behavioral therapy that he developed
became known as "relapse prevention." This would, surprisingly, be quite
rapidly incorporated into most twelve-step/Minnesota Model treatment
programs, albeit in somewhat adulterated form. The idea was to understand what experiences might "trigger" relapse and learn ways to manage
these risky situations while staying abstinent.

Of course, relapse prevention, by its very name, does not threaten the
supremacy of abstinence, since the whole point is to help people maintain
it. However, it also includes information on how to minimize damage in
the extremely common event of a slip—aka harm reduction.

In fact, one of its key concepts is the "abstinence violation effect," or more colloquially, the "fuck it" response. This refers to the idea that once you've had one drink or broken your diet or otherwise lapsed, you may as well continue since you've already blown it. Research shows that having this belief, especially if you also see yourself as "powerless" once you start engaging in the behavior you are trying to change, leads to more severe relapses. The phenomenon could be seen during the early days of AIDS, when without good information about risk, gay men would alternate between celibacy and sexual extremes. It recurred during COVID, when, again, people with little good information on moderating risk flip from going overboard with measures like double-masking and seeing no one to simply taking no precautions at all.

In contrast to the relatively widespread acceptance of relapse prevention therapy, however, Marlatt's support for what became known as "controlled drinking" stirred far more conflict. The idea that some addicted people can return to moderation is far more threatening to the core idea of the Minnesota Model, which is that twelve-step abstinence is the only—or, at least, the best—way to recover. Both relapse prevention therapy and the controversy over controlled drinking, however, ultimately helped spread harm reduction into whole new areas of addiction research and practice.

At the first harm reduction meeting, Marlatt described the colorful history of the cultural war over controlled drinking. The drama—in which he himself played a part—involved claims of research fraud, Congressional and university investigations, and the firing of a leading treatment doctor who was seen to be on the wrong side. There were arguments over who was to blame for a drunk driving crash that killed two people. At one point, Marlatt even received death threats.

The first round, he explained, took place in the late seventies and early eighties. In 1973, two researchers, a husband and wife team, published controversial data on alcohol moderation. Mark and Linda Sobell had found that training people with severe alcoholism to control their drinking led to better life outcomes and functioning, compared with abstinence treatment. And in a three-year follow-up, the results remained consistent: the controlled drinking program was superior.[10]

This, of course, made abstinence supporters crazy and furious. It was simply not supposed to be possible for anyone with alcoholism, especially not severe cases, to cut back rather than abstain—just as people who inject drugs were seen as incapable of reliably using clean needles or moderating their use. Marlatt's BAR lab research had undermined the idea of "powerlessness after the first drink." But the Sobells' work put the terrifying notion into practice with real people who were undergoing addiction treatment. Minnesota Model supporters and many twelve-step group members thought that the research simply couldn't be true.

And so the data and the researchers were attacked in a massive media blitz culminating in a 1983 60 *Minutes* investigation. A dramatic portion of the show included footage shot at the graves of several of the study's participants. The exposé was based on a ten-year follow-up of the controlled drinking study, conducted by a different set of authors. To top it off, this new research was published in one of the most prestigious journals in the world, *Science*.

In their media appearances, the follow-up authors revealed that four out of twenty participants in the controlled drinking group had died, a full 20 percent. Before the *Science* paper was even publicly available, they claimed that the Sobells had faked their previous publications and lied about the positive outcome data for the earlier years of the study. And this deceit, they implied, had been fatal.

"Beyond any reasonable doubt, it's fraud," one of them told the *New York Times*.[11] The actual journal article was more cautious in its claims: *Science's* lawyers had almost certainly toned down its shrill language about the Sobells for fear of being sued for libel. Ultimately, whoever made these changes would deserve every bit of their paycheck.

At first, however, the coverage was positive. Other media proclaimed that *Science* and 60 *Minutes* had revealed a deadly scandal, in which the Sobells had essentially killed some of their research participants. AA was right: people with alcoholism could never achieve control over their drinking.[12] Soon the Sobells were subject to a research integrity investigation by their employer. They were also investigated by Congress, because the National Institutes of Health had funded the study. Marlatt, who was a friend of the couple and had been given access to their data during the investigations, stood by them.

And when the truth finally came out, it was shocking, particularly given the zeal with which the Sobells had been attacked. First—and astonishingly, given the journal's reputation—*Science* had made a freshman-level research error when it published the attack paper. The article only included ten-year outcome data for the moderate drinking group, not for the control group, who had received typical abstinence treatment. Without ten-year data from the comparison group, the claim that the Sobells had done harm was unsupportable.

In fact, as it turned out, the abstinence group had done even worse. Six of these participants had died, compared to the four who died after the Sobells' treatment. And all of those who died had also tried abstinence programs after the moderation treatment had failed. Clearly, neither approach had been especially successful in these severe cases. However, the Sobells had not faked anything. All of the investigations exonerated them. They had not been the ones who'd made dishonest claims.[13]

When Marlatt wrote about the controversy in 1983, he noted that of the twenty-two then-published controlled drinking studies, twenty-one had found that it worked, producing successful outcomes in around 65 percent of participants who were followed for at least a year.[14] Little of this background had been mentioned in the media. And research since then has only continued to support the idea. Indeed, by 1990, the highly respected Institute on Medicine—in a report that Marlatt co-authored—recommended that alcohol treatment programs across the U.S. expand to include options like moderation. That's because, even though people with the most severe alcohol problems are less likely to succeed at moderation, most cases of alcohol use disorder do not fall into that category. It's also because when people choose their own treatment goals, they do better.

Incredibly, however, when the issue came to public attention again in 1995, it replayed almost identically. I had a small role in the resulting skirmish, when I wrote an article for *New York* magazine that was wildly misinterpreted. Marlatt had tried to calm the media storm that resulted.

My piece had been intended to highlight the progress made by a prominent Minnesota Model program in New York, which had added an evidence-based controlled drinking option for those who didn't agree to its abstinence approach. Instead, what I actually wrote was ignored and my story was interpreted as having claimed that the program no longer supported abstinence at all.

The resulting panicked attention from the *New York Times* and elsewhere led to the firing of the program's director, basically for providing therapies supported by the most prominent and respected national experts on the research!

To make the controversy even more intense, around the same time, the woman who had founded a self-help group aimed at teaching controlled drinking, known as Moderation Management, relapsed. She drove drunk and crashed, killing a father and his twelve-year-old daughter. When she was arrested, her blood alcohol level was three times the legal limit.[15] Most journalists assumed that the conclusion to be drawn from this catastrophe was self-evident: surely, here was proof that it was unethical for alcohol treatment and self-help groups to do anything but demand full abstinence.

But again, a big element of the story was simply ignored in most of coverage. The founder of Moderation Management had written explicitly in its literature that if moderation fails, people should go to AA or other abstinence programs instead. And indeed, two months before the crash, she'd started attending AA regularly.[16] As a result, her story could just as easily have been used to illustrate the failure of AA—if that's how journalists had wanted to play it.

Throughout the eighties and nineties, this was the hostile climate harm reductionists faced, whether they were working with alcohol or other drugs. The media reflected the culture—and it was deeply committed to abstinence. When recovery was shown—whether in the news, on stage, in films, on TV—it was almost always via the twelve steps. Indeed, twelve-step programs were so popular in the early nineties that a major film, *The Player*, had a storyline about Hollywood producers who didn't have drinking problems going to AA—because that's where the deals were being made. Around the same time, *New York* magazine suggested that AA was so hot that single non-alcoholic women should go there to meet men.

Celebrities touted the program; when they went to rehab it was Betty Ford or Hazelden or Eric Clapton's program in the Caribbean, all Minnesota Model. When journalists tried to write or broadcast stories about other approaches, the response of editors was often dismissive or the piece would be played as a contrarian novelty, not exactly to be taken seriously.

Just as journalists tended to see support for the war on drugs as "objective" because both political parties favored it, the media also tended to reflexively favor twelve-step abstinence—again, because alternatives were just not visible to the mainstream. Marlatt helped change that.

Engaging with pop culture, he wrote about how the 1994 suicide of grunge god Kurt Cobain had been immediately preceded by a tough-love intervention, arranged by his then-wife, Courtney Love. Living with chronic pain, Cobain couldn't face the idea of total abstinence, but quitting all opioids, including methadone, was presented as his only option for recovery. This made him feel even more hopeless. And as the connection between his death and the lack of harm reduction options became clear, Cobain's record label planned to support a "Come as you are" harm reduction center in his memory, to be led by Marlatt. (Unfortunately, when the company was sold, these plans fell through.)[17]

Further, one of his colleagues noted that Marlatt's work on college drinking alone "made harm reduction the paradigm in college health"—at least insofar as the counseling they receive.[18] (Campus alcohol policy is another story.) Marlatt's relapse prevention program was also one of the most important conduits of harm reduction ideas into traditional addiction treatment.

THE FINAL SPEAKER AT THE FIRST HARM REDUCTION CONFERENCE, FITTINGLY, was the psychedelic guru Ram Dass. In his pre-drug life, he'd been known as Richard Alpert and was an assistant professor of psychology at Harvard. Working with Timothy Leary, he'd conducted some of the earliest research on LSD, psilocybin mushrooms, and spirituality in the early sixties.

Critically, Dass helped develop the concept of "set and setting," which is important in many types of harm reduction. Originally, this was the idea that psychedelic experience is determined not just by a drug's pharmacological effects, but also by the user's emotional state and expectations and the cultural and physical environment where the drug is taken. Understanding set and setting is important because it allows people to recognize dangerous situations for psychedelic use and avoid them.

But the concept has also been highly influential beyond hallucinogens, because it turns out to apply to all substances: for example, the effect of alcohol expectations that Marlatt found studying drinking. And within harm reduction, a movement focused specifically on psychedelic drugs developed in conjunction with other organizing, starting in Liverpool and Manchester's ecstasy rave scene, during the late 1980s and early nineties.[19]

Dass's own psychedelic experience, which led him to visit India and become a spiritual leader, had made him intimately familiar with the harms related to the war on drugs. In his talk, he noted the importance of listening to people who take drugs when setting policy related to them. "I look at harm reduction as relieving the maximum amount of suffering," he said.

Then he went on to make a more subtle but just as important point. Explaining that lack of human and spiritual connection causes much of our pain, he noted that a great deal of this suffering is linked to our attachment to specific identities and the social status we believe we get from them. This attachment can cause serious problems, especially within political movements like harm reduction.

"It's perfectly fine if you are an administrator to administrate," he said. "Just don't get caught in thinking you are an administrator . . . If you are a junkie, God bless you, but don't get caught in being a junkie! It's not interesting enough, there is no role identity which is *that* interesting." He added, "If you are recovering, recover, by God, recover! But don't get caught up in the drama of being a recoverer."

This wisdom about identity would be greatly needed as harm reduction grew. In order to center people who use drugs, the movement had to come up with a way to determine who could legitimately speak for such people. Was it only people who injected drugs? What about abstinent former users—or those who took psychedelics? A group fighting for the human rights of drug users clearly shouldn't be dominated by those without drug experience. However, if people's social status within harm reduction relies on their continued use of dangerous substances, that could also obviously pose problems.

Here was yet another situation in which the concept of drugs had to be deconstructed. Answering the question "Who speaks for drug users?" would be at least as tricky as trying to redefine addiction and recovery.

fifteen

Nothing about Us without Us

HEATHER EDNEY WAS SOMETIMES UNCOMFORTABLE WITH BEING A POSTER child for active users within harm reduction. The raven-haired California native who, in the early days, wasn't even old enough to drink legally was often asked to speak at national and international conferences to represent the user's perspective. Her youth, relentlessness, and fervor made her particularly popular. Consequently, because of her deep commitment to empowering people who use drugs, she often agreed to do it.

At these events, she spoke powerfully about the stigma she was subjected to as a target of the war on drugs. She discussed specific examples, like overdosing, being revived, and then being left in severe withdrawal in a hospital's janitorial closet. She described how, in that closet, she'd been seated in a disused dentist's chair with an IV and ignored for hours, while nauseated, sweaty, and shaking. Occasionally, a nurse would stop by and berate her, telling her she should be ashamed of herself and saying things like "This is what you get" for being addicted. She made the need for more respectful and appropriate treatment vivid.

In her talks, however, Edney didn't just dwell on how she'd been harmed. She also noted her privilege—and how, as a rich white girl, she never got arrested even when police had clear evidence of crimes like driving while impaired. She made her experience of being someone who injects drugs—and the need for harm reduction—real to many who tended to look at the issue as an abstract policy question. She also made clear that far more than one voice was needed.

Occasionally, however, she just couldn't bring herself to do it. Her experience was too raw. She didn't feel like she was in control of her own story or what other people might make of it. At least once, she overdosed before a planned presentation and required someone else to do the speech as she recovered.

Her fear wasn't linked to doubts about harm reduction—nor did she have concerns related to the need for representation of active users. Instead, she was plagued by the problem that Ram Dass had raised, which is the stickiness of identities and the social status associated with them—and how this can sometimes trap people in unexpected ways.

This would become a serious issue for Edney when her own drug use began to spin out of control. She'd staked out a position—along with people like John Marks in Liverpool—entirely rejecting the need for abstinence. She'd argued that regaining control was pretty much always possible for everyone. She'd also made the case that people who were abstinent couldn't speak for active users; they had a different agenda and were no longer in touch with the immediacy of the experience and the needs people had during it. Consequently, she began to feel that her role in the movement required her to continue to use.

But over time, she began to question this. She started to suspect, in fact, that she might really need to quit some drugs entirely in order to survive. Initially, she didn't know how to reconcile her personal conflict over abstinence with the political views she remained convinced were important. At first, she thought that being a true harm reduction radical meant rejecting abstinence entirely. Her journey would show the dangers of that perspective—and illustrate why the harm reduction movement had to ensure that it was carefully defining its own positions, not just reacting against everything associated with existing approaches.

Raised in an upper-middle-class home in Thousand Oaks, California, Edney had a childhood that looked great on its glossy surface. Just twenty miles from Malibu Beach, Thousand Oaks has long been an emblem of the wealthy California suburbs. Edney herself has lush, wavy hair, big hazel eyes, and a Hollywood smile—a glamorous look suited to a glamorous place.

Underneath, however, was chaos. Her stepfather, who had post-traumatic stress disorder associated with his service in Vietnam, could be unpredictably violent. Her mother, while loving, was often checked out. In fact, she gave Heather her first drug, Miltown, a tranquilizer, in order to keep her calm for her grandfather's funeral. She was fourteen or fifteen at the time.

"It was a revelation," Edney said of the experience. "As soon as I got home from the funeral, it was straight to the medicine cabinet and it was on." Not long afterward, she began smoking crack with an older man, whom she describes as "super-high functioning" who binged with her every weekend. Since she lived in such a moneyed community, she said, "There's a lot of access to drugs, good drugs." She began injecting before she completed high school.

At this point, Edney's drug use didn't much get in her way. After a stint at a community college, she transferred to the University of California–Santa Cruz. Always drawn to helping people, she wanted to fight the growing HIV epidemic. She started working in a hospice program. At eighteen, she became a home health aide to a woman with AIDS who had become infected via an unsterile syringe. Her client's son had been born with the virus—and as his mother declined, Edney became one of the baby's primary caregivers. The boy was three when his mom died and Edney took on even more of a maternal role, helping his grandmother raise him.

During this time, some of her colleagues at the hospice had begun bringing home excess needles to supply local IV drug users and protect them from HIV. Having seen the damage done by lack of access to clean works, Edney immediately joined them. In 1989, still in college, still a teenager, still helping raise a younger child, and still injecting drugs herself, she helped found the Santa Cruz Needle Exchange. She came of age in harm reduction when it was a very young movement itself.

Within six months, she'd become the exchange's executive director, as they operated illegally and underground. "We had this stroller and you put the needles in the stroller. I don't know who we thought we were fooling, late at night on the hooker's stroll," she said. The exchangers would visit the houses and apartments of people they knew were injecting and go to shooting galleries and dealing spots. "Looking back, that's kind of crazy," she said, "but everyone was amazing and lovely and appreciative."[1]

Unlike many other exchanges, the Santa Cruz program skewed young—its teenage founder and its mobile guerilla operation were able to reach kids who remained invisible to services that were created and run by a different generation. Soon they added fixed sites and times, setting up in places where people congregated, such as under the Barson Street bridge.

Right from the start, Edney was defiantly out as a young IV drug user. She was also out about being one who didn't want to hear from so-called experts about what she could and couldn't do. After she met George Clark of Prevention Point in San Francisco, she was invited to join the working group.

With enough attitude to intimidate critics and friends alike, Edney began proudly giving a voice to young injectors. She was openly disdainful of abstinence and unapologetic about her own use. "I learned from people like Edith Springer how to be a high-functioning opiate user," she said, explaining one tactic. "You take pills during the day and shoot up at night."

And, for about fifteen years, she made it work: running the needle exchange, attending conferences, helping harm reduction grow. In collaboration with exchange participants, she created a zine called *junkphood*. An exemplar of punk style, it included poetry, distinctive artwork, and photo illustrations—along with interviews with needle exchange participants about their experiences. Some of the covers included dead-on parodies of sugar cereal boxes, with the green frog who usually sells Sugar Smacks now pitching plain old smack. Frosted Flakes' Tony the Tiger was appropriated for amphetamine—and in the *junkphood* world, the cuckoo was going crazy for "Coked-Up Puffs" rather than Cocoa Puffs.

Junkphood soon won national acclaim and media coverage for its frank portrayal of the lives of young heroin users and their ambivalent feelings about drugs, death, and risk-taking. (Locally, it was not always so popular: when a copy was found near the body of a young man who had overdosed on heroin, the health department and the police tried and failed to shut the needle exchange down.)

Its manifesto, which was reprinted at the front of each issue, expressed its distinct mix of bravado and realism:

Being a young injection drug user and asking for information, generally from adults, means that you have to put yourself lower than them, and admit that you're a fucked up, ignorant kid. That's an ego-busting experience, it's terrible, and we won't do it.

Instead of asking adults for help, we make up our own information and our own ethics. That's what makes being a kid the awesome experience that it is. But sometimes, our actions are really misguided and lead us to do something dangerous . . . The point of this series is not to tell other users what to do, but to get people talking about their drug use, what we love about it, what we hate about it, and what we wish was different.[2]

By expressing both arrogance and fear—and detailing young users' complex mix of desire for drugs, longing for a better life, and ambivalence about risk—*junkphood* was able to reach youth who (apparently literally) wouldn't be caught dead with a pamphlet from the health department.

For Edney personally, however, over time, her feelings about drug use and its place in her life began to change. She'd dealt with many of her own traumatic experiences by self-medicating with opioids; she'd kept her feelings about the losses her childhood and her work had exposed her to mostly hidden, even from herself. She had many close calls with overdoses. And then, when she began shooting methamphetamine instead of heroin, her ability to balance her drug use with her work was lost.

"I was strung out on opiates, and I did what so many of us do," she said. "I had this brilliant idea that I would replace opiates with meth and then kick meth." But while she'd been able to keep her opiate habit reasonably regular, with meth she lost control. At first she believed she could handle it and that, as she'd argued so many times herself, there was always a choice. She just had to try harder. It didn't work, though. She became more and more erratic and unreliable. Realizing that she might damage her own organization, she left in 2003.

Without her work, however, she was undone. Edney lived on the street in Los Angeles for months. "I could not really pull that off very well. It's hard to be homeless," she said. It got to the point where nearly every time she injected, she would overdose—a phenomenon that has been described by researchers, but is not yet understood. Somehow, for some people, having one overdose makes it more likely that you will soon have another.[3] For people like Edney who are affected, it gives every shot worse odds than Russian roulette.

By the end of the year, realizing that she would probably die if she didn't stop, she entered abstinence-based treatment. In rehab, she even started attending and embracing Narcotics Anonymous meetings, though she continued to disagree with much of their rhetoric. She remains a proud harm reductionist, but these days, she regrets having ever dismissed the need for abstinence as part of the spectrum of recovery.

"It breaks my heart that I was a part of conversations when I did not know what the fuck I was talking about," she said. Just as abstinence ideology that rejects harm reduction can do real damage, so can harm reduction ideology that rejects abstinence. Politically, Edney also recognized how the debate itself had been unproductive: it could make enemies of allies who were united in their opposition to the war on drugs, but also committed to their own abstinence-based recovery.

"If I had known better, I would never have spoken disparagingly about people in traditional recovery," she says now. "We cannot afford to be separated. There's not enough of us."

FROM THE START, ISSUES OF IDENTITY HAVE BEEN COMPLICATED WITHIN THE movement. Beyond questions of race, class, gender and sexual orientation, harm reduction has an identity dilemma that is unlike those faced by most other activists: that is, the changeable nature of people's relationships to their own and to other people's drug use.

A racial identity like being Black isn't mutable. As Lisa Moore put it, "That's what daddy always said, 'You were born Black and you're going to die and stay Black.'" The same is true for other ethnic identities and, in most cases, for sexual orientation and gender identity. Moreover, being Black, gay, trans, or female isn't inherently harmful. Harm associated with those identities is due to other people's prejudices, not the identities themselves.

With drugs, however, people have many and varied relationships with substance use. Although only a minority ever develop addictions, this is the group that is by definition at the most risk of being harmed. Moreover, among addicted people, many completely alter the way they think about drugs and drug use in order to recover. This makes the question of who can speak authentically as a drug user extremely vexed.

Harm reductionists had to think deeply about these issues in order to appropriately represent those it was designed to serve. The main questions are these: who truly does represent the user voice? Can it be someone who is abstinent—or must the person still be using drugs? Can it be a user who sticks to psychedelics and dance drugs—or must it be someone who shoots drugs like heroin or cocaine? What about marijuana? And what about frequency of use—surely, the people most oppressed by the drug war are those who inject daily, so only this group should count, and not folks who use only occasionally?

The future of the movement would depend on finding a way through the thicket of identities created by the concepts of "drugs" and "addiction" and "recovery." And that was difficult because these had been skewed not only by the legal status of specific drugs, but also by the racism that helped create that status—and by ongoing debates over the nature of addiction. It was yet another area where drugs needed to be undone.

Further, as in other disability rights movements—particularly those involving mental illness and developmental disorders—harm reduction would also have to face the question of which behaviors that are currently stigmatized are genuinely harmful and should be discouraged and which are harmful only because mainstream society has tried to suppress or doesn't accept them. For example, it's clear to the autistic community that while autistic hand-flapping might be annoying or distracting to neurotypical people, it doesn't hurt anyone. Consequently, autistic advocates argue for its acceptance. In contrast, behavior that could harm others is not just a violation of social convention, and it does need to be managed. Similar issues in relation to drug-related behaviors would need to be elaborated.

Also, as with the early days of the gay rights movement, harm reductionists had to contend with the fact that the behavior around which the movement was organized was not just stigmatized, but also actively criminalized. Keeping drug use hidden was not just about shame or fear of embarrassment. Being open about it could lead to serious consequences ranging from job loss to prison.

This creates real problems for people who want to be "out" about their status. It is one thing to proclaim on national TV, as I had, that you are a person in recovery who hasn't taken drugs for years. It is quite another to speak in front of an audience that might include your employers or the police and say that you still inject heroin and would likely do so again in a few hours. This is obviously even more difficult for Black and brown people and other minorities.

Gay rights activists could wholeheartedly fight against anything and anyone that pathologized homosexuality because it absolutely is not a disease and indeed does no harm at all. But harm reduction had to contend with genuine issues around drug-related impairment and addiction, which can be deadly.

The first point that advocates tend to make here is that most people who use most drugs—legal or illegal—are not harmed by them and do not become addicted. Research shows that around 10 to 20 percent of those who use alcohol, cocaine, and methamphetamine become addicted, even though these drugs vary widely in legal and medical availability.[4] Depending on what measures are used, the percent of users who become addicted can be slightly higher for heroin and slightly lower for cannabis. The drug that addicts and harms the highest proportion of its users is nicotine in the form of cigarettes, with low-end estimates starting at 30 percent. In other words, harm is not inherent to most drug use in and of itself.

The second and related point that is made is that most of the harm that we tend to think of as being "drug-related" is actually drug-policy-related. For example, if clean needles are legal and people are educated about sterile technique, blood-borne illness is not a "natural" or automatic consequence of injecting. Recognizing the safety and non-exceptional nature of most drug use is part of harm reduction.

But so too is acknowledging the harm that is associated with some drugs and with addiction, regardless of a drug's legal status. And, in terms of user perspectives and identities, these facts mean that people who have never had problems controlling their drug use are the wrong people to represent the experience of those who have.

The question of whether former problem users can speak for current ones is also difficult. Critically, many early American harm reductionists came to it after being abstinent themselves for years, often with the support of twelve-step programs. Edith Springer herself spent many years as an abstinence advocate, as did Imani Woods. What this meant was that even after they became harm reductionists, these activists saw abstinence as part of a continuum of harm reduction strategies and tactics. On one end was "any positive change" within continued drug use—like safer injection practices or cutting back on days of use or reducing doses. But on the other end, for some people, with some substances, this group argued, abstinence might really be the only way they could avoid harm.

Harm reductionists like Springer and Woods didn't think abstinence was for everyone, nor did they argue that everyone who ever had a problem with one substance needed to abstain forever from all the rest. They saw recovery using medications like methadone, buprenorphine, and even heroin as being as valid as any other type. Abstinence supporters within harm reduction tried—not always successfully—to argue that they weren't saying that their approach was a superior option for everyone, just that it should be *an* option. For this group, being nonjudgmental applied not only to how they saw active drug use and prescribed medications, but also to their view of any form of abstinence—from quitting cocaine and still using marijuana to never ever eating sugar or taking psychoactive substances, even caffeine.

Others, however—particularly in the U.K.—took a stance every bit as absolutist as that of the abstentionists. They insisted that drug use was always a choice, even when it might be a bad one and lead to harm. At the start of the movement, this perspective became popular among some in the American harm reduction movement as well, sometimes advocated by leaders like Edney. For years these arguments raged, often taken to extremes. And they had serious implications for how people managed their own drug use and who they saw as authentic user voices.

Indeed, throughout the history of harm reduction, people have tended to move between these camps—frequently as a result of changes in their own relationships to drugs. In my own case, in my early recovery, I was rigidly in favor of abstinence and the twelve steps, but supported needle exchange because "dead addicts don't recover." I saw harm reduction, basically, as a way to get to abstinence—just as Edith Springer, Yolanda Serrano, and most of the members of ADAPT had originally. Over time, however, I came to see that harm reduction was important whether or not it ever led to abstinence and that there was no reason to believe abstinence was best for everyone. But I still thought it might always be needed for some.

Fortunately, as the movement grew, many people who'd initially been on one extreme end or the other drifted toward the center. It became clear that respect for all pathways was needed—and that while some people can recover while still using occasionally or in a less harmful way, others very much did need to abstain from certain substances in order to have a life that they wanted to live. Representation of a variety of perspectives would be required.

Paul Cherashore, a heroin user who became one of the first employees of the Harm Reduction Coalition, offers critical insight on this issue. Like Edney, he was open about his drug experience from early on—and as in Edney's case, this didn't always serve him well.

Cherashore, who grew up in a middle-class home near Philadelphia, had gotten into heroin as a punk college dropout in San Francisco in the 1980s. He discovered harm reduction after moving to New York and first participating in and then working as a user organizer for the Lower East Side Needle Exchange. Thin, with dark hair and eyes, he brought intense passion to his work and, through it, was able to stabilize his drug use over time.

At the first two harm reduction conferences, however, he had to jump in at the last second to give a plenary talk. At least once, he replaced Edney. Cherashore used his second unexpected opportunity to discuss exactly why representing active users is so hard—and what harm reduction needs to do about it.

He began by joking about his repeat experience as an understudy. But his point was also serious: the fact is that being out in public as a drug user in the U.S., even within harm reduction, is something very few people are able or willing to do. He personally had spent at least thirteen years hiding his use. For him, he said, this had meant that he had to "fragment myself into private and public personas," in a far more extreme way than more privileged people can do when they move between spheres. At first, he felt that the only way he could be fully out was to put his drug use behind him. And so he became involved with twelve-step programs.

The experience of being out is quite different for those who identify as recovering addicts or former users, he explained. "It's okay to talk about your past use, especially when you're remorseful," he said. "People will forgive and forget the most horrible things that are over and done with. But the same person talking about those same activities in the present tense will get flayed alive. The active user who is not apologetic for his/her sins will not receive redemption."

Sadly, this reflects one of the drug war's most successful tactics, which is to shame active users into silence. Being unable to talk about such a critical part of their lives keeps people who use drugs from finding solidarity in shared human experience. "As we remain silent," Cherashore said, "we are isolated and alienated from each other and from ourselves. When we speak up, we see that we are not so different: that many others have common experiences and problems and have chosen similar methods of dealing with them, i.e., self-medication. By lifting that veil of secrecy, we feel better about the decisions we have made, and that in turn gives us additional strength to fight against oppressive drug policies and laws."[5]

Conveniently, staying quiet also allows drug warriors to frame users as liars—and to reinforce all types of other stereotypes because the people who could refute them are afraid that they will lose what stability and relationships they have if they do so. In fact, Cherashore lost at least one job and several friends when he began to talk about current use.

At the same time, however, being identified within harm reduction as an active user can also be something of a snare. "We are cultivated because as users we lend legitimacy to programs that crave just that," he said, "and we bring a point of view that is desperately needed, the 'privilege of experience.' The downside of such a relationship is that our contin-ued use is necessary to fulfill our part in the bargain." For obvious reasons, this is not always helpful for personal health and growth.

Cherashore's conclusion, however, was heartening. The issue is not fundamental to harm reduction itself, he explained. Instead, it results from the fact that users remain marginalized within it, valued primarily for their experience rather than for the wisdom and skills they gain as they do the work. The solution is to make lived experience a commonality, not a rarity—and value everyone not only for what they bring due to past and present experience, but for other gifts and skills as well.

One person's skill might be at managing—and, yes, she also uses drugs; while another brings artistic talents to the table. Someone else might be good at writing or outreach or mediation—and if all or most are also current users, that doesn't have to be the main or ongoing reason that they are valued. Former users also bring real value to the table.

"We need to create an environment where it doesn't matter whether you use or not, where we can go beyond the labels," Cherashore said.

sixteen

Undoing Tough Love

B Y 1999, Gretchen Burns Bergman was done. Her oldest son was struggling with heroin addiction—and she'd had it with Al-Anon, the twelve-step program for partners and family members of people with addictions. The mother of two was tired of being told she was "codependent." She'd had enough of hearing that her efforts to help were just "enabling" and that she needed to practice "tough love" so that he would "hit bottom" and recover. She was especially sick of the idea that she had no control over anything related to her son's addiction: how could it be true that she could make him worse by "enabling" but, at the same time, she was also "powerless" to make him better?

These contradictions infuriated the petite, blond dancer and dance instructor from Southern California. She had married a doctor and was successful in a series of ventures ranging from creating infant swimming programs to producing fashion shows. She had access to what was supposed to be excellent health care, and yet what she was seeing in the world of addiction treatment made little sense to her.

"I was realizing that I wasn't buying everything," she said, describing how she began to question Al-Anon. Bergman was especially distressed by its ubiquitous and apparently unquestioning support for using the criminal justice system to fight drugs. Although twelve-step groups are not supposed to have opinions on "outside issues" like public policy, at Al-Anon meetings, members would applaud and cheer when parents talked about having their children arrested or cutting off all contact with them—

events that she saw as reason for distress, not matters for celebration. If these parents genuinely believed that addiction was a disease, as Al-Anon claimed, why would social rejection and jail help?[1]

While harm reduction was beginning to spread more widely in the U.S. through Dan Bigg's naloxone work, Edith Springer's trainings, and the efforts of the Harm Reduction Coalition, parents like Bergman were beginning to come to many of the same conclusions about addiction and the drug war. This confluence of events would make harm reduction much more visible—and seriously threaten drug warriors, whose dominance had historically relied on strong support from parents. In the U.S., early harm reduction efforts like needle exchange had had very little input from parent activists—largely because such activism around drugs in the eighties and early nineties was focused on bolstering the drug war, not questioning it. And so moms like Bergman had virtually no political representation at all.

Bergman had seen her son worsen as the punishments imposed on him became more severe. An exceptional student, he was nonetheless kicked out of high school for smoking marijuana. When he was twenty, an arrest for cannabis possession only exacerbated his problems. Shortly thereafter, he had his first shot of heroin—not on the streets, but in a jail cell. Marijuana hadn't led him to heroin; the punishment intended to stop his drug use had. To make matters worse, incarceration and conviction also interfered with his ability to get work and, she felt, damaged his ideas about who he was and who he could be.

His drug use had started at thirteen. Since then, he'd gradually given up or been forced to give up all of his other interests, which included surfing, tennis, and his career goal of being a sportscaster. He struggled with depression and suicidal behavior. All of the policies seemingly aimed at changing his drug use instead just took away his alternatives to it, she realized.

Bergman had grown up in an upper-middle-class family on a sixty-five-acre avocado farm in Escondido, in Southern California. Unlike so many people who are ground down by the war on drugs, she was well-connected and empowered. And, as a white suburban mom, she wasn't used to being told that she just had to accept whatever the judicial and health care systems wanted to do to her child. She didn't have to contend with systemic racism or issues around "respectability" that Black mothers in the same situation faced. Her resources gave her an enormous advantage.

"I knew that my son was a good person," she said. "I knew that the criminal justice system was mishandling it and that was destroying families." And yet at every Al-Anon meeting she attended, she felt she was being told that there was no other way. "The whole idea of the Serenity Prayer was to have the strength to accept the fact that my child had a substance use disorder, which is not what they called it then," she said, pointedly avoiding the stigmatizing phrasing of "my son was an addict."

At first, she asked herself all the questions society poses: What did we do wrong? What's wrong with him? Why can't he just stop? But ultimately, she just couldn't accept what she was being told. "I had the strong sense that my maternal instincts were being disrespected and ignored," she said. "I felt like I knew my son. I loved my son. I didn't believe that love was a bad thing."

The codependence model, however, which Al-Anon supported, taught otherwise. From this perspective, trying to help and being kind to your addicted child was not good parenting; it meant that you, too, had a disease. And this disease, codependence, was seen as a genuine mental illness in which people use someone else's addiction and their own attempts to control that person as a way to distract themselves from their own serious emotional problems.

The concept turns normal human interdependence on its head. Your desire to nurture your child isn't love—it's twisted and selfish. You aren't really trying to help; you are getting a high from attempting to control your child, in this view. The idea is that "codependents" are addicted to drama and so they unconsciously strive to keep their loved ones sick in order to dodge their own issues. The result is that, in stark contrast with other illnesses where parental support is seen as admirable and those who *don't* provide it to their kids are suspect, with addiction the opposite is the case. Parents are applauded for throwing their addicted children out on the street—and actually shamed for being supportive.

Bergman wasn't going to accept it anymore. If addiction is a disease, why would loving care be contraindicated, unlike with literally all other mental and physical illness? When her younger son also became addicted to heroin, the more she thought about the advice she'd been given, the angrier it made her. "I think that's sort of my tenacity and my stubborn streak, which maybe has served me poorly and well at the same time," she said. "I think if you can look inside yourself and say, 'Hey, wait a minute, am I a good person? Am I really doing the right thing? Is this self-serving? Or is this really because I love my children?' And then that's what gave me the power to speak out."

She began to think about the second part of the Serenity Prayer, which asks for "the courage to change the things we can." After one Al-Anon meeting, she cautiously revealed her concerns to a few other members, whom she suspected might be simpatico. "I had already tried everything that people told me to try," she said. Soon, she found out that she was far from alone in her frustration.

Like her, other Al-Anon members were starting to question whether tough love and incarceration were the right answers. Like Bergman, they'd previously questioned their own sanity and whether they were just "in denial" of their codependence—or whether the whole idea was simply wrong and the people at the meetings were the ones who weren't facing reality. The drug war was supposed to be protecting their children—but what if it was really making their problems worse?

With those who agreed, Bergman founded a group called A New PATH, or Parents for Addiction Treatment and Healing. "I tried to totally debunk the whole codependent model because it's not based on science or anything else," she said. Indeed, research shows that codependence is not a reliable concept; it is not an accepted psychiatric diagnosis, let alone a diagnosable brain disorder.[2] Though parents, children, and partners can and often do have dysfunctional relationships with people with addiction, this is far from the only way to have an abusive, controlling, or harmful love. Bad relationships with people with addiction are as varied as bad relationships with anyone else. The notion of codependence serves only to sustain addiction stigma by adding stigma by association to friends and family.

As Bergman began organizing events and giving lectures, she found that simply speaking publicly about being a mother whose child was both addicted and in the criminal justice system helped free others to get involved. "I feel like I gave permission to so many parents to start speaking out, because they were in the closet with the shame of it," she said, describing how sharing this experience helped them start to question why addiction was treated so differently from other conditions.

That, in turn, helped many decide to take political action, which would result in a surprising victory. That triumph showed just how disillusioned most people were becoming with the drug war. Independently at first, and then in collaboration with other harm reductionists, she began to mobilize parents.

BY 1999, WHEN BERGMAN BECAME AN ACTIVIST, THE RAW FERVOR OF THE drug war was finally starting to die down. Reporters and politicians had begun to grow tired of constantly banging the drum for ever greater crackdowns: the headlines were now about Bill Clinton and Monica Lewinsky and the resulting impeachment scandal, not the horrors of crack. As early as 1995, Walter Cronkite—long considered the "most trusted man in America" as he anchored the *CBS Evening News* for decades—compared the failure of the drug war to the failure of alcohol prohibition. Cronkite was notably the reporter whose shift of position on the Vietnam war caused President Lyndon Johnson to say, "If I've lost Cronkite, I've lost Middle America."

At this point, too, American drug incarceration rates were in the midst of an exponential rise, going from around 19,000 inmates in 1980 to over 237,000 by 1998. And these numbers don't even count the many thousands more who were incarcerated for crimes associated with the high price of drug use under prohibition. Annual federal drug war spending (overwhelmingly on law enforcement) skyrocketed in tandem, rising from around $437 million in the late 1970s to more than $17 billion in 1999. State drug law enforcement spending increased in a similarly explosive way, costing billions. Nothing else in the domestic budget had been given this sort of blank check. By 2010, a stunning trillion—that's 1,000,000,000,000 or 10^{12}—had been spent.[3]

Needless to say, despite all of this, drugs had not gone away. By 1998, more high school seniors were reporting that cocaine and heroin were easy to get than at any time since national survey data were first collected in 1975. Drug-related deaths (mainly overdose) had doubled between 1979 and 1998—long before any attention was being paid to an "overdose crisis."[4]

Moreover, it wasn't like Al-Anon or other twelve-step groups were short of potential members with illegal drug issues—and certainly, none of Bergman's or her fellow parents' kids seemed to have any difficulty getting the substances they wanted. In contrast, it was almost impossible for them to find effective, affordable treatment and good information about what genuinely worked. Parents became enraged.

Their discontent helped fuel the drug policy reform movement. This movement had begun to grow slowly, starting with the founding of the Drug Policy Foundation in 1986 by Arnold Trebach and Kevin Zeese (who later became a member of the Harm Reduction Working Group). But its real momentum into the mainstream began in 1994, when billionaire George Soros became committed to the cause.

That year, Princeton politics professor Ethan Nadelmann convinced Soros that the American drug war was a serious threat to his ideals of an open, democratic society. Courts and politicians had for years carved out what Supreme Court justice Thurgood Marshall derided as a "drug exception to the Constitution," allowing violations of privacy, liberty, free speech, property, and civil rights that had previously been rejected as un-American. As a Holocaust survivor, Soros was concerned about erosion of these crucial aspects of democracy. His philanthropy was aimed at preserving what he called "open societies" around the world.[5] And so he listened to the Harvard-educated Princeton professor.

With Nadelmann's encouragement, Soros began funding the Drug Policy Foundation (DPF). He also created a new drug policy think tank—and Nadelmann left Princeton to run it.[6] Soros would soon be a major financial supporter of harm reduction, including HRC, in the U.S. and internationally. Both HRC and DPF recognized that voters were ripe to question the continual escalation of the drug war—even as politicians remained terrified of any measure that might get them labeled "soft on crime." They would work together for change.

To get around politicians' fears and try to show them that the public was ready for new thinking, DPF began to create and support state ballot initiatives. They started with easier and more popular ideas like medical marijuana and moderate shifts away from the drug war more generally, such as sending people who got arrested to treatment rather than jail. They worked with allies like groups already pushing for marijuana reform. The year 1996 was the turning point: California voters legalized medical marijuana and Arizona began to go even further.

In Arizona, DPF had organized a campaign for a state ballot initiative, which would both legalize medical marijuana and provide for "treatment, not punishment" for people arrested for any kind of drugs. Instead of incarceration, Proposition 200 mandated probation and treatment for the first three drug offenses, with some exceptions. It also guaranteed a parole hearing to give nonviolent drug offenders serving long mandatory sentences an opportunity for release. But, bowing to the get-tough climate of the times, the initiative also mandated that violent prisoners serve 100 percent of their sentences.

Gathering an unlikely coalition of liberals (who wanted compassion for addiction), libertarians (who ultimately wanted legalization), and fiscal conservatives (who wanted to spend less on something that clearly wasn't working), DPF hired people on the ground to organize, collect signatures, and do the work needed to get the initiative onto the ballot. A local billionaire, the founder of the for-profit University of Phoenix, led the fight. In the months leading up to the November 1996 election, the campaign ran hard-hitting TV ads, one featuring a former senator who was also an ex-prosecutor, another spotlighting a retired cop. In the ads, these law enforcement experts discussed their experience of the failure of the drug war and expressed concern for their children should this disastrous policy continue.[7]

Politicians across the board expressed universal horror. One state representative said it sent the message, "Do drugs, so what?"[8] In possible violation of the federal law that prevents administration members from engaging in state politics, Clinton drug czar Barry McCaffrey actively campaigned against it. A retired four-star general with no medical or public health expertise, he called the initiative "a stalking horse for legalization" and "cunning public policy manipulation."[9]

But despite his efforts, Prop 200 passed overwhelmingly. The margin was two to one. This victory was the first real proof that the drug war was not as popular as it had seemed.

DURING THESE SAME YEARS IN THE NINETIES, ANOTHER CRITICAL FORCE WAS also starting to have a real impact: the internet. Google had been founded in 1998. By that year, 41 percent of American adults were already online.[10] And, of particular relevance here, the very earliest internet users—some of whom had been dialing up as far back as the 1980s—were primarily a mix of libertarians, academics, geeks, and Grateful Dead fans, with significant overlap among those categories. Many saw themselves as outsiders. Few were fans of drug prohibition, to put it mildly.

I got online in 1990, before the World Wide Web and browsers even existed, dialing up to a text-only "bulletin board" discussion group founded by a friend. In fact, much of my own harm reduction education came via an email listserv, which was intended to be an "academic and scholarly" discussion of addiction. Founded in 1995, the list known as "addict-l" became instead an online brawl. Counselors and others, who like me were steeped in twelve-step-based treatment programs, joined. We thought we were highly educated about the nature of addiction because of what we'd been taught by one another. But we were not.

Often for the first time, we were confronted by leading researchers in the field, who had data that pretty much contradicted every single thing we thought we knew. When I joined this list, I already supported harm reduction. However, I didn't realize just how much misinformation I'd imbibed, at meetings, from the media, on the street, and during treatment. Myths about drugs are part of our education, our mainstream press and entertainment, our politics, our arts and literature, and our medical system. Part of the reason this is so hard to change is that it means that many people don't know what they don't know. Journalists, for example, frequently do not check "conventional wisdom" because it's been repeated so often that they don't think it needs checking. On addict-l, we were forced to check.

Over time, this meant that I became acquainted with most of the important research in the field. Not infrequently, I changed my position after being flamed and battered over the head with conflicting data. No one could survive for long on addict-l without having to think carefully about pretty much every assumption they'd ever made about drugs and addiction. If you couldn't back your argument with data, you would be certain to be humiliated (not that I recommend this as a teaching tool). It was quite an education—and was especially useful for being extremely cross-disciplinary and including many people with real-world experience of addiction and treatment. Sociology, criminology, psychology, psychiatry, epidemiology, and history were all represented. This meant that we had to learn about methods across different disciplines, too.

Critically, the early arrival of scholars, harm reductionists, and other drug policy reformers online provided a significant advantage when new-fangled "blogs" and other internet publications began to threaten the mainstream media. The networks, newsmagazines, and newspapers had had near-monopoly control over drug-related information for most of the twentieth century. When that began to change, simply by getting there first, drug war critics dominated online dialogue about substance use. They led this conversation long before many establishment drug war supporters had even heard of the net. For example, websites like Erowid that provided both user-informed and scientific information on drugs had been up and running for several years with thousands of views per day before the drug czar's office even had a website.[11]

Further, unlike what is now called legacy media, blogs, email lists, and other internet discussion groups tended to share a culture of backing up their arguments with data. The beauty of the internet, after all, is its ability to connect people and all types of information previously hidden away in libraries and universities. No one needed to worry about limited space and word counts—that's why there were links.

This meant that from the start these conversations and publications frequently provided direct access to previously obscure scholarly articles and medical research. Sometimes, the papers' authors would answer questions by email, often flattered to see that new people outside their tiny field were reading their work. And, of course, much of the data and analysis in academic scholarship directly contradicted drug war truisms. Previously, drug warriors rarely had to face strong opposition, never mind fierce opponents armed with data to support their claims. Nor had they been required to provide citations to back up their own statements to the press. Now it was different.

Drug prohibition, it turns out, relies heavily on monopolizing the media. Its claims don't hold up well when people can easily obtain a full range of alternative perspectives, often straight from scholarly sources, with full citations and methods. With its empirical base, harm reduction, for once, held the advantage.

IN OCTOBER 1999, SHORTLY AFTER FOUNDING HER PARENTS' GROUP, Gretchen Burns Bergman published an op-ed in the *Los Angeles Times*. It described her older son's counterproductive experiences with the criminal prosecution system and argued for treatment, not punishment. After reading it, the Drug Policy Foundation contacted her. The group was working on a California version of Arizona's reform initiative. Introduced as Proposition 36, the new law would require that drug possession offenders be given at least three chances at treatment before jail or prison could even be considered. It would also provide significant funding for that treatment.

The group wanted to know if she'd consider joining them. Soon Bergman had agreed to become the state chair for the initiative, essentially its key spokesperson. This was an inspired choice: since the war on drugs was supposedly being fought to protect children, having a mother argue that it did more harm than good was an especially potent way to undermine those claims.

Women—and mothers in particular—are a critical and often-overlooked constituency when it comes to drug policy. Their fears about their children have often been exploited to pass and strengthen drug prohibitions. Consequently, undoing such laws also requires their mobilization or at least assuaging their concerns.

In fact, the only major prohibition that the U.S. has completely over-turned so far is that of alcohol, which was driven both to passage and to repudiation mainly by women. In the early twentieth century, many newly enfranchised and progressive female voters believed that banning alcohol would protect families. Men would no longer be able to drink up their paychecks. They'd no longer become violent when disinhibited by booze. Crime and domestic abuse would virtually disappear, Prohibitionists ar-gued. Anti-Black racism and anti-immigrant animus also played a big role in the Prohibition movement—many of its most enthusiastic supporters were members of the KKK, as noted earlier. But women, both racist and otherwise, strongly favored the policy, at least at first.

Once they began to see how it played out, however, many of the same women began to have second thoughts. As Bergman later wrote, "[I]t was also women who were instrumental in repealing Prohibition because this 'noble experiment' had failed. Millions of women came to oppose Prohibi-tion because it was corrupting morals, eroding liberties, creating violence, destroying lives, and endangering their children." She described seeing a 1920s poster of an idealized mother holding her child, captioned, "Prohi-bition Failed! Please do something about it."[12]

Critically, the current iteration of the war on drugs was also initially powered by angry mothers. Before these moms raised the alarm, there had been a trend toward liberalizing policy, which was borne by the re-bellious sixties into the mid-1970s. The "Parent Movement" put a stop to that. These proud drug warriors first organized in Atlanta in 1976. A previously liberal woman who went by the name of Keith Schuchard had discovered open marijuana smoking at her daughter's thirteenth birthday party. Horrified by what she saw as the drug-driven change in her teen's behavior, she decided that tolerance had gone too far.

By 1980, Schuchard and other moms had helped organize some 300 parent groups in thirty-four states. Earlier, in 1977, President Jimmy Carter had spoken out in favor of national decriminalization of cannabis. But he soon dropped the idea, in part due to a drug scandal involving an aide—and in part due to the growing outcry from parents. His successor, of course, sided completely with the anti-drug mothers. Then, buoyed by

First Lady Nancy Reagan's soon-ubiquitous "Just Say No" campaign—and President Reagan's own passion for tougher policies—these parents supported more and more draconian measures.

Most of them, however, were personally focused on prevention. Few had real experience with or knowledge of what it's like to live with illegal drug addiction. Since they were overwhelmingly white and middle class, their own children rarely had any significant negative encounters with law enforcement. In fact, the one major Black leader involved in the Parent Movement—who had promoted the "Just Say No" slogan long before Nancy Reagan did—was expelled from her own organization after the first lady picked up the idea and sought to commercialize it.[13] Essentially, these privileged parents seemed to want policing to deter their kids before they ever tried drugs—by making examples of others.

But at least one set of parents who shaped the movement did have actual drug experience, both personal and with their own children. That was a couple named Phyllis and David York. Although Phyllis herself had gone so far as to try heroin, she saw her youthful experiments as spiritual exploration. Kids today, she said, were just selfish.

In 1977, the Yorks organized a group for parents who wanted to "take a stand" against their rebellious drug-using teens. Called ToughLove, it would have an enormous impact on both addiction treatment and self-help for many decades. By 1981, it had 250 chapters in North America and had been featured in *People* magazine. That same year, ToughLove was endorsed by beloved advice columnist Ann Landers.[14]

In their 1982 bestseller by the same name, the Yorks claimed that, just by laying down the law, they had solved their daughter's addiction. Being nice hadn't helped; what worked, they argued, was letting her sit in jail and refusing to have anything to do with her until she quit. The book and related support groups similarly advocated expelling drug-using teens from the family and having them arrested when possible. They soon flooded Al-Anon with parents who saw these harsh tactics as the only way to stop "enabling." Before long, parents who *refused* to practice tough love were seen as exceptional and problematic—not parents who followed their usual instincts to be supportive.

By the time that Bergman began to question these ideas in 1999, all of them had congealed into conventional wisdom. Tough love had become popular despite the fact that it had never been studied scientifically and despite its clear potential to do harm to both family relationships and to abandoned children themselves. It was based on a single anecdotal story. Nonetheless, through the concept of tough love, the ideology of the drug war had come to completely dominate not just the criminal prosecution system, but also the treatment system, with its tight connection to twelve-step groups. A punitive mindset now fully permeated every institution and system intended to help people with addiction.

Like the anti-Prohibition mothers before her, Bergman knew that she and the other parents who were increasingly joining her were engaged in a fight for the lives of their children. The drug war was doing more harm than good—and it was more important to reduce harm than to seek some ideal of a drug-free America. That's why she was so excited about leading the charge for California's Proposition 36.

AS WITH ARIZONA'S INITIATIVE TO TRY TREATMENT BEFORE PUNISHMENT, THE opposition from drug warriors was intense. After all, California was the nation's biggest state, and trends that start there notoriously tend to spread nationwide. Proposition 36 had to be defeated to ensure that no one would get the crazy idea that any lenience whatsoever was acceptable in the drug war.

And once again, drug czar McCaffrey, probably illegally, led the charge. He claimed that the proposition was part of a legalization agenda. He argued that treatment couldn't work without the threat of incarceration. He was joined by many supporters of twelve-step-based treatment, including actor Martin Sheen, who was working for the anti-reform cause with the Betty Ford Center. These opponents were so stuck in drug war thinking that they couldn't imagine any way to get people to seek treatment that didn't involve the police.

This was, it must be noted, a very peculiar form of logic for people who supposedly supported treating addiction as a disease. Here was the Betty

Ford Center—at the time, the nation's pre-eminent rehab for alcohol and other drug addiction—opposing putting treatment ahead of punishment. By doing so, it was seemingly rejecting its own mission. The center was also apparently ignoring its own financial interests, which would clearly be bolstered by increased treatment funding. Nonetheless, in an op-ed for the *Los Angeles Times*, Sheen wrote that in order for people to get into recovery, they needed the "consequences and accountability" of the threat of a jail or prison sentence.[15]

This, too, did not make sense. The rehab's namesake, the former first lady, had struggled with alcohol. But she had become sober without facing jail time, as had the founders of AA, which was the basis for the Betty Ford Center's program. Sheen seemed to believe that coerced treatment was essential to his son Charlie's recovery (a fact later belied by his repeated relapses). However, he had no way to explain why so many others did just fine without legal pressure. The argument was absurd on its face. Blind allegiance to the drug war completely subsumed any pretense that addiction was a medical rather than moral problem.

"I would have loved to have had an audience with him. Just to try to convince him, parent to parent, what are you talking about?" Bergman said. She didn't get the chance. But she was able to debunk his claims in the press, especially noting Sheen's apparent disregard for the lack of treatment opportunities among people who didn't have his advantages and his failure to consider the harms associated with incarceration and having a criminal record.

On November 7, 2000, Republican George W. Bush lost the popular vote to Democrat Al Gore, while winning the electoral college. But in California, Proposition 36 won by an indisputable margin, without any need for an asterisk. It received the support of 61 percent of voters.[16]

The initiative ended a period in which the number of people incarcerated in California's state prisons for drug possession had quadrupled in twelve years. It cut that sector of the prison population by about a third almost immediately after taking effect. And, in the seven years that it was fully funded, it saved the state some $2 billion, while 84,000 people completed treatment. Around half of those who received treatment via the initiative had never previously received help. Though funding was cut starting in 2007, since its implementation the number of state drug prisoners in California has fallen by 55 percent.[17]

AT THE SAME TIME THAT BERGMAN WAS STRUGGLING WITH HER RELATIONSHIP to Al-Anon and the idea of codependence, the harm reduction movement was facing a peculiar challenge. Drug warriors had launched an attack on the phrase itself, as it gained ground internationally in the early nineties. They claimed that it was, like Arizona and California's state initiatives, a stalking horse for legalization. They weren't totally wrong: certainly, some of the same people who supported harm reduction also supported legalization, though many did not. But the fact that drug warriors immediately saw the phrase itself as a mortal threat spoke volumes.

After all, if the drug war was working, the concept of harm reduction should be innocuous: an effective policy, pretty much by definition, will prevent more harm than it causes. Advocates for a failing policy, however, *should* be concerned by the idea of focusing on harm first and foremost. If prohibition was helping, an alternative called "harm reduction" wouldn't be needed. And they knew it.

This reasoning meant that the spread of the term—and not just the movement—terrified drug warriors. As the evidence favoring harm reduction began to increase, proponents of punitive policy became increasingly shrill. Even on its own terms, the drug war hadn't ended drug use or reduced addiction or overdose. But it had certainly racked up massive costs and fueled an enormous rise in incarceration rates.

If the drug war was to be judged on its capacity to reduce harm, rather than on the number of arrests or drug seizures, it would almost certainly have to be declared lost. And if the racism at the core of the drug laws became widely understood, the moral position of drug warriors would shift from being seen as on the side of all that is good and pure to being seen as, at the very least, accidentally abetting evil. The power of harm reduction was in flipping this script, in undoing the idea of drug use as the ultimate immorality and simply providing a better goal. That made it terrifying.

Rather than face the facts, however, prohibition supporters tried to suppress them. For example, in 1998, Clinton's Health and Human Services (HHS) secretary was preparing to lift the ban on federal funding for syringe exchange. The original legislation had included a provision that said that the policy could end if the president's HHS secretary declared that the data showed that needle exchange prevented HIV without increasing drug use. A campaign to get Clinton to end the ban was led by the Harm Reduction Coalition.

By that point, the data did indeed show beyond doubt that needle exchange was both safe and effective. Essentially every expert committee that ever examined the research objectively came down in favor of it, from the Institute of Medicine (now the National Academy of Medicine) to the Centers for Disease Control, the World Health Organization, the National Commission on AIDS, the National Institutes of Health, and the American Medical Association.[18]

But here, drug czar McCaffrey was unfortunately effective in stopping reform. He got to Clinton on Air Force One on a trip to Latin America. He claimed, falsely, that he was the only person who had read "all three studies" of syringe exchange—which would likely come as a shock to the experts who not only had conducted many dozens of studies, but read and compiled extensive reports on them and found the opposite of his "review."[19]

According to Clinton, McCaffrey also insisted that, politically, allowing the funding of needle exchange would harm Democrats. The president caved. Years later, in 2002, he said that yielding to McCaffrey was one of the policy decisions that he most regretted. At the very minimum, it had costs hundreds, if not thousands of lives: a 1997 study showed that earlier expansion of syringe exchange could have reduced the number of AIDS cases by 15 to 33 percent, preventing up to 10,000 infections.[20]

Notably, the attempt to suppress harm reduction wasn't just localized to the United States. The U.S. had always been a bully in both the initial creation of the international drug control regime of the United Nations and in maintaining support for it. One reason for this long-term dedication was that drug control was one of the few issues on which the U.S. and the Soviet Union could agree, which made it useful throughout the Cold War.

Nonetheless, in much of the rest of the developed world, harm reduction had caught on quite quickly, at first largely driven by concern about
HIV. By 2000, twenty-eight European countries had government-approved
syringe exchanges, with all of them expanding access to methadone as
well.[21] The U.K. continued with its ongoing heroin prescribing, with Switzerland starting a pilot program in 1994 and the Netherlands in 1998.[22]
As the Liverpool group spread the word—with the internet amplifying its
messaging—the broader philosophy began to take off as well. All of this
stirred up a massive reaction.

Because it was seen as such a threat to the world consensus on prohibition, American drug warriors fought hard against harm reduction. They
sought to preserve and bolster the treaties that are the foundation of the
drug war. They tried to ensure that countries would not experiment with
policies like marijuana legalization, by insisting that they were illegal under this body of international law. These groups regularly used threats from
the U.S. state department to get all types of liberalizing policies stopped.
And they had some big victories, at first.

In fact, after Liverpool's Allan Parry and John Marks appeared on
60 Minutes touting heroin prescribing and needle exchange in late December in 1992, their city immediately received greater scrutiny from the
Thatcher government. By 1995, Marks had stopped prescribing. Many of
his patients died shortly thereafter, though some were picked up by the
rare doctors who would agree to continue their prescriptions.[23] At various times, pressure was also applied successfully to stop both Jamaica
and Mexico from decriminalizing cannabis possession within their own
borders.

Within the bureaucracy of the United Nations, American drug warriors, often with the support of Russia, spent much of the 1990s trying to
keep the phrase "harm reduction" out of documents, unless the goal was
to disparage or ban it. Attendees at meetings spent long days negotiating
about the minutiae of language in various guidelines and public statements, often only to be frustrated at the last minute by rigid American
demands related to the concept. "There was a charade for years in which
the U.S. fought against using the term 'harm reduction' and went after

other countries for doing so," said Sanho Tree, director of the Drug Policy Project at the Institute for Policy Studies.[24]

But the late nineties and early 2000s would also see the start of a slow turn away from the excesses of the drug war, led by moms like Gretchen Burns Bergman whose children had been harmed by them. Initiatives like those passed in Arizona and California at this time can seem reactionary to harm reductionists today, with their continued acquiescence to the lead role of the criminal prosecution system in drug policy. At the time, however, even speaking out as a mother opposed to the drug war—especially as one whose own child had been incarcerated—was rare and brave. Genuinely winning concessions against ever more punitive policy, as she'd done with California's drug treatment initiative, was even less common. "A big form of harm reduction is keeping people out of jail, because jail is really harmful," Bergman explained.

Unfortunately, for people who use drugs—particularly opioids, even medically—the situation was about to get worse before it got better.

seventeen

Undoing Pain Care

O N A CLEAR BUT CHILLY SPRING DAY IN 2005, AROUND TWO DOZEN PEOPLE gathered at a social club in the lakeside city of Erie, Pennsylvania. They were not there to celebrate, conduct business, or raise money; they had come together to speak to the press about their doctor, who had been arrested for illegally prescribing opioids.

"I have no quality of life," one man said. At age forty, he added, "I'm either on the couch or the recliner." A thirty-six-year-old woman spoke of having attempted suicide, while others lamented their loss of ability to care for their families or work.

Typically, media coverage of such cases overwhelmingly favors law enforcement officials. Federal and state prosecutors give lurid, if clichéd, quotes, labeling accused doctors as "pushers with a pen" and accusing them of operating "pill mills." One of the more florid described a defendant as "no better than a street corner crack dealer" who "dispenses misery and death."[1] Typically, patient press conferences regarding the prosecution of doctors are arranged by prosecutors. Generally, they feature people who claim that physicians caused their devastating addictions—as well as those who have lost loved ones to overdoses linked to their prescriptions. Rarely mentioned is the fact that some of the speakers have a hidden agenda: if the addicted patients decry their former doctors, criminal charges against them may be dropped or reduced.

In this particular case, the prosecution had portrayed Dr. Paul Heberle's practice as a "drive-through" for prescriptions. They alleged that he distributed "powerful and addictive prescription medication to patients for no valid medical reason." In their press release, they also included a mock-up "wanted" style poster, with a picture of the accused, unshaven and smiling, wearing sunglasses and the words "Overprescribing Controlled Substances" and "Medicaid Fraud" in bold letters beside it.[2]

But the patients gathered at the Siebenbuerger Club on May 3, 2005, had a very different mission. They were there to support Heberle—not blame him for their plight. From their perspective, it was law enforcement who had done wrong. Their disability and lost quality of life was not due to addiction to opioids—it was because those medications had been cut off. Now they wanted to tell their side of the story.

Unfortunately, such voices were rarely heard as coverage of Oxy-Contin, "accidental addicts," and a ceaseless rise in prescription drug overdoses began to dominate the media in the early 2000s. In the media, it was common to see articles on the issue quote only addiction experts and people who'd had problems with prescription opioids. In contrast, pain patients and their doctors were silenced or relegated to competing with the trolls in the comments.

Siobhan Reynolds, who had organized the press conference, wanted to change that. Like Gretchen Burns Bergman, she was a mom who'd been radicalized by the harm done to her family by the war on drugs. In her case, however, that harm didn't involve addiction—but instead, misguided and misinformed fears about it. A legal crackdown on doctors driven by such concerns was causing harm to patients who were being denied appropriate pain relief. Reynolds knew that if the patients she organized could be heard, prosecutors would have a much harder time justifying their crusade against doctors.

Shockingly, many of the patients who spoke out in Erie—a small, working-class town on Lake Erie in Pennsylvania—were not facing or experiencing withdrawal and loss of access to their pain medication due to an arrest of their doctor for the first time. Heberle had been the only one willing to take on patients of another local physician who had previously been targeted for his prescribing of pain medication. Now that doc was in prison, serving thirteen to twenty-nine years.[3] And the prosecutors wanted Heberle to face the same fate.

Inside the social club, one woman described being turned down by no fewer than thirty-seven other doctors after she told them the name of her former prescriber. The physician who was now accused was the only one who'd agreed to try to help. These patient stories were strikingly similar: each had a litany of complex chronic pain issues, ranging from back pain to pain from lung surgery gone wrong to pain from disfiguring car accidents and on-the-job injuries. Each had been through multiple treatments, surgeries, injections, and alternative treatments, and all had tried many different types of medication. None had a history of addiction.

However, opioids were the only thing that helped their pain. One patient described how when he had access to an appropriate dose, he could coach his son's baseball team and do housework and yard work—but now he was restricted to his bed or the sofa. The woman who'd attempted suicide had done so not because she felt like she was hopelessly addicted—but because she'd lost access to the only drugs that touched her pain. Reynolds put it this way: "This is a battle for the hearts and minds of the public. We want to shine some light on this matter now, not when the doctor gets to court and his fate is sealed."[4]

With dark blond hair, big blue eyes, and the implacability of a lioness protecting her cub, Reynolds was hard to ignore. She foresaw the disaster that awaited both pain patients and people with addiction as media attention on OxyContin and overdose led to sharp cuts in the medical opioid supply. Her activism brought important new thinking into harm reduction, by helping to clarify how the drug war turns doctors into cops who harm both pain patients and people with addiction—and how a false narrative about the causes of the overdose crisis was promoted and continues to do harm.

Politicians and many others at the time thought that simply cracking down on prescribing would solve the overdose crisis. But harm reductionists saw right away that this would only increase damage all around. They knew from both data and experience that if a policy just stops opioid maintenance for addiction or opioid treatment of pain—without providing effective and available alternatives—more people become disabled and more die. Pain and addiction don't go away just because you take away people's medications. In fact, typically, driving people from a medical source of drugs to a street source increases overdose and suicide, rather than preventing addiction or reducing fatalities. Unfortunately, these warnings went unheard. But the Cassandra-like accuracy of harm reductionists would ultimately elevate the movement as their dire predictions came true.

"The question, is, Where are we going to go? What kind of a country are we going to be? Are we going to have law enforcement deciding who does and does not get pain care? Are we going to be having law enforcement punishing physicians—which is what we have now—for not being good law enforcement officers? Or are we going to be a free country?" Reynolds asked rhetorically at a Congressional briefing she'd arranged in 2004, to bring attention to these issues. Her work often involved connecting journalists and politicians with pain patients and their doctors whose stories were not being heard—but who were suffering at least as much as addicted people under the lash of the drug war.

Reynolds was a cousin of the Kennedys—and her life unfortunately adhered to their public narrative of wealth, public service, and tragedy. Her father had been a Los Angeles defense attorney, who had served as one of Robert F. Kennedy's groomsmen at his wedding. As a public defender, he was later randomly assigned to defend RFK's assassin, Sirhan Sirhan, but recused himself.

Reynolds herself started but did not complete law school. However, she brought a fine legal mind to her activism, which involved the law as it relates to prescription opioids. As the Drug Enforcement Administration and state prosecutors began to target and arrest physicians who prescribed OxyContin, she recognized the way that the drug war set doctors, pain patients, and people with addiction against one another. She devoted the rest of her life to trying to improve care for patients and provide a legal safe haven for their doctors.

Reynolds was moved to this type of activism for deeply personal reasons. Her husband, Sean Greenwood, had severe chronic pain. Eventually, the couple learned that it was caused by a rare congenital connective tissue disorder. Because this condition makes the joints flexible in ways that they should not be, it constantly causes injuries that produce many types of pain. Greenwood was only diagnosed after decades of agony, because

their son was found to have the same disorder, which is genetic. And once
Reynolds knew that her child was at risk for the suffering that had disabled
his father, she became determined to ensure that he would not have to
struggle to get relief.

Greenwood was a large man who had been in severe pain for many
years. Both of these factors—physical size and the length of time pain
has gone without successful treatment—as well as various metabolic and
genetic variations can affect the way opioids work. Unfortunately for him,
only very large doses of opioids could successfully tame the intractable
pain his condition caused. When he was appropriately medicated, he
could function and help raise his son; when he was not, he was incapaci-
tated and unable to get out of bed. But as the overdose numbers rose and
media attention to OxyContin grew, doctors became increasingly afraid to
prescribe what patients like Greenwood needed.

REYNOLDS WATCHED AS THE MEDIA CREATED A FALSE NARRATIVE ABOUT THE
causes of what it first labeled the "OxyContin epidemic." She saw how
almost no attention was given to pain patients—except when they were
seen as having been "turned into accidental addicts" by doctors. She saw
a nice, neat story being told that completely excluded critical facts—and
pushed legal crackdowns and monitoring of doctors and prescriptions as
the best way to solve the problem. She saw how patients like her husband
were either defined as already addicted and denied care as a result—or
denied help because they might instead one day get hooked, regardless of
what worked to fight their pain. "At the beginning, it was sort of a press
campaign, this Oxy hysteria," she said.[5]

There is a great deal of misinformation about the real roots of the overdose crisis—and it needs to be clarified in order to shed light on the rise
of harm reduction. In addition, this story is yet another example of how
racism shapes drug policy in the U.S.—and how the desire to see white
users as innocent while Black people are viewed as criminals warps our
response.

The most well-known version of the overdose tale begins in 1996.
That year, Purdue Pharma took advantage of recently relaxed FDA over-

sight to heavily promote its new product, OxyContin, to doctors for the treatment of chronic pain. The drug itself wasn't actually new: OxyContin was simply a reformulation of the opioid oxycodone that made its effects last longer. Still, in 1996 alone, Purdue sold $48 million worth of Oxy—and by 2000, annual sales had reached $1.1 billion.[6] However, as early as 2001, there were clear signs of trouble. OxyContin began to be tagged with the offensive term "hillbilly heroin" with media reports spotlighting increasing rates of addiction and overdose death in Appalachia.[7] Unlike in the crack epidemic, however, this time the people who got addicted would largely be seen as victims, not perpetrators—and the drug companies and doctors would get most of the blame.

Here's how that happened. First, Purdue exploited a community of well-intentioned patient advocates and doctors, who had long argued that pain was significantly undertreated. This was true: research showed that even with end-stage cancer, a person's odds of receiving adequate pain relief were only around fifty-fifty in the nineties and 2000s.[8] Care for intractable, chronic pain that wasn't associated with the end of life was even worse. And this data remains undisputed. At least in this way, Purdue did not distort the facts.

But as advocates made their case for better end-of-life care, chronic pain patients and their doctors began to argue for greater relief, too. They began to wonder why, if it was okay to have opioid pain relief for cancer when you were at death's door, it wasn't acceptable to have it if your equally severe suffering would last decades.

Here, Purdue stepped in, saying that the chronic pain patients were asking the right question—and there really was no reason not to reduce their suffering, preferably with a long-term prescription of brand-name OxyContin. Their marketing included amplifying some of these patient voices and exaggerating the number of patients who could be helped by opioids. It also included active selling to doctors, with quotas for salespeople to hit to get bonuses if they increased prescribing, which, bizarrely, is legal. Purdue and other drug companies funded nearly every pain group and advocate in the field—with the exception of Siobhan Reynolds.

The result was this: between 1999 and 2010, the number of opioids prescribed per capita more than quadrupled, while related overdose deaths tripled. In 1999, roughly 5,000 deaths were linked to prescription opioids each year. By 2010, however, there were some 15,000 such deaths.[9] The media told this story as a simple morality tale, in which evil pharma had led complacent or greedy doctors to hook innocent patients on a deadly and devilish drug.

But that account fails to encompass many inconvenient facts. For one, the majority of the Americans who died of overdose did not become addicted during treatment for pain. And conversely, the majority of people treated with opioids for pain, even long-term, do not ever develop addiction. While media reports frequently state that opioids do not work at all for chronic pain, this contention, too, is as unsupported by data as the exaggerated drug company marketing material that made the opposite case. The truth is far more complicated.

One reason that we think otherwise is because human beings—especially the click-hungry media—prefer simplicity. A second and perhaps equally important one is that drug warriors who promoted what became the dominant narrative had no non-racist way to explain why they wanted to treat today's opioid-addicted people with compassion, but previously argued that people with crack addiction were criminals who required incarceration. The only alternative was to admit they'd been wrong last time—but yet should be trusted to provide the best solution now. And that didn't seem exactly like a winning message.

The real facts are these. Research conducted for the government's own National Institute on Drug Abuse shows that 80 percent of people who start misusing prescription opioids do not have a doctor's prescription for them. Their pills come from family, friends, and dealers—or from their parents' medicine cabinets—with few initially getting them directly from medical practitioners.[10] Moreover, at least two-thirds of people who become regular opioid misusers have previously taken psychedelics and/or illegal stimulants like cocaine or methamphetamine.[11] In other words, they are already experienced drug seekers, not naïve children unwittingly having their first experience of drug euphoria because of a careless doctor. The overwhelming majority of drug use that leads to addiction is not medical use. Or, to put it bluntly, if you must divide drug users into "guilty" and "innocent," white drug users belong in the former category at least as often as Black ones do.

Most of the pills that were misused, then, weren't taken by pain patients—even when they had been legitimately prescribed to them. Ironically, these drugs were available precisely because most people who use opioids medically do not have any problem stopping. As a direct result, the rise in prescribing resulted in a torrent of leftover medication. In fact, between 67 and 92 percent of patients given opioids after surgery or dental work don't even take their whole prescription[12]—largely because prescribers typically provide more doses than needed to avoid midnight calls for refills. People also tend to keep opioids in their medicine cabinets rather than throwing them out "just in case" they suddenly have terrible pain. It was these leftovers—far more than medication taken as prescribed—that drove the initial crisis. They provided a ready supply for curious teens and young adults, who are the group at highest risk for new addiction.

Moreover—and again, contrary to the media narrative—the risk of addiction from medical use genuinely is low, albeit with one important caveat that Purdue Pharma and many doctors ignored. Among *carefully screened* adult patients, who do not have current or former addictions, the odds of developing new opioid use disorders are less than 1 percent, according to a Cochrane Review, which is considered the highest standard of medical evidence.[13] Unfortunately, such screening is rarely done in actual practice. And, because people who are addicted deliberately seek doctors in order to get drugs, any population of patients taking opioids long-term will almost inevitably include a large percentage of them.

In our current system, doctors are presumed to be able to detect patients who are faking pain easily. But in reality, like most people, physicians are terrible lie detectors. Moreover, even though doctors are often taught to disregard this when it comes to alcohol and other drugs, good medical care requires believing patients—not treating them with continual contempt and suspicion. The result is that some of the best and most compassionate doctors will almost inevitably attract some people who are already addicted and seeking drugs, while looking from the outside as though they are the cause of those patients' problems. And then, to top it all off, family members and people with addiction themselves often prefer to tell their story in the least shameful way possible. This makes a narrative that blames the doctor even more appealing.

One further issue also completely confounds the white innocence narrative. That is, economics. As prescribing loosened, some pain patients discovered that those extra pills that they now had lying around had a street value of thirty dollars or more for a single pill. And so, for white people in financially desolate communities where decent jobs were rare, OxyContin and other opioids became both a way to manage distress and an alternative way to make money—just as crack had been previously in many lower-income Black communities.

Another parallel between crack and prescription opioids is apparent here as well. That is, the exponential rise of overdose deaths didn't actually start when Oxy was introduced. Instead, the increase began far earlier, as economic conditions in specific communities declined. The recent leap in overdose fatalities began in 1979—not 1996—according to a study published in *Science*.[14] Not coincidentally, that's around the same time when economic inequality began its own exponential growth in America and when cocaine use was already rising.

Pharmaceutical marketing and regulatory failure certainly supplied the product that first rang national alarms around the turn of the twenty-first century. It is absurd that America permits the type of pharmaceutical marketing that it does—and equally shocking that the Drug Enforcement Administration allowed a massive rise in the quota of pills it allowed manufacturers to produce, without doing its job and determining whether such an increase in the medical supply was warranted.

But the crushing despair that underlies overdose and addiction had begun moving through different communities and driving various types of risky substance use long before Oxy was ever marketed. As drugs like crack, methamphetamine, heroin, and prescription opioids waxed and waned in popularity during the 1980s and 1990s, the hopelessness that accompanies shrinking opportunities, stagnant wages, and lingering unemployment continued to metastasize into new areas.

This despair was spurred by the loss of middle- and working-class jobs and other resources, region by region and community by community.

It became visible in the U.K. in the eighties when British and Scottish youth turned to heroin as local factories shut down. It could also be seen in the United States during that decade, when many Black American city dwellers were being hit by deindustrialization and turned to crack. The same phenomenon recurred when job loss and economic stagnation came for rural whites in the nineties and 2000s—and they took up meth-amphetamine and/or prescription opioids.

At first, this trend wasn't readily apparent, in part because of the way exponential growth works—and in part because politicians, experts, and journalists tend to focus on problems with specific drugs, rather than on addiction, which tends to involve multiple drugs. It would take an under-standing of harm reduction—and the way that despair rather than indo-lence drives addictive drug use—to make these truths visible.

In the meantime, in the absence of this vision within the mainstream, most of the media created an entirely different version of what happened. We've heard about the "opioid epidemic" primarily as a simple story of good guys and bad guys. The bad guys are Big Pharma, which sold evil drugs to greedy doctors, who then addicted innocent patients. The good guys are those innocent white people who, unlike the Black folks who'd taken illegal crack, had no idea that the legal pills they were taking could turn them into criminals. And the whites who sold these pills—unlike those vicious crack dealers—were just doing what was economically nec-essary to support their families.

Our continual drive to create false distinctions between "innocent" and "guilty" drug users is yet another reason that harm reduction calls us to undo the concept of drugs. The differences between substances that people can legally use for pleasure, substances that we can legally use only to relieve pain, and all other drugs that might produce comfort or joy are artificial. While some substances clearly fall into the medical or nonmed-ical bracket, others simply do not.

Nonetheless, this false dividing line cuts through the heart of medi-cine, recruiting doctors to police the use of opioids by their patients—or face criminal prosecution if they fail to discern whether people's pain is acceptably "physical" or whether it is an illegal seeking of unearned emo-tional comfort. It's not a scientifically justifiable legal boundary. Physical and emotional pain blend inside the brain. The sting of social rejection literally activates many of the same regions that respond to a bee sting. This means that the only way to evaluate another's pain is subjective. But physicians are somehow supposed to reliably and consistently determine what drug use is legal and what use is criminal—without a clear standard.

Meanwhile, racism, sexism, and other biases also profoundly influence whose pain is seen as "real" and therefore worthy of medical relief. In fact, it was these prejudices that helped create the legal/illegal and medical/nonmedical distinctions between psychoactive drugs in the first place. All of this is what Siobhan Reynolds began to try to undo.

As THE OVERDOSE CRISIS AND THE MISGUIDED ATTEMPTS TO CRACK DOWN ON it without providing care for either people with addiction or pain patients progressed, Reynolds and her husband tried to find relief. It was an increasingly desperate quest.

"We went from doctor to doctor," she said. "We were maligned. We were abused. I've been hit by nurses . . . All pain patients who come to emergency rooms are treated as drug seekers. And the assumption, I suppose, among emergency room personnel is that pain patients get their medicines from doctors, and if they were legitimate, they'd be getting them from doctors. So, the very fact that they're there proves that they're not legitimate, and hence it's okay to abuse them."[15]

It wasn't just patients who were feeling the heat, either. One after another, physicians who did prescribe began to be targeted by medical boards or even arrested and charged with drug dealing offenses that carried decades-long sentences. Federal and state prosecutors only took on a few dozen such cases each year—but that was enough to drive away many more doctors, who tend to be risk-averse by nature. One expert told me that each local prosecution led at least fifty or sixty other doctors to stop prescribing.[16]

Worse, once a patient like Reynolds's husband, Greenwood, was associated via medical records with "bad" doctors and high doses, getting effective care became more and more difficult. Simply knowing the names of the medications that worked best was itself seen as evidence of addictive obsession; going from doctor to doctor to try to get real help became the crime of "doctor shopping." This was unlike anything else in medicine.

Nearly everything that doctors are not supposed to do—from dropping patients without providing alternative care to harming them by requiring unnecessary and invasive procedures, surgeries, and tests—is common in chronic pain treatment. And all of this policing—whether it involves expelling a patient whose opioid use might lead a doctor to be prosecuted or doing medically unnecessary procedures to be sure that law enforcement will see opioid use as legitimate—is a result of the laws that criminalize addiction.

Reynolds dug deep into law and history books to find out why this poor treatment was apparently legal and even condoned by many doctors. Noting that drug prohibition began with the Harrison Narcotics Act of 1914, she saw that few people still alive had experienced anything else— and that most of us now see criminalization as a natural fact, rather than a policy choice. She said, "Americans today are inured to the violence, the corruption, and the conflation of the roles of law enforcement, parents, and medical professionals that current drug policy engenders."[17]

She also discovered the history of early American maintenance treatment in the first decades of the twentieth century, which is little known outside of drug policy nerd circles. What happened was this: After the Harrison Act went into effect in 1915, doctors and pharmacists were at first allowed to continue to supply cocaine, morphine, and heroin to people who had become addicted when those drugs were legal. There was no requirement for these folks to become abstinent: the idea was to keep them functioning until an addiction cure was invented and became available, which was seen as imminent.

The practice was similar to what John Marks would later do in his harm reduction prescribing in Liverpool; indeed, the early "British system" that allowed Marks to prescribe this way had first developed in the U.K. during the same period to deal with exactly the same problem. And it worked just as well in America as it had in England.

In the U.S., however, the 1919 Supreme Court decision in *Webb et al. v. United States* basically outlawed maintenance prescribing by doctors, except for short periods of tapering. In *Webb*, the Court ruled that continuing to supply "a habitual user" with morphine merely "to keep him comfortable"[18] without trying to end the addiction was illegal. This flew in the face of precedent. Prior rulings had determined that federal regulation of the specific details of the practice of medicine was unconstitutional because the power to determine what lies within the bounds of professional practice is not mentioned in the Constitution. Under the Tenth Amendment, such "unenumerated" powers are reserved for the states.[19]

Nonetheless, the court ruled that maintenance could not be medicine. The *Webb* decision states that labeling a doctor's order to provide an addicted person with a drug like morphine as an appropriate prescription "would be so plain a perversion of meaning that no discussion of the subject was required." And so, without any actual evidence or reasoning beyond presumed universal agreement about this "perversion," the Supreme Court allowed the federal government to regulate medicine when it came to controlled substances. In 1970, sociologist Troy Duster was among the first to analyze the harm this had done. As a direct consequence of *Webb*, he wrote, "the medical profession abandoned the drug addict."[20]

And to this day, the *Webb* decision continues to haunt both pain and addiction care. Its interpretation of the law—and the regulatory updates that codified it—assumes that doctors can accurately distinguish between "addicts," whose use of opioids for "comfort" is not allowed, and pain patients, for whom greater comfort is the entire point. It assumes that making these distinctions is always possible to do and medically justifiable—neither of which is true. It further presumes that doctors can safely and effectively police this border and that those who don't detect patient lies about their needs for drugs are corrupt, not compassionate. Essentially, the law demands that doctors act suspicious about all claims of pain, which is antithetical to patient-centered care. Simultaneously, it makes addiction into the one medical condition for which abandonment by doctors—and even having patients arrested—is seen as appropriate.

Moreover, *Webb* and related jurisprudence and regulation assumes that addiction can be clearly defined. The law does not distinguish between people who are simply physically dependent on a substance to function and those whose lives are being destroyed by their inability to stop using a drug despite harmful outcomes. This meant that until the federal government began to allow the use of methadone in 1965—under the strictest regulations of any legal drug on both the federal and state levels—prescribing opioids to people with addiction for anything other than the brief treatment of pain was completely verboten.

Even treating formerly addicted people for pain was questionable. Many doctors simply refused, some because they saw any potential "enabling" of addiction as worse than allowing suffering; others held back for fear of crossing an unclear line into criminality. Basically, most doctors felt safest simply avoiding anything that could run afoul of the law. Legally and therefore financially as well, it was clearly better to stay away from opioids when treating anyone for any significant period of time, even if they were close to death. This accounted for many decades of undertreatment of pain until activism and then Purdue's marketing began to make doctors feel more comfortable with prescribing.

Due to these early twentieth-century court decisions, the question of whether long-term opioid prescribing for chronic pain is legitimate medicine now lies in a sticky thicket of legal interpretation that tends to change with fashion. For patients, how these laws are interpreted can mean the difference between living comfortably or being disabled by pain. For doctors, it can be the difference between having a thriving practice and spending multiple decades in prison. For people with addiction, it determines the ease of access to medications like methadone and buprenorphine—and whether or not they will be considered to be "in recovery" if they continue to take them. And all of this rests on how addiction is defined medically, which has changed over time as it has become better understood.

Until at least the 1970s, addiction was defined as merely a physical problem. If you needed more to get the same effect over time (tolerance) and became visibly ill with predictable symptoms when you tried to quit abruptly (withdrawal), you were addicted. Drugs that weren't associated with obvious physical withdrawal syndromes—like marijuana and cocaine—weren't seen as addictive. But this definition turned out to be both too broad and too narrow.

For one, few would try to argue post-crack that cocaine isn't highly addictive, even though people who quit it don't start vomiting and shaking or show other obvious physical symptoms when they stop. The main symptom of cocaine withdrawal is psychological: craving for more cocaine. Secondly, conflating addiction and dependence also errs in the opposite way, wrongly characterizing drugs that have no addiction potential as being addictive. For example, certain blood pressure and antidepressant medications produce absolutely no high. But you can become severely ill—or even die, in the case of the blood pressure drugs—if you try to stop taking them too quickly.

Addiction, instead, needs to be defined psychologically. Top experts now agree on this, including psychiatry's *Diagnostic and Statistical Manual* (DSM) and the leading scientific authority on addiction in the U.S. government, the National Institute on Drug Abuse.[21] The essence of addiction is compulsive drug use that continues despite negative consequences. What this means for pain patients is that while anyone who takes opioids daily for long enough can be defined as dependent, unless their use of the drugs is destructive, it should not be called addiction. The editors of the latest edition of the DSM felt so strongly about clarifying this distinction that they rejected their former term for the diagnosis of addiction—substance dependence—and replaced it with "substance use disorder, moderate to severe" as of 2013.

Harm reductionists have also incorporated this view of addiction into their work. It is part of seeing recovery as "any positive change." Obviously, from this perspective, if someone goes from out-of-control bingeing that precludes employment and healthy family life to being stable and productive but still physically dependent on buprenorphine or heroin, this counts as progress. Addiction by definition involves harmful drug use; physical dependence is not necessarily detrimental if the benefits of the drug outweigh the risks and it improves quality of life. For many pain patients, physical dependence on opioids is a far better bargain than agony that causes disability.

However, while psychiatry has gradually come to recognize these distinctions, the legal system still doesn't. Said Reynolds, "The government wants everybody to believe that if you take a medicine every day, and it happens to be opioids, you're an addict. But that's not true." Nonetheless, the DEA still defines an "addict" as a "habitual" user of (illegal) drugs who has "lost the power of self-control with reference to [their] addiction" or whose use somehow "endangers the public morals, health, safety, or welfare."[22]

Reynolds realized that it was this highly confusing area of law that kept doctors afraid of prescribing the doses of medication that her husband needed. She began to consider the implications of a body of legal thought that allows courts to decide whether a doctor's prescription is criminal or acceptable, with only vague and subjective standards for doing so.

These days, this determination is supposed to be based on the 1970s Controlled Substances Act (CSA). That law consolidated drug prohibition by creating five categories ("schedules"), which are supposed to represent the relative dangers of drugs and whether or not they have legitimate medical uses.

The degree to which science or politics lies behind the CSA may be understood by considering that both heroin and marijuana are included in "Schedule One." This means that these extremely different drugs, each of which actually does have demonstrable medical uses, are considered equally dangerous and equally addictive and without any conceivable medical use. As Reynolds put it, "Contrary to public assumptions, the Controlled Substances Act is not a public safety measure; it is a blunt instrument by which the federal government exercises police powers that were explicitly denied it by the founding fathers."[23]

Under the CSA, a prescription for a substance that is permitted only for medical use must meet certain standards. The law says that a prescription is only authorized if it has been written "for a legitimate medical purpose by an individual practitioner acting in the usual course of his professional practice."[24] However, if physicians and police disagree about the nature of "legitimate medical purposes" and what lies within the "usual course of professional practice," this poses a severe problem. The doctors' intentions don't matter: physicians might believe that they are practicing in good faith when they prescribe opioids, but if law enforcement doesn't see their practices as "legitimate," they can be criminally convicted.

Essentially, *Webb* and the decisions that followed that supported the constitutionality of the Controlled Substances Act allow the DEA to determine the boundaries of addiction and pain medicine, regardless of changes in data and standards of care. This functionally criminalizes certain types of malpractice, because normally, when a doctor is out of bounds in terms of care, civil law determines liability. If a bad doctor kills you on the operating table, he can't be charged with murder unless there is clear evidence of premeditation and intent. But if you fatally overdose after taking a drug that the very same doctor prescribed because he incorrectly believed you needed it for pain, he can be charged with homicide, defined as drug delivery resulting in death. The presumption is that addiction is always obvious, people with addiction can't have genuine pain conditions, doctors have effective lie detectors, and they only prescribe to addicted people if they are acting as dealers, not doctors.

The result is that, in the eyes of the law, doctors can turn into drug dealers without even being aware of it if police view their prescribing practices as illegitimate. And this, of course, makes them want to avoid dealing with either chronic pain patients or people with addiction. For patients, it creates a terrible situation, too. It means that a doctor's default attitude toward pain should not be compassion, and if you are someone like Sean Greenwood, whose pain is only relieved by high doses of opioids, you will be likely labeled an addict and expelled from care repeatedly, without recourse.

And as the media was flooded with stories of OxyContin addiction and overdose in the early 2000s, that's exactly what happened to him. Reynolds decided that the best way to fight back was to focus on changing the interpretation of the law. To do that, she began working with doctors who were accused of "overprescribing," starting with a Stanford-educated physician, William Hurwitz. He had been arrested in 2003 and charged with forty-nine separate crimes, including drug trafficking resulting in death and running a criminal enterprise. Reynolds's husband was one of his patients.

The sheer number of charges in this and similar cases is designed to intimidate doctors into accepting plea deals and avoiding trial: with that many counts, jurors will naturally think that the physician must have done at least something wrong. But this is misleading. The essence of the prosecutors' cases is that ordinary events in a doctor's office become criminal the moment the doctor steps outside of what they consider "legitimate" medicine.

Instantly, every action is transformed into one or more crimes. A single prescription can be several counts: in addition to drug dealing or distribution, it becomes fraud when the patient is billed, because such transactions are obviously not covered by insurance or Medicaid. If the prescription is mailed, add a count of mail fraud. If one of the patients sells a prescription to someone else, now the doc is involved in a drug conspiracy. Depositing a paycheck? Money laundering. And most seriously of all, any fatality that can in any way be connected to the use of the prescription can become a charge of drug dispensing resulting in death or serious injury—even if the person who died lied to get the drug, used it with alcohol or other drugs, injected or snorted a drug meant to be taken orally, or had a fatal illness or injury that was just as likely to have been the real cause of death.

"In other words, these were purported to be criminal cases, but were essentially government-generated malpractice cases where they can hire a witness to come in and say the doctor shouldn't have done this or that," Reynolds said, summing up how the CSA basically criminalizes actions by doctors that more typically would be dealt with through civil charges. Even the term "overprescribing"—which is often used to describe these offenses—would seem to suggest a mistake or an outlying practice, rather than an intentional crime.

In his first trial, Hurwitz was convicted on all charges and sentenced to multiple concurrent twenty-five-year prison terms. With Reynolds's help, however, that conviction was overturned, because he hadn't been allowed to present a defense that showed that he had practiced in good faith. And he did much better on appeal. The only convictions that stood were associated with patients who sold their drugs so obviously that the judge simply couldn't believe Hurwitz was unaware of it. But from the bench as she announced the verdict, she said that most of his care had been legitimate medicine and that the high doses some patients received that she'd originally described as "absolutely crazy" were instead supported by "an increasing body of respectable medical literature and expertise."[25] He was resentenced to less than five years.

In 2003, Reynolds founded an organization called the Pain Relief Network to help defend pain doctors and their patients (its acronym is PRN, which is the medical term for having the patient choose when to take the medicine). One of her advisors was another MD whom she had helped to win one of these cases. Like Hurwitz, Frank Fisher, a Harvard-educated physician, had been charged with drug dealing and homicide—again, based on the idea that prescribing high doses of opioids cannot be legitimate.

However, the case against him rapidly fell apart. For example, one of the homicide charges involved a woman who died as a passenger in a van accident that completely severed her spine. The state's argument was that she'd actually been killed by OxyContin, due to the high levels of the drug found in her blood. Just trying to devise a plausible scenario in which this gruesome death was really an overdose demonstrates how ludicrous the charge was. The rest of the case against him also collapsed upon examination. In pretrial hearings, it was revealed that no fewer than seven attempts by undercover agents to get drugs from him had failed. None had succeeded. "I had a screening process for those who tried to get controlled substances," Fisher said. "I screened out sixty percent of those and apparently, the agents were amongst them."[26] In January of 2003, the judge dropped all of the charges.

Reynolds and PRN began highlighting cases like these to the media, aiming to get journalists to recognize that not everyone prosecutors labeled a "pusher with a pen" or a "pill mill" was guilty—regardless of claims about high dosages or dubious tactics like giving the physician the presumably shameful status of being the "number one opioid prescriber" in the state (there's always going to be one, because math). She also drew attention to the horror that the drug war was causing for pain patients, in a climate where journalists were claiming that OxyContin was basically being given to anyone who so much as stubbed a toe or broke a fingernail. In fact, many people were suffering tremendously.

For example, a Florida man whom Reynolds helped free had been sentenced to twenty-five years in prison for "trafficking." He used a wheelchair and had pain from both multiple sclerosis and a mutilating failed back surgery—but prosecutors couldn't believe that he was truly taking the dosage of drugs he'd been prescribed. Even after surveillance failed to show that he was selling, he had been convicted based on the weight of the pills alone.

The Erie, Pennsylvania, case was another one of her victories. The press conference and other efforts she organized to support Dr. Heberle paid off. Expert testimony from Dr. Fisher explained to the jury why large doses of opioids were medically necessary for some patients. And, by getting the perspective of pain patients included in the press and during the trial, Reynolds was able to flip the prosecutors' story on its head. Rather than telling the tale of a vicious pill pusher profiting by getting people addicted, she offered an account of a brave healer who took on patients rejected by everyone else and made them better—at least until the law came for him.

"The government position is that the doctor wasn't cruel enough," she said, explaining that if these prosecutors had their way, doctors would be required to treat patients with unrelenting skepticism, forcing them to jump through numerous hoops to get their medication, regardless of how well he knew them and how well they were doing. However, she added, "By making the pain patients real, we made the good guys and the bad guys change places."[27]

It was another example of how a compassionate view of drug use and related harm could change everything. However, Reynolds and PRN were fighting an uphill battle. For every victory like this, there were countless losses. For one, over 90 percent of criminal cases end in a guilty plea rather than a trial,[28] and of the few that do go to trial, prosecutors win at least 75 percent of the time.[29] By organizing the patients of doctors who were targeted for prosecution, Reynolds was sometimes able to help them beat the odds but, in many instances, she wasn't.

In a Kansas case, for example, she tried to support a doctor by paying for a billboard that proclaimed his innocence. Law enforcement had publicly described him as a villain: she believed that she had the First Amendment right to do the opposite. However, this so infuriated the lead prosecutor that she got the court to impose overwhelming fines, claiming that Reynolds had obstructed justice. Before long, this bankrupted her and her organization. Her appeal of these fines went all the way to the Supreme Court—but, bizarrely, they were upheld in a decision that has unaccountably been kept secret.[30]

And as the overdose death toll rose, doctors, afraid of legal conse-quences, simply began to stop prescribing. While the total number of pre-scriptions didn't fall that much initially, high dose prescribing for chronic pain dropped dramatically as doctors began to reduce the amount that they gave to patients like Greenwood in order to avoid being legally tar-geted. Many simply refused to see such patients.

By 2016, after the Centers for Disease Control introduced guidelines that were widely perceived as a mandate to decrease opioid prescribing, 70 percent of general practitioners said they had reduced both the number of patients that they prescribed to and the doses they used. A full 10 percent stopped opioid prescribing entirely. Between its peak in 2011 and 2017, overall opioid prescribing fell by 29 percent. And suicides of chronic pain patients—some from overdose after hoarding their pills because they knew they wouldn't get any more—seem to have increased in concert.[31]

While little research data on this has been gathered until very recently, a study of patients whose opioids were discontinued nonconsensually found that half wound up in the emergency room or hospitalized with an opioid-related problem like an overdose within weeks.[32] Another study, which included more than 500 veterans who had their opioids cut off, found that 9 percent developed suicidal thoughts and 2 percent actually made an attempt.[33] In a cruel irony, the risk of overdose for patients whose pain medications are stopped is three times higher than for those who continue to receive opioids.[34] This is yet another example of measuring drug policy success by the wrong metric. Politicians, regulators, and law enforcement all crow about achieving big reductions in prescribing and punishing dirty doctors. But doing so without providing help for patients, whether with pain, addiction, or both, only increases disability and death.

Another tragic example of the negative effect of cutting supply with-out helping patients also marks this same period. In the late 2000s, Oxy-Contin was reformulated, in an attempt to prevent misuse by making it harder to snort or shoot. The new version debuted in 2010, and the old pills were quickly removed from pharmacy shelves. Not surprisingly, this did nothing to end existing addictions, but rather pushed people toward substitutes. One study found that 80 percent of the threefold increase in heroin overdose death that occurred between 2010 and 2014 was due to this reformulation.[35]

In an attempt to prevent overdose and addiction, the reduction of the medical supply of opioids has significantly worsened both problems. For people in pain, this tends to increase suicide risk, rather than push them to buy illegal drugs. For one, usually, if you haven't taken street drugs previously, you typically don't know how and where to buy them. Negotiating either the darknet or an open-air dealing scene without getting ripped off as a novice isn't easy. In contrast, people with addiction simply return to their other sources of illegal drugs: it's rare (and dumb) to rely on just one dealer with no backups.

Consequently, in many rural areas where heroin had never previously been available, it popped up everywhere. The free market abhors a vacuum. Overdose rates increased because street drugs—unlike pharmaceuticals—vary in purity and dose. Without knowing how much you are taking, it's hard to protect yourself. Also, any period of abstinence, voluntary or otherwise, lowers tolerance and increases overdose risk; this is why staying on medications like buprenorphine and methadone is so protective and why coming out of prison or an abstinence-only rehab are both linked with dramatically elevated overdose rates.

Worse, as the internet made more potent and far cheaper synthetic drugs available, heroin became increasingly contaminated with various kind of fentanyl: the group of synthetic opioids that can be hundreds to thousands of times stronger than heroin. For cartels, making this shift was something of a no-brainer. Producing fentanyl-like drugs or getting them from a lab in China cuts both labor costs and the risks associated with employing people who could wind up becoming informants. With opiates like heroin, which are made from poppies, kingpins need farmers, farm workers, labs, and technicians to process it as well as smugglers before it even gets to street sellers—a supply chain that can include hundreds of people, any one of whom might turn on them. With fentanyl and similar drugs, in contrast, all they need is a few chemists to mail a tiny packet that can supply hundreds of dealers and thousands of users. The business case for synthetics is overwhelming.

The rise of fentanyl or something like it was also completely predictable in the wake of a supply cut. It's such a common occurrence in drug policy that it has a name, which is the "iron law of prohibition." The principle is simple. Crackdowns and prohibitions typically lead to the rise of more potent forms of drugs, which are easier to smuggle. From the predominance of more potent liquor over wine and beer during alcohol Prohibition to today's fentanyl crisis, the outcome is nearly always the same: harm production on a massive scale.

Reynolds's husband's health began to deteriorate as, one after another, his doctors stopped prescribing to him. In 2006, he was traveling with Reynolds to Arkansas, where a new pain doctor had agreed to see him. By this point, his blood pressure was extremely high, which can be a consequence of severe, unrelieved pain. He died in his sleep in a hotel room. Reynolds refused an autopsy, fearing that regardless of what had killed him, his death might be blamed on any drugs that remained in his system.

She would continue the fight—for her son and everyone else suffering intractable pain. But tragically, right before the most intense attacks on opioid prescribing for chronic pain began, she died in an accident. A small plane piloted by her then-boyfriend crashed for unexplained reasons in good weather on Christmas Eve in 2011. Her work would have to be taken up by a new generation of activists, connected to and within the harm reduction movement.

eighteen

Undoing Overdose, Part 2

A T TWO A.M. ON AN EARLY AUGUST EVENING IN 2008, DENISE AND GARY Cullen's doorbell rang insistently. On the doorstep of their Orange County, California, home was a man from the county coroner's office, bearing the news that parents spend their lives hoping that they will never hear. Their only child, Jeff, was dead. His body had been found on a lawn outside an apartment building. The young man had apparently been lying there for at least four hours, while people walked and drove by without checking on him. Finally, someone who'd passed twice while making a round-trip journey realized that help was needed.

The Cullens later learned that their son had overdosed on a combination of the anti-anxiety drug Xanax and morphine. He died less than forty-eight hours after Denise had driven him home from jail, where he'd served four months on a nonviolent drug crime charge. Upon release, Jeff had put himself on a waiting list to get treatment; he'd been enthusiastic that he was going to start a program that would, for the first time, allow him to use medication to treat his attention deficit/hyperactivity disorder (ADHD), rather than requiring him to abstain. But the rehab couldn't take him immediately. When he died, he was just twenty-seven years old.

Research has long shown that one of the most dangerous periods of time for people with opioid addictions is their first week or two after being released from jail or prison. During these weeks, the risk of death is three to eight times greater than their already elevated odds of dying.[1]

The danger is so great that, at least in one state, a study found that 15 percent of all overdose deaths occurred among people who had recently been incarcerated.[2]

However, few lockups have programs to educate people about these risks and either provide naloxone or immediate treatment entry to reduce them. Nor are parents like Denise—or patients themselves—required to be given true informed consent for treatment. Ongoing use of either buprenorphine or methadone is the only approach proven to significantly reduce the death rate from opioid addiction. Yet two-thirds of all rehabs ban these medications, often along with others that help conditions like ADHD. Such programs aren't required to tell consumers that their abstinence-only approach for opioids has twice the death rate seen in people staying on medication, nor are they required to inform them about other medications that might help pre-existing disorders. Denise is a highly educated social worker who didn't know these facts—and if someone like her wasn't informed, it's unlikely that the average parents without such an education would be any better equipped to protect their child.

Jeff's death would turn his parents—and thousands of others like them—into outraged harm reduction advocates. Like Gretchen Burns Bergman, they would no longer be content to be told what to do by a system that was clearly broken. And this second wave of parent activism, by those who had suffered the ultimate loss, would bring harm reduction to a whole new level.

Denise called her son's addiction "the roller coaster from hell"—and her family had ridden it for many years before he died. Every time they'd start to get some hope, it would be dashed yet again—often by a relapse linked to being expelled from rehab for violating a minor rule or to being arrested for a petty crime. They'd first learned that Jeff had started drinking and taking other drugs when he was in junior high school. Later, he would become addicted to both heroin and methamphetamine.

Jeff bore a distinct resemblance to the actor Ben Affleck, with dark eyes and a dimpled chin. Standing six feet, four inches, he took after his father, Gary, who is also tall with dark brown hair and a full mustache. Denise, in contrast, is just five feet tall, a California blonde with blue eyes and plenty of freckles.

Both father and son struggled with symptoms of ADHD. For Jeff, the condition was first diagnosed when he was nine. Soon, Gary recognized that he, too, likely would have been given the same diagnosis as a child if he'd been evaluated. It had been ADHD, he saw looking back, that probably accounted for why he'd dropped out of high school and joined the army. The condition may also help explain why his career took off only after he was able to be his own boss, a common experience for people with ADHD.

In fact, ADHD—aside from at least doubling the risk for addiction—is linked with success in challenging, risky endeavors like creating a start-up. But infuriatingly to parents and teachers, many people with the disorder are only able to focus well when they are deeply interested in a subject or activity. For Jeff, this had made most schoolwork a nightmare. He wasn't defiant, but many times he just didn't seem to hear his teachers' instructions and frequently forgot to do assignments or didn't finish them. Despite struggling with grades, however, he was popular and athletic, enjoying surfing, soccer, snowboarding, skateboarding, and BMX riding.

The first sign of trouble came when he was fourteen—and got arrested for smoking pot on the roof of an abandoned building. The Cullens immediately put him into a thirty-day rehab, but this only seemed to expose him to other kids who did more dangerous drugs. Before long, he was using pretty much anything he could get and was in and out of jails, counseling, and rehabs.

Unfortunately, the courts and most of the treatment programs never seemed to take into account his disability and how ADHD can make perfect compliance with strict rules almost impossible. As a result, he constantly risked getting thrown out of treatment and into jail or onto the street for single incidents like not attending a twelve-step meeting or being late. "Jeff battled for twelve years with periods of recovery followed by relapse," Denise said. "We were always waiting for the shoe to drop."[3]

After their son died, both parents felt that they needed to do something to make sense of what happened, perhaps by finding some way that they could make a difference to others with similar experiences. Denise learned that another couple had started a group specifically for parents who had lost children to overdose. It was called Grief Recovery After a

Substance Passing (GRASP). There wasn't a local chapter, so the Cullens decided to create one—and seventeen people came to their very first meeting. By 2010, the Cullens found themselves in charge of the whole organization.

But both Denise and Gary soon felt that they also needed to do something more, something to try to change the treatment and criminal prosecution system that had utterly failed Jeff. They didn't want any other parents not to know how to protect their addicted kids.

By the year that Jeff died, more than two dozen community-based naloxone programs already existed in the U.S.[4] Some states had instituted rules to make the drug easier to get, with a few allowing doctors to write a "standing order" so that anyone could be provided with it rather than requiring an individual prescription.[5]

But the Cullens hadn't even known that naloxone existed. Now they wanted to ensure that other parents were better informed and to organize them so that they could fight against a war on drugs that didn't provide any real help. They didn't want politics to intrude on their grief support group. But they also felt that for some, like them, it would be an essential part of healing. And so they created a parallel group called Broken No More to help themselves and others channel their anger and anguish to fight for political change.

IT WASN'T WIDESPREAD OR ESPECIALLY TENACIOUS PUBLICITY THAT HAD ALlowed the Cullens to attract so many parents to their very first meeting of GRASP. By the late 2000s, the national overdose rate was indeed a crisis, reaching every part of the U.S. Orange County alone already probably had at least dozens of potential members.

In 2009, for the first time, overdose deaths outpaced car accidents as the top cause of accidental death. Part of the reason for this shocking statistic was good news: harm reduction practices have made driving itself much safer. With the advent of the "designated driver" and greater social disapproval of drunk driving, the proportion of crash deaths related to alcohol fell from 46 percent in 1982 to 30 percent in 2009. Other harm reduction measures like seat belts and laws to encourage their use, as well as airbags, meant that the total number of vehicular deaths had declined as well, falling from around 53,000 in 1980 to just over 36,000 in 2009. The rate of deaths per mile driven has fallen even more dramatically: it was cut by more than half during that period.[6]

But harm reduction access for overdose was still far from being as ubiquitous among people at risk. And the cuts in the medical supply of opioids that led people to heroin and then street fentanyl and similar compounds made addiction increasingly deadly. In 1999, the number of overdose deaths in the U.S. was just under 17,000.[7] By the time Jeff died in 2008, however, the total had more than doubled, rising to around 36,000. Meanwhile, although the number of naloxone programs was certainly growing and states were trying to expand access to it, at least three-quarters of the states with the highest overdose rates had no naloxone programs at all as late as 2010.[8]

Coincidentally, Denise Cullen had been taught the basics of harm reduction by Edith Springer, many years before she knew it would have any application outside of her professional life and long before naloxone education and distribution had become a well-known part of its tool kit. At the time in 1993, she was a clinical social worker at the University of California–Irvine. "I came back from this conference just blown away by her," Cullen said.

That year, Jeff was just twelve and had yet to even experiment with drugs. But as his addiction worsened, Cullen kept in mind some of what Springer had taught. For example, once she knew that Jeff had started injecting, she made sure that there were clean needles in the house. In Orange County, there was no syringe exchange. Denise also refused to practice tough love, recognizing that shame and stigma drove addiction rather than ending it. So she did her best to make sure Jeff made it through the times when he was using and not ready for or able to get treatment. "All I 'enabled' Jeff to do was to be with us longer. And to know he was loved," said Cullen.[9]

Nonetheless, she was furious that even someone as well-informed as she was had not learned about naloxone and the risk associated with being released from incarceration until it was too late. With Broken No More, she set out to change that situation.

IN 2009, SOME OF THE MOST INVOLVED MOTHERS WITHIN THE HARM REDUC-
tion movement decided to join forces. Sitting at a table drinking coffee
during a break in that year's drug policy reform conference, Gretchen
Burns Bergman was talking to her friend Julia Negron. Negron was a mom
and activist who'd once been married to the drummer for the Doors.
She later married an Allman brother—and then the singer for Three Dog
Night. She had the drug history you would expect from such a rock and
roll résumé. She said, "It just kind of dawned on us that we should totally
use our mom credibility."

The result was a group called Moms United to End the War on Drugs.
Denise Cullen, Joyce Rivera (a member of the Harm Reduction Working Group), and Diane Goldstein, a former police lieutenant, were also
among the founders. They all agreed that change was needed, and that
criminalization certainly hadn't helped their children. They wanted to
massively expand access to naloxone. By 2018, they would have members
in thirty-six states and six countries.

If a mother whose child had been incarcerated during the drug war,
like Gretchen Bergman, was a powerful voice for change, the mother of a
child who had been lost to overdose, like Denise Cullen, was even more
compelling. Supported by those whose children who had been less grievously harmed, moms like Cullen began to take the case for naloxone and
for harm reduction more generally into the mainstream.

"I have talked with hundreds of people who have been the one to
find their friend, their loved one, experiencing an overdose," Cullen wrote
in HRC's newsletter in 2011. "They tried all the usual 'remedies'—cold
water, ice, slapping them. However, all these actions do is waste precious
time. If they had access to naloxone and knew how to use it, their loved
one could have been saved."

Can anyone say to a mom like Cullen that if it was their own kid turning blue and close to death, they wouldn't want naloxone and someone
trained to use it nearby?

IN 2012, THE FOOD AND DRUG ADMINISTRATION HELD HEARINGS TO DETER-
mine whether naloxone should be made available over the counter—a

policy that harm reductionists had called for ever since Dan Bigg first made his case for expanded access back in 1996.

The OD mortality rate per capita had more than tripled since then, while an extremely safe and effective drug to treat it was, for the most part, still locked up in the government's medicine cabinet. Pushed by Bigg and CRA, Illinois and a few other states had passed laws that meant that an individual prescription was no longer needed to get naloxone. But in the rest of the country, the only way to obtain it was via harm reduction programs.[10] Meanwhile, drugs that can do far more damage—for example, acetaminophen (Tylenol), which can cause fatal liver failure—can be purchased without a prescription by millions of people every day.

Addiction stigma and fears about "enabling" were among the biggest obstacles to change. There was also a bit of turf-claiming by medical professionals, who often don't like it when amateurs try to seize tools that they believe can't be handled safely without their own group's extensive training. Sheer bureaucratic inertia also sustained the status quo.

At the hearing, however, it was stupendously obvious that failing to make naloxone far more accessible was scientifically unsupportable and was costing lives. Megan Ralston, who worked on the issue for the Drug Policy Alliance (formerly called the Drug Policy Foundation), had written and been quoted extensively about overdose reversals. Thanks to Google, this meant that she constantly heard from anguished parents who had learned about the antidote only after having lost their children to the poison.

"I have had more gut-wrenching conversations with moms and dads who lost their children to opiate overdose than I can remember," she testified. "[They] aren't just dealing with the trauma of losing their loved one but dealing with the added grief of discovering the existence of naloxone only after the death."[11]

One of the most shocking and ironic instances of such an experience is the story of Joy Fishman, the second wife of pharmaceutical researcher Jack Fishman, who literally invented naloxone. When her son from an earlier marriage fatally overdosed in 2003, she was not even aware that there *was* an antidote—let alone that her current husband had devised and patented it. Jack's drug development work had mainly been on cancer drugs and, being retired, the couple hadn't talked much about the specifics.

But when a *New York Times* article about the famously posh building where they lived in Manhattan mentioned her husband's invention, Fishman was stunned. Soon she was contacted by DPA head Ethan Nadelmann, who convinced her that her family's story needed to be told. She became committed to the harm reduction movement, saddened to learn about alternatives to tough love and better ways to protect her child only after he was dead.

There are thousands of similar stories. At the hearing, DPA's Ralston mentioned having spoken at a national conference of grief support group leaders, all of whom had children who had died from overdose. "I was explaining that [naloxone is] affordable, safe, effective and has been used to reverse opioid overdose for forty years," she said. "A man in the back row raised his hand. 'Wait,' he said. 'So if naloxone is so safe, and works so well, and is so affordable, and it can't be abused, and you can't get addicted to it, why didn't I know about this when my son was still alive? Why can't we get this?'"

That was the question of the day. One grieving mother from Freeport, Illinois, testified about the loss of her only son. She said, "He was a good son and my greatest joy and he never lost hope for recovery." She added, "I live with the certain knowledge that had my son suffered from cancer, doctors would have exhausted their skills and tried every possible drug to save his life. But no doctor ever mentioned naloxone to me . . . It makes me livid. I have the rest of my life to live without [my son], and I cannot describe that kind of loss to you."[12]

Being in that packed hearing room and listening to parent after parent describe the same experience was almost unbearable. And yet, when I pressed the FDA panel, they would not say when or even whether they would act. Only one speaker out of more than two dozen had actually opposed the idea of making naloxone widely and easily available. He was a representative of the American Society of Anesthesiologists, who said the organization was concerned that people wouldn't be able to handle naloxone administration safely on the street.

This doctor didn't seem to know about the data showing that not only could it be done, it had already been done by thousands of people—nor did he seem aware of the study that showed that taking the person to the hospital afterward didn't have any added benefit. He also ignored the testimony of one of his colleagues, who said that 700 times the recommended dose could be given to a person who wasn't physically dependent on opioids without negative effects, adding that pharmacology texts list only a few possible side effects, "in contrast to a dangerous drug like ibuprofen" (Advil).

Despite the moving testimony, the agency's response to my question instantly made it clear that any action by the FDA would be slow. Although the media had been extensively focused on the "opioid crisis," there seemed to be little interest in a proven antidote: I was the only journalist present, writing for *Time*.

And so, back in the community, parents like Cullen, Bergman, Negron, and many others stepped up. They offered training for parents on naloxone and called on states to pass "Good Samaritan" laws so that witnesses to overdose could call for help without fear of being arrested for drug possession. By 2017, forty states and the District of Columbia had enacted such laws, although they do not always provide complete protection from the most serious legal consequences.[13]

But while the government moved slowly, public opinion changed much more quickly. Unlike with needle exchange, there has been no organized opposition to naloxone distribution. Here's an example. I have written about naloxone since Bigg first went public about distributing it, publishing the first story about an overdose reversal in the national media in early 2000. In it, I included some concerns about the idea from a doctor.

However, while I could always easily find someone to denounce needle exchange in the eighties and nineties, by 2012, it had become nearly impossible to find a genuine expert to dismiss expanding naloxone access. Certainly, you might hear the odd paramedic grousing about "repeat customers," and in the comments of any naloxone article, there is often a troll chorus chanting, "Let them die." But there were no legitimate organizations or outspoken physicians who would agree to be quoted by the media. I suspect that none of them wanted to face the question of whether they would want the antidote available if their kid was at home and not breathing—and then have to either lie or rationalize denying it to others in the same situation.

This shift in attitude toward harm reduction was reflected in and was certainly due, at least in part, to changes in the views of parents, especially mothers. In the nineties, they had not come out in any significant way for needle exchange. In fact, they were often among the voices of the opposition. Tough love parents and their organizations like the Drug Free America Foundation actually advanced and publicized many of the attacks on harm reduction in its early years.[14]

By 2012, however, the voice of the parent in drug policy was increasingly that of someone like Bergman or Cullen. The drug war certainly hadn't helped their children: they had personal experience of specific policies that had harmed them or even hastened their death. Millions of parents had children who were at risk—and at least a million had actually lost a child since the turn of the twenty-first century. "We get so many new people," Cullen said, noting that while she used to know everyone in the grief support group she'd founded, this was now impossible because of the sheer increase in numbers. By 2015, they had 100 chapters in thirty-one states, which met at least twice monthly—as well as a Facebook group that connected thousands of people.

The growth of harm reduction and its increasing acceptance by parents was also facilitated by the way naloxone itself works. In contrast to the case for naloxone, the argument for needle exchange is abstract. If you give someone clean needles, they can avoid HIV. But the results are rarely visible to anyone other than their intimates—and some of them might not even know. Ten years later, when that person who might otherwise have died of AIDS is thriving, his past as an IV drug user may not even be known to any of those around him. And it's completely invisible to the general public.

Naloxone, on the other hand, unmistakably brings people back to life right in front of your eyes. One minute they are blue, not breathing, unconscious, and nonresponsive; the next, they are sitting up, their color has returned, and they are talking. It's hard to oppose something that so dramatically and directly saves a life. When parents and family members begin to see this, it makes the concept of harm reduction concrete and compelling.

Naloxone is like a gateway drug—if gateway drugs were really a thing and not just a drug war myth—to harm reduction.

nineteen

Undoing Divisions

WHILE RUNNING TO CATCH A BUS, CIVIL RIGHTS ATTORNEY MICHELLE Alexander passed a bold orange flyer stapled to a telephone pole. It was some time in the late nineties. In strident capital letters, the poster said, "THE DRUG WAR IS THE NEW JIM CROW." In smaller print, it advertised a meeting at a Bay Area church, where an activist group planned to discuss crime and drug policy. Alexander's reaction to this sign would become the catalyst for a stunning new policy analysis—and her work would soon forge a much stronger connection between harm reduction and other progressive movements, especially around racial justice.

In 1998, the thirty-one-year-old lawyer was working for the ACLU in northern California. She had recently been hired to lead its Racial Justice Project—she saw the poster not long after she'd started her new job. Disagreeing with its claim, she continued on her way. She didn't even consider stopping to get more details, let alone attending the meeting. Alexander, who is Black, had no idea how much that sign was about to change her life.

At the time, she writes, "I sighed and muttered to myself something like, 'Yeah, the criminal justice system is racist in many ways, but it really doesn't help to make such an absurd comparison. People will just think you're crazy.'"[1] Before long, however, she found herself starting to think that there might be something to it.

As she began to understand just how absurdly disparate the criminal "justice" system was, the grinding daily experience of working within it began to change her mind. She studied the history of the drug laws. She learned about their lack of connection to the harms of specific substances and the utter disconnect between rates of drug use and sales by various races and arrest numbers. Not surprisingly, whites use and deal just as much as everyone else—and with certain drugs, far more.

Soon Alexander reconsidered not her own sanity, but that of those who *didn't* recognize what was truly going on. Over time, she began to agree that the statement made by the orange sign was accurate; in fact, its phrasing became part of the title of her 2010 book, *The New Jim Crow: Mass Incarceration in the Age of Colorblindness.* Alexander's work brought the idea that drug policy is an instrument of racism to mainstream, widespread attention—and in the process transformed harm reduction and the debate over drug policy reform.

The New Jim Crow was not an immediate bestseller. Alexander spent years on a relentless speaking tour, often at small churches like the one that had advertised the meeting that initially drew her attention. She spoke at countless conferences, gave readings and talks, and participated in panels at events held by various activist, drug reform, civil rights, and criminal justice–focused groups. She made her argument at colleges and universities and in almost any media she could get.

Finally, nearly two years after it had been originally published, the book hit the *New York Times* bestseller list, following its paperback release in 2012. It is hard to overestimate its impact. By demonstrating that the drug war was not—and could never be—"colorblind," Alexander had changed the terms of the debate forever.

"She gave me language," said Monique Tula, a long-time harm reductionist who became the first Black executive director of the Harm Reduction Coalition in 2016. "It was the stuff that we've known, but she tied it together in one place . . . honestly, it was life changing."

The current fight against what we now recognize as "mass incarceration" frequently uses Alexander's phrasing, language, and arguments and recognizes drug policy as a critical part of systemic racism in law enforcement. *The New Jim Crow* brought together horrifying statistics that demonstrated the escalation of the drug war, focusing on its extreme racial disparities. Noting that the U.S. at the time imprisoned a larger proportion of its Black population than South Africa did during the worst of apartheid, the book goes on to describe an America where one in three young African American men at any given time is either in prison or jail or on probation or parole.

Alexander then shows how, for much of recent history, criminal justice and drug policy reform were rarely framed in the mainstream as racial justice or civil rights issues. For example, she describes a 2009 letter from the Congressional Black Caucus to community groups asking them to identify their priorities, listing some three dozen topics as options—not one of which was criminal justice reform. Essentially, civil rights groups fighting racism tended not to focus on crime and the drug war—while drug war opponents tended not to center race.

The New Jim Crow "provided the intellectual basis for merging the harm reduction movement with the criminal justice reform movement," said Ricky Bluthenthal, a Black member of the Harm Reduction Working Group, who is associate dean for social justice and professor of preventive medicine at the University of Southern California, as well as cofounder of the Oakland Needle Exchange. While harm reductionists have long recognized the role of racism in drug policy, Alexander's arguments spotlighted it in a way that made it impossible to ignore. Previously, many harm reduction arguments had been made on the grounds of individual human rights, but, Bluthenthal said, Alexander brought the focus back to systematic oppression.[2]

Her book also demolished the "respectability" case for Black support for harsh drug policy. Since the criminal justice approach was neither effective at nor really designed to reduce drug problems, there was no way to continue it without a continuing racist outcome. As she put it, "Saying mass incarceration is an abysmal failure makes sense . . . only if one assumes that the criminal justice system is designed to prevent and control crime. But if mass incarceration is understood as a system of social control—specifically racial control—then the system is a fantastic success."

Within two decades, the drug war was able to quadruple the prison population and put a tremendous proportion of Black people into the criminal prosecution system, leaving millions with criminal records and blighting their lives by reducing their ability to get decent jobs, housing, and other benefits. "One could argue this result is a tragic, unforeseeable mistake," she wrote. "But judging by the political rhetoric and the legal rules employed in the War on Drugs, the result is no freak accident."[3]

Of course, once current drug policy is understood as an oppressive and racist campaign, it becomes hard to find any reason whatsoever that Black and brown people should support it. Consequently, Alexander's book and its conclusions allowed many more African Americans and Hispanic people to comfortably embrace harm reduction. If the drug war was racist, opposing it wasn't "pro-drug"—and attacking it didn't imply that you were ignoring the damage that addiction itself can do. If the real purpose of the drug war was to maintain white supremacy—and not to save children, as its supporters claimed—then the antiracist position was to oppose it.

Further, before *The New Jim Crow* came out, it was much easier to dismiss calls for decriminalization and legalization as the special pleading of white people who just wanted to get high and didn't care about the consequences that this might have in minority communities. That argument had often been used to dismiss drug reform advocates, who frequently were overwhelmingly white.

Tracie Gardner, who is Black, was a policy associate at the Minority Task Force on AIDS in the early nineties and a harm reduction pioneer at Gay Men's Health Crisis and the Legal Action Center. "We'd have these meetings talking about harm reduction," she said. "And it's like 'These are wealthy white boys who want to be able to use heroin in peace . . . That's what this is all about. They want to be able to use drugs and not suffer the consequences that folks of color do. So that's why harm reduction is bullshit, because they just want permission.'"

From this perspective harm reduction was seen as a step toward permissive legalization, which would create new industries to prey on Black communities, in the same way that the alcohol and tobacco companies already do. Alternatively, as needle exchange opponents so frequently claimed, it was a Band-Aid that was a cheaper and inadequate substitute for the comprehensive services that were really needed.

Once Alexander had demonstrated that the drug war was, in and of itself, an attack on African Americans, however, that argument held less force. If the message sent by the drug war wasn't "don't do drugs" but rather "here's a way we can be tough on people of color without admitting it," then there is no need to worry about the signals sent to children by changing to "softer" tactics. A message of compassion, sent by harm reduction programs like needle exchange, did not have to conflict with racial justice. In fact, it was essential to it.

"Michelle Alexander made what we all knew accessible and palatable," said Gardner, noting that there were people in harm reduction and drug policy reform—like whoever had written that sign that first inspired her—who had made such claims for many decades. "She definitely pulled it all together in a way that helped people who couldn't make the connection, make the connection," Gardner added.[4]

The publication and success of *The New Jim Crow* laid the groundwork for new coalitions among activists, across the racial spectrum. And this, in turn, helped expand the growing cracks in the façade of the drug war into a genuine threat to the integrity of the edifice itself. Without turning people of color against each other, it would be impossible to make the racist war on drugs look like anything other than racism. Without middle-class Black and brown support for a policy that was clearly devastating minority communities and was not solving drug problems, it would be much harder to sustain.

By seeing the drug war itself as a profound racial injustice, harm reductionists now had a way to bring their ideas to new, more receptive audiences. Many hadn't ignored the role of racism earlier. But understanding just how central race is to the results of the drug war both sharpened the harm reduction argument and helped expand its coalition.

The New Jim Crow was also perfectly timed. It came out as attention to opioid addiction and overdose as a problem among white people was escalating after the 2008 economic crash. Clearly, the drug war had not prevented this catastrophic rise in overdose deaths and addiction. And, after decades of declining crime rates, the American appetite for always getting tougher and spending more on police and prisons finally had started to wane.

The decline in both crime and the frenzy to "get tough" on it also meant that more conservative groups were becoming receptive to rethinking drug policy. Libertarians had been a part of the drug policy reform movement from the very start, because it fit much of their philosophy. They had always recognized the drug war as a threat to civil liberties. Early proponents of legalization, in fact, included former Reagan secretary of state George Shultz, who came out for legalization in 1989, and Nobel Prize–winning economist Milton Friedman, who made the case in 1991.[5]

As the 1990s turned into the 2000s, however, other types of conservatives also began to see drug policy as a money pit that didn't provide the benefits it claimed. And after Alexander made a convincing case that it was racist, unusual coalitions could form more readily between groups who differed completely on other policies but could come together on criminal justice and drugs. Criminal justice policy became perhaps the only area where the conservative Koch brothers and liberal George Soros actually agreed.

In 2015, the Kochs joined with the ACLU, Families Against Mandatory Minimums, the NAACP, and other liberal groups to form a coalition.[6] Ultimately, their work resulted in legislation, the First Step Act, which passed in 2018. While the law disappointed those seeking much more radical change, the rare bipartisan legislation did help free thousands of drug war prisoners, the vast majority of whom were Black.[7]

Throughout the debate over the drug war, one group of activists had been especially vulnerable to the critique of being privileged white college kids who just wanted to get high: marijuana reformers. Some had tried to highlight the role of racism in the origins of cannabis prohibition and the disparities in policing and incarceration. But as a white-led movement, they didn't have much credibility when they attempted to make these arguments to Black people, especially in the context of "respectability" concerns. In contrast, a Black Stanford-educated civil rights attorney like Alexander—with impeccable credentials and no whiff of joints being passed in dorm rooms—wasn't going to be as easily dismissed.

With all of these factors and groups coalescing, the long-stagnant debate finally began to change. None of this was without conflict or friction, particularly among groups that had not previously had to face their own racism. But harm reduction had provided a vision of workable alternatives to the drug war—and a language to bring them together in an easily understandable way. Then Michelle Alexander and *The New Jim Crow* brought the racism of the drug war out of the realm of academic and specialized history and into the public eye.

Meanwhile, white, empowered parents with opioid addicted children were becoming a large and growing constituency. Parents' organizations like A New PATH and Broken No More were expanding, and a new group, Families for Sensible Drug Policy, joined the effort in 2015, founded by a New Jersey mom who had lost two of her three sons to overdose. In 2015, the *New York Times* headlined a story on the issue: "In Heroin Crisis, White Families Seek Gentler War on Drugs." Legal scholar Kimberlé Williams Crenshaw was quoted, saying that while greater compassion was welcome, "one cannot help notice that had this compassion existed for African-Americans caught up in addiction . . . the devastating impact of mass incarceration upon entire communities would never have happened."

The ground began to shift in two ways, as Hemingway said about going bankrupt: gradually and then suddenly. After many decades of long, hard work—and much tedious repetition of the same arguments—public opinion was finally catching up.

POLITICAL AND SYSTEMIC CHANGE COULD BE SEEN IN MANY DIFFERENT AREAS as the 2000s moved into the 2010s. In terms of needle exchange, the number of programs in the U.S. nearly tripled between 1995 and 2008. President Obama was briefly able to lift the ban on federal funding for it between 2009 and 2011, after overdose first outpaced car accidents as the number one cause of accidental deaths. Then, however, Republicans in Congress inserted the measure back into the budget, forcing Obama to re-instate it because Democrats were not willing to face a government shutdown over the issue.[8] Once again, politicians had used drug policy to send a message and to get budget negotiating points, not to save lives.

By 2015, though, there was new debate over the issue. That year, the deep red state of Indiana faced a stunning outbreak of HIV among IV drug users. After Oxy was reformulated to deter injection in 2010, users in the tiny town of Austin had shifted to another prescription opioid, Opana.

When that, too, was redesigned in supposedly "abuse-resistant" form, injecting actually increased in the rural town. This led to needle sharing and then to HIV rates in the local population that rivaled those seen at the peak of the epidemic in sub-Saharan Africa.

Then-governor Mike Pence was told that the only way to end the crisis was to legalize needle exchange. He demurred, with the usual arguments about messaging and morality.

Here, however, is where it became clear that attitudes toward harm reduction truly had changed. Unlike in the 1980s and nineties, Pence wasn't immediately embraced by a chorus of drug war supporters eager to "send the right message." From that quarter, there was mostly silence. Instead, he was attacked by a unified group of health authorities across the country—including at the federal level—for resisting this quite obviously proven approach. Even local Republican legislators spoke up in support of the exchange. Eventually, after praying on it, he decided to allow a highly restricted, emergency-only program.

A study later estimated that Pence's indecision allowed the number of cases to rise by 40 percent between the time the epidemic was discovered and the time he began to allow syringe exchange.[9] Nonetheless, for the first time, the issue of needle exchange had been framed decisively by the media as a case of politics interfering with science, rather than simply a "controversy" with two intellectually and morally equivalent sides. Between the first round of debate on syringe exchange when I first covered it in the nineties and the 2015 replay in Indiana, the idea that "sending the right message" was more important than saving lives had almost been vanquished. (The fact that these were white lives, however, was not irrelevant.)

As a result, in 2015—at least in part due to the rural Indiana outbreak—the federal funding ban for syringes was, at last, permanently lifted. The legislation that accomplished this still contained the absurd proviso that federal money can be used for anything but the needles themselves[10]—a lingering legacy of the "message" issue. Regardless, needle exchange has finally become an established public health intervention, no longer a matter for serious debate.

And during these same years, naloxone access expanded even more explosively. In 2007, only three states had "standing order" legislation for the drug, which basically makes it available without an individual prescription from community-based groups or health departments. By 2013, such orders were in place in seventeen states. That number had more than doubled just two years later. And, as of 2017, a variety of different laws to expand naloxone access had been enacted in all fifty states.

Further, at the same time, cannabis law and policy were also being revolutionized. Initially, harm reduction activists and workers hadn't focused much on marijuana, in large part because the drug wasn't linked to the spread of AIDS. At the same time, however, they knew from either being or working with drug users that weed was far less harmful than most other substances, legal or illegal. This meant that the war on marijuana was in and of itself an argument for the necessity of harm reduction.

Beyond this, however, marijuana decriminalization and legalization further engendered support for harm reduction in a more subtle way. When the sky doesn't fall down after drug policy is liberalized, the lack of dire outcomes itself threatens support for punitive prohibition. And when prohibitionists' predictions of widespread loss of productivity, youth depravity, increased mental illness, and violent crime do not come true, this tends to demolish their credibility. This connection is another reason why the two movements grew together and expanded at the same time, helped along by the New Jim Crow argument made by Alexander. Bolstered by activists across racial lines, Alexander had flipped the script on marijuana reform—making support for it both respectable and antiracist.

Medical marijuana legalization began on a state level in California in 1996, with a ballot proposition that passed by a significant margin, fifty-six to forty-four. By 2010, when *The New Jim Crow* was first published, thirteen other states had followed suit. But 2012 was the real turning point. That was the year that Colorado and Washington state legalized recreational cannabis use.

At this point, *The New Jim Crow* had already sold some 200,000 copies. Bowing to what was clearly becoming a new political reality, the Obama administration's Department of Justice sent out a memo emphasizing that it would not prosecute marijuana cases in these states, so long as sellers followed state laws. This was the first evidence that real change might be possible on the federal level. Also, in 2012, national support for recreational legalization hit 50 percent for the first time ever in Gallup polls. By 2018, ten states had legalized recreational use, which gave legal access to a full quarter of the U.S. population. Today, some two-thirds of Americans favor legal weed.[11]

There were other watershed moments as well. In 2014, President Obama appointed Michael Botticelli to be "drug czar"—the first person who was out about being in recovery to ever hold the job. That year, while awaiting Senate confirmation, he gave the keynote address at the national harm reduction conference. "I hope that my presence here reflects the Obama administration's continuing commitment to drug policy reform," he said, similarly noting support for naloxone and needle exchange, as well as medication treatment.[12]

It was extraordinary to see the head of an agency that had once worked to stamp out the very phrase—and had actively blocked President Clinton's plans to end the ban on federal funds for syringe exchange—give clear, if qualified, support to people in the field.

And all of the progress made by needle exchange, naloxone programs, and marijuana reform efforts would be consolidated and advanced by the arguments made by Michelle Alexander in *The New Jim Crow*. Her work drove rapid change across all fronts of drug policy reform. Civil rights activists, racial justice organizations, and criminal justice policy reformers are now united in their opposition to the war on drugs. And it had all started with a little orange sign in Oakland that outraged the right reader.

twenty

Redoing Organizing

"**O**RGANIZING THE UNORGANIZABLE"—THAT'S HOW DEAN WILSON DE-scribed his work and that of Ann Livingston, who is the co-founder of the Vancouver Area Network of Drug Users (VANDU). Wilson, who injected heroin for many decades, and Livingston, who seems to get high on organizing itself, were leading a session at a major drug policy conference in Edmonton, Canada, in 2018. The couple have a teenage son together.

At the event, they were finishing each other's sentences, bickering and interrupting gleefully in the way that only people who have known each other forever can. They had been asked to provide their insights on drug user activism from what is almost certainly the most successful and sustained example of it in the world. The conference room was packed.

Livingston, who has long, center-parted gray hair, wore big round glasses with a black button-down shirt and jeans. Her manner is intense, and she speaks rapidly. Wilson, who seems at least somewhat more laid back, has a slight graying beard and short brown hair. He sported a long-sleeved, brightly flowered shirt over a black tee. That shirt bore an image of a syringe that is the logo of Insite, the safe injection space that is one of VANDU's crowning achievements.

Safe injection facilities, now known as overdose prevention sites (OPS) or supervised consumption sites—are basically needle exchanges where people can use their street drugs under medical supervision rather than outside or at home. They provide all the support, referrals, and benefits that needle exchanges do, but also fight overdose, because help is immediately available if one occurs. Some are also set up for harm reduction related to other routes of administration, like smoking crack or heroin. Ironically, in many, tobacco smoking is not allowed due to other public health laws.

VANDU fought hard to create Insite in the midst of a dual overdose and HIV crisis in British Columbia. They modeled their site on European programs, which had begun as far back as 1986 in Switzerland and had spread as the idea of harm reduction gained currency across the continent. Now there are at least 100 OPS in ten countries, including Australia, Denmark, France, Germany, and Switzerland[1]—and the most important thing to know about them is that although thousands of people have taken millions of injections in them, no one has ever died of overdose in one. There are at least thirty-three in British Columbia alone.[2]

Insite would ultimately provide critical data on these programs—but it never would have opened without the activism of Livingston, Wilson, and VANDU. Indeed, Insite and many other crucial "first in North America" harm reduction achievements are either directly or indirectly linked to the organization and its members. VANDU provides a real-world example of both how to organize people who use drugs and how to sustain such activism. It is now more than twenty-three years old.

A 2003 documentary on VANDU turned Wilson into a minor celebrity: in the film, he appears as a skinny, brown-haired, blue-eyed charmer with the look of a debauched rock star. Titled *Fix: The Story of An Addicted City*, the doc made him "the most famous junkie in Canada," he's said. In fact, he was once stopped and searched at an airport after someone recognized him from it and security officers overheard the conversation.[3] The film contains many scenes of him injecting, most of which occur when he is purportedly trying to quit heroin.

Wilson began his presentation with a tribute to Livingston. "Ann has supported me though twenty years, good and bad, and when I say bad, I mean really fucking bad, when most people would have deserted me, she hung in," he said, adding, "I can't say enough about saying thank you to Ann, and enough of that or I will actually cry."

He then turned to the matter at hand, noting that the most important lessons that VANDU can teach about the current opioid crisis come from Vancouver's history of drug user organizing. "If you have good drug policy in your city, it's because you have good drug user voices in your city," said Wilson, "There is no other way of doing it."

But while harm reduction aims to ensure that these voices are heard, harm reduction organizations themselves are often led by health professionals or former users and not those who are currently addicted. This has long been a source of tension within the movement. Users rightly argue that harm reduction programs should be by and for them, and that professionals frequently take over when real funding becomes available. Once this happens, the new leadership often relegates the people with lived expertise to unpaid or underpaid "peer" positions.

It's not an easy problem, though—and it's not only an issue of the typical professionalization that occurs when money floods into a field aimed at helping a vulnerable group of people. In this specific case, not surprisingly, funders are wary of giving money to people who are open about having current illegal drug addictions to support, especially if any of that money comes from taxpayers. There have been real disasters where groups led by current or former users collapsed because a leader lost control over an addiction and the organization did not have a strong enough structure to manage associated problems successfully.

Simply surviving as an active drug user seeking a daily supply in a criminalized market is a challenge. It certainly doesn't make it easy for people to show up on time in a regular manner to do activism or other work. Nonetheless, since harm reduction is for people who currently use drugs, it should be primarily run by—or at the very least be fully accountable to—them. VANDU's story holds crucial information for those trying to thread this needle.

The group is indeed led by current users, and they do most of its actual work. However, they also have critical support from concerned non-users and ex-users, as well as a democratic structure designed to prevent any single person from having the kind of financial power that could destroy the group. As Wilson once put it, "We have twenty-five board members because you never knew who was going to be alive at the next meeting."[4]

In VANDU's case, the outside support began with Livingston, who was especially attuned to ensuring that she was not the only one who would benefit financially or otherwise from the work. She is principled and committed, often to the point where others find her difficult. When the group received its first grant of $50,000 from Canadian health authorities, Wilson said, "We thought that Ann would just take thirty-five or forty thousand dollars for her salary and we'd pick up the pieces, but she said, 'No, what are we going to do with this money?'"

Livingston was born in Nelson, British Columbia, the child of a mining engineer and a social worker. She seems to have gotten her activist streak from her mom, who was always trying to improve her community, whether by organizing clothes swaps or other support for indigenous people or by guiding women who sought abortions to safe care when it was practically illegal.[5] If a law or policy was doing harm, she was taught that it was her job to fight against it.

As a single mother of three herself, Livingston came to Vancouver in 1993. She and her kids moved into a nonprofit mixed income co-op apartment in a building in the Downtown Eastside neighborhood. Since at least the nineties, this area has been a stark illustration of rising inequality, ten to twenty shrinking square blocks of concentrated poverty amidst ever-encroaching extreme wealth.

These days, luxury condos, high-end furniture stores, and upscale restaurants overlook streets filled with homeless people or others of little means. Even in broad daylight, some are visibly shooting up; some smoke crack; others are drunk or otherwise visibly disturbed, moving disjointedly as though in some seething dance. Some sell sex, some offer loose cigarettes, illegal drugs, or various assorted possessions, few of them valuable. It can be hard to tell who is high, who is withdrawing, who is struggling with symptoms of mental illness, and who is just odd or intensely stressed. The neighborhood is redolent of trauma—but also of spirited resistance to it.

Not long after she moved in, Livingston began to see people overdosing in the street, just steps away from her apartment. She called for help and was dismayed by the sluggishness of the official response. She started to invite street people, often homeless, to her place—sometimes to stay, which did not go over well with some of her neighbors. As she later told the panel in Edmonton, "My method of organizing was taught to me by my mother, which was, 'Oh, there's a community problem, why don't we do something about it?' And she invites the affected population over."

Livingston didn't realize that most people wouldn't even consider offering such a welcome to homeless folks, let alone those with addictions. "I was actually inviting drug users into my home, and it took many years of analysis to understand that that's a very powerful message to people who aren't invited into anyone's homes, ever," she said.

During this time, she began meeting with other local activists, who had also become concerned about the sheer numbers of people dying in the street from overdose and the rising toll of AIDS. Between 1991 and 1993, the overdose rate in Vancouver had tripled.[6] Within that short period, life-threatening overdose went from being a relatively rare event to a common experience that was killing hundreds of people. By 1997, nearly one in four of the city's roughly 10,000 injection drug users would be HIV-positive,[7] a rate that would hit 40 percent at its peak. Indigenous Canadians, who make up 6 percent of British Columbia's population,[8] were grievously overrepresented among the dead and the dying.

Vancouver didn't lack a syringe exchange program. One of the first—and for a while, the largest in North America—had been founded there by a former injector in 1988. It was even funded by the government. But this program insisted on a "one for one" exchange—in other words, in order to get a new needle, people had to first bring in an old one. There was also a limit on the total number that could be distributed. While extras could be obtained in some circumstances, this kept a limit on the supply—with the good intentions of both reducing needle litter and making frequent contact with participants.

And at first, the program did seem to keep HIV under control. A critical factor that helped was that it was already legal in Canada to buy needles at a pharmacy without a prescription. Along with these sales to users who could afford them, Vancouver's needle exchange kept rates of infection in the primarily heroin-injecting population low in the late eighties, at around 1 to 2 percent.

Unfortunately, two major factors changed by the early nineties. For one, the cocaine supply increased, which meant lower prices. Secondly,

rising pressure from gentrification shifted sex workers and the street cocaine scene into the same small area that had once been dominated by
heroin.[9] The virus took off in parallel with the comingling of these two
groups and the associated rise in cocaine smoking and injecting by heroin
users. To top it all off, methadone treatment was not easily accessible,
with many barriers to getting care.[10]

Pharmacology helps explain why the rise in cocaine use was so disastrous. People who inject heroin tend to do so around three or four times
a day; the drug's effects last for four to six hours and are calming and sa-
tiating. Cocaine, conversely, lasts just ten to twenty minutes at best when
smoked or injected, and each dose amps up excitement and desire for
more. This means that if, like I did, you have access to a big supply, you
can easily shoot up dozens of times a day.

As Wilson, who as a dealer had a similar experience, put it, "When I
was on a coke run, I'd go through a full box of needles a night, myself. Like,
what, am I going to make a hundred trips back and forth?"[11] And worse, because of cocaine's effects on desire, it can also increase risky sexual activity,
including sex work by those who finance their addiction that way.

Essentially, the curbs on the Vancouver needle supply meant that the
massive increase in injection frequency associated with cocaine led to
much more sharing—and this sharing occurred mainly among the poorest,
unsheltered users who were already at highest risk for infection. (Research
on this group was what had given American drug czar Barry McCaffrey
the basis for his misleading claims to President Clinton about syringe exchange spreading HIV.)

All around her, Livingston was seeing the death and illness that resulted. Her own neighbors and people she knew from community meetings
were overdosing or dying from AIDS. Through her activism, she became
involved with a poet named Bud Osborn, who had long, flowing locks and
looked like Oscar Wilde in an especially dissipated phase. Osborn had
fled from the U.S. in the 1970s to avoid the Vietnam draft. When he met
Livingston, he was homeless and addicted to heroin.

A shocking story that Osborn heard in 1997 spurred them both to
action. He had met a friend on the street, on her way to visit her family.
It wasn't going to be a happy reunion. The relatives were meeting to try

to figure out who could take in her cousin's small child. The boy's mother had overdosed. After his father found her dead, he hanged himself using the bedsheets where she'd lain, leaving the toddler looking on.[12] And this was far from the first family member that Osborn's friend had lost to overdose.

Osborn couldn't take it anymore. "That's enough, that's it—that is just too much death," he said. Along with Livingston and other activists, he organized a demonstration that stopped traffic in the Downtown Eastside. On July 15, 1997, around 200 demonstrators took over Main and East Hastings Street, a central intersection known for flagrant drug activity.

Flanked by dozens of IV drug users, they unfurled a banner across all six lanes. It read "The Killing Fields." After burning a set of what they saw as useless government reports on the crisis in a trash can in the middle of the street, the group marched to a nearby park. The organizers had stayed up much of the previous night hammering pieces of wood into crosses at a local carpentry shop. Now, they set up 1,000 of them in the grass, to represent those who had been lost in the past five years.

Spontaneously, people began writing the names of their dead, one by one, on each cross. Some were crying as they recalled the lives of loved ones they'd lost. The dramatic images of mourning, along with the earlier traffic disruption, made the media and politicians pay attention. During the demonstration, Osborn recited a poem he'd written for the occasion, which said in part, "And so we are all abandoned if one is abandoned/So we are all uncared for if one is uncared for."[13]

By that September, Livingston and Osborn had decided that a more permanent activist organization was needed. Via his connection to the needle exchange, Osborn had managed to get a seat on the local health board, where his role was to represent the views of street drug users to policy makers in city hall and other officials. He wanted to be sure he was conveying more than just his own concerns.

So Livingston posted signs in the park, asking people to attend a community meeting. On September 9, a few dozen turned out. Before long, they'd managed to wrangle some funding out of the health board and a space to meet at a local church. Soon they had a name: VANDU. And not long after that, in early 1998, they began developing a proposal for a place where people could go to get clean needles and inject safely, with medical supervision to prevent overdose and infections.

Over the next few decades, VANDU would win what can seem like unimaginable victories to Americans in harm reduction. Though it took years of battles, they won the right to open North America's first legal safe injection site in 2003. Then they fought all the way to Canada's Supreme Court to keep it running after national-level politicians tried to shut it down. They also pushed for a trial of heroin prescribing, which again became the first on the continent. That research began in 2005.[14]

But they didn't stop there. After the study was completed, VANDU won ongoing access to legal heroin for all who had taken part in it; the original plan had been to just leave participants to go back to the street, even though the research they'd participated in had shown that being able to get heroin in a known, regular pharmaceutical dosage had dramatically improved their health and quality of life.

VANDU also helped win expanded access to hydromorphone (Dilaudid), a prescription opioid around twice as strong as heroin, which had showed similar success as an alternate medication in the heroin trial. One stage of the research had been blinded so that injectors did not know whether they were receiving heroin or hydromorphone and—at least in those circumstances—they seemed to find the drugs equally acceptable.

But VANDU didn't just make specific or piecemeal changes. Along with supportive researchers, public health officials, and even some politicians, they were able to transform Vancouver's official drug policy and influence thinking on the issue across Canada and around the world. This began in 2001, when, with input from the group, the city adopted what it called a "four pillar" approach to dealing with drug issues. They were following the lead of Zurich, Switzerland, which had introduced the idea in 1989.[15] The first three pillars are the traditional ones: treatment, prevention, and law enforcement. The fourth and coequal pillar, however, is harm reduction—and the policy requires that all of the other strategies recognize that preserving the life and health of people who use drugs overrides other goals. As the document laying out the strategy states:

The principles of harm reduction require that we do no harm to those suffering from substance addiction, and that we focus on the harm caused by problematic substance use, rather than substance use per se.

Harm reduction involves establishing a hierarchy of achievable goals which, when taken step by step, can lead to a healthier life for drug users and a healthier community for everyone. It accepts that abstinence may not be a realistic goal for some drug users, particularly in the short term. Harm reduction involves an achievable, pragmatic approach to drug issues.[16]

So, what is the secret to VANDU's success? Some of it is down to the usual factors of having the right dedicated activists pick up the right cause at the right time with the right connections. Some of it is linked with being able to get financial support from health authorities and nonprofit groups. Some of it is due to VANDU having a transparent structure and process for decision-making, including its board, which protects it from being too dependent on any one member who could run into trouble.

But, surprisingly, one important thread that runs through sustainable drug user organizing—from the Dutch junkiebonden to VANDU—is providing initial small incentives for participation, like meals and stipends. That was what drew Dean Wilson in originally—and when I say small incentives, I mean small. In his case, it was three dollars Canadian, the amount that was then offered to people simply for showing up and staying through a meeting. Those selected to take on specific roles within the organization can be hired for paid positions; people who just attend a particular meeting can get quick cash, along with a free meal, simply for being there.

Wilson's involvement began in January of 2000, when he needed money to buy a bag of dope. Born in Winnipeg, Canada, he'd had a difficult childhood and started injecting heroin at twelve. He managed to go relatively straight in his twenties—becoming an IBM salesman with a kid and a four-bedroom house in a leafy suburb. But by 1996, he was re-addicted and living in a single room occupancy hotel on the Downtown Eastside, selling cocaine and getting high on his own supply.

On that winter day in 2000, he was short three dollars he needed to buy his "paper," as street bags of heroin are called in Vancouver. And so he and a friend walked into VANDU's church basement meeting space, which was especially crowded at the time. The group happened to be holding its annual elections for some of its paid positions.

"We walked into this room and there are 200 fucking junkies just going wild," he said.[17] These days, the group has approximately 2,000 voting members overall and dozens turn up regularly for meetings.[18] The funding that supports the stipends, meals, and meeting space comes mainly from the government, through its health agencies—just as it does for the Dutch junkiebonden. And similar to those groups, VANDU collaborates with health authorities, representing the voice of drug users on questions of policy that affect them.

At that first meeting, Wilson immediately set his romantic sights on Livingston. He told his friend, "I'm going to get that girl." Unfortunately, sitting behind them as he spoke was Osborn, the poet, who was Livingston's partner at the time. He warned Wilson off. Within several months, however, Wilson had become president of VANDU—and he hooked up with Livingston eventually, too.

Just as in other aspects of harm reduction, enticing people rather than coercing or hectoring them works best in spurring activism and improving health. While future activists may originally come for the money or the food or the needles or, yes, an attractive potential partner, over time they start to be motivated by the cause itself. As Osborn described it, "If we're off demonstrating, we're having board meetings, deciding what to do and thinking about what our actions could be . . . all that's taking you away from being totally fixed on 'I got to get a drug, I got to get a drug.'"[19]

Several other elements were also important to VANDU's success. For one, the obvious failure of the war on drugs had gotten the attention of the city's conservative mayor. He had met an American reform leader who helped introduce him to harm reduction and to American conservatives who supported more rational drug policy.[20] In the spring of 1998, he held a conference on the issue and learned for himself how European cities had begun working together to create and implement effective harm reduction. Amsterdam and Liverpool had led the way—but now there were many other continental examples. A harm reduction collaboration between municipal governments had helped spread these policies across Europe.

Ironically, one city in the collaborative—Zurich, Switzerland—was long used as a cautionary tale by American prohibitionists. They liked to talk about how the city's 1987 "Needle Park" experiment had turned into an orgy of violence, public injecting, dealing, and other crimes not long after the city decided to simply allow drug activity in the area in order to focus on fighting AIDS. "It had become a 'no go' area without law: people were shot, stabbed and thrown into the River Limmat," one author wrote.

The problem was that creating an island of legalization within a sea of prohibition attracted users, dealers, and criminals from all over Europe. But what drug warriors don't like to talk about is what happened next. In 1992, police rousted the drug scene from the park. It didn't go away, however, just reorganized nearby in an abandoned train station. During these years, Bern, the capital of Switzerland, was also facing similar problems. And so the cities decided to try a different tack.

Switzerland's injectors had been hit early and hard by HIV: transmission via needles accounted for half of the country's AIDS cases at the time. This meant that Bern had begun experimenting with safe injection facilities that offered syringe exchange as early as June of 1986. Their program, which became the first safe injection site in the world, originated as a coffee shop and drop-in center. At first informally, it tolerated injection—and then it began officially supervising it. Like Zurich's "four pillars," Bern's safe injecting site would be a model for Vancouver.[21]

But Switzerland didn't stop there. Swiss policy makers and physicians met with Liverpool's harm reductionists and visited John Marks's heroin prescribing clinic. Inspired by what they'd seen, in 1992, the Swiss federal government approved a large trial of heroin maintenance. Concurring with other data, the research found that not only did prescribed and supervised heroin consumption improve the health of users and reduce other drug use, it also helped stabilize people's lives and move them into more traditional treatment, including abstinence.

As before, fears that "enabling" addiction by providing heroin would lengthen disability or attract new users did not materialize. In 1997, more than two-thirds of Swiss voters rejected a referendum that would have banned heroin prescribing—and they again supported the policy by a similar margin in a 2008 vote (oddly, they simultaneously rejected marijuana legalization). And, along with expansion of methadone, heroin prescribing had dramatic results. Between 1991 and 2009, overdose death rates were cut in half. The number of new heroin users fell by 80 percent, and HIV rates fell by 65 percent.[22]

In the fall of 1998 in Vancouver, VANDU members and others[23] helped organize a second conference that served as a bookend to the mayor's event earlier that year. Experts from European cities that had led on harm reduction were invited to speak.

This conference was held in a large party tent outside in the same park where the crosses had been staked the previous year. It was a cold, rainy November day. But inside the tent were some 800 people, including the mayor, the drug squad, council members, local and national health officials, and local business owners. They were sitting among the drug users, other activists, and homeless people of the neighborhood. The *Vancouver Sun* marveled that a meeting of "often antagonistic groups" turned out to be "a remarkable scene full of mutual respect." As the organizers had hoped, listening to drab, gray, bureaucratic European mayors and police chiefs touting safe injection sites and heroin prescribing made the ideas seem far less radical and far more possible.

Another significant advantage that VANDU had in its organizing is that Vancouver is a relatively small city, with a population of just under 700,000. This made local politicians and health officials far more accessible than they are in larger cities, where just getting attention is much more difficult. Small-scale activism at the city level and below has been critical to harm reduction's spread; it's one more example of the power of the idea that activists should "think globally and act locally." It also didn't hurt that, because the overdose crisis had gotten so bad in Vancouver, there was real interest in hearing from foreign city officials who had faced similar problems and solved them.

After listening to their European counterparts, Vancouver's city government became far more open to the ideas being pushed by VANDU. Nonetheless, it would take ongoing lobbying for them to win the policies they wanted, particularly since the local Chinese community and real estate interests were adamantly opposed to efforts like safe injection facilities. VANDU members frequently attended city council meetings, often carrying a coffin or dressed as ghouls to emphasize the deadly nature of the ongoing crisis. They were as much of a thorn in the side of the city of Vancouver as ACT UP had been in New York. And like ACT UP, they got results.

Although the original proposal for a safe injection site had been put forward in the late nineties, it took a huge fight in order for it to finally come to fruition. While Canada does not have the Harrison Act and its legacy to contend with, it does have its own prohibitions. They had to be negotiated both legally and politically in order for Insite to open.

Before it did, VANDU, Livingston, and various members went through quite a few underground iterations, providing informal spaces for people to come in off the streets, take their drugs, and get medical attention if needed. Finally, a plan for a pilot site was included in the mayor's 2001 "Four Pillars" agenda. And, although there were bumps, the new mayor who was elected the following year also supported it. He was a former coroner who had attended the conference in the park. He'd actually made a campaign promise that he would ensure that the site would open in 2003.[24]

Then, however, the Americans tried to step in. The nonprofit that had been funded to launch Insite was asked to send staff to the American consulate. There, they were met by George W. Bush's deputy drug czar who told them that, regardless of the fact that Canada is a sovereign country, the U.S. would not allow a safe injection site. They listened—and then ignored the threat. Nothing happened.

As with much in activism and harm reduction, there were also many arguments over details. The researchers and health officials wanted a clean, hospital-like setting, while the users and activists wanted warm and homey. They compromised on a "hair salon" look. It has booths and mirrors that resemble a place where you might gossip with your barber or beautician—but there are also sterile medical surfaces and nurses watching. After people have completed their injections, however, they can stay in a more welcoming "chill out" room, complete with cushioned seats and a large, mainly purple mural by a local artist.

Moreover, in the same Hastings Street building, one floor above Insite—which is simply a contraction of the words "injection" and "site"—the group opened Onsite. Here, there are beds and medical support for people who want to kick opioids entirely and need a safe place to manage withdrawal symptoms. Help finding housing, mental health care, other addiction treatment, and additional services is available as well. These days, an average of about 1,000 people use the injection room each month. Since it opened in 2003, about 3 million injections have taken place at Insite—and not a single person has died of overdose there.[25]

IN OCTOBER 2018, I VISITED THE DOWNTOWN EASTSIDE TO MEET THE PEOPLE who had actually made user activism sustainable. Though writing a history of harm reduction had taken me on a tour of some of the most troubled and impoverished neighborhoods in the U.S., I was nonetheless shocked by overt and incongruous inequalities in Vancouver. Perhaps it was because I expected better from Canada, a place that, to an American at least, seems to have a far better social safety net, including, of course, national health care.

Still, I live in Manhattan, which has some pretty extreme inequities itself. Here at home, I've seen homeless people steps away from some of the most expensive real estate in the world. I've witnessed public injecting in San Francisco literally in the doorway of a high-priced department store. I've seen encampments under bridges in Philadelphia, which vary from relatively neatly organized to wildly chaotic and filthy. But nowhere else had I ever seen anything like Vancouver's sleek glass luxury towers with elegant balconies, literally looking down onto a street where dozens of people were openly injecting themselves, staggering around high or smoking crack.

Walking down Hastings Street, it would be easy to question how well harm reduction is actually working here. But I knew that what I couldn't see just by exploring the neighborhood were the risks that had been averted and the lives that have been and are being saved. Critically, people who have stabilized and recovered just aren't as visible: they blend back into the city and look just like anyone else. And the solidarity between activists and their neighborhood that produced VANDU and Insite and all the rest takes time to observe and experience. The surface is deceiving.

Between 1998, when VANDU started raising hell, and 2008—when Insite had been open for five years and the clinical trial of heroin had been ongoing for three—overdose death rates were cut by more than half. Treatment for HIV also made that illness far less deadly. But unfortunately, in around 2011, a new and far more rapidly deadly foe had hit the streets.

Like the U.S., Canada had increased its opioid prescribing for pain during the nineties and 2000s—and like us, they had a similar media and political freakout around overprescribing and began cutting the medical supply. Not surprisingly, in Canada the outcome was the same: addicted people and even some pain patients shifted to heroin when they could no longer access a safer medical supply. And, as in the U.S., that supply began to be contaminated with cheaper, stronger street fentanyl. It was another example of the "iron law of prohibition" in action.

When fentanyl and similar strong synthetic opioids first hit the Downtown Eastside, they caused the worst overdose crisis the city had ever seen. Back in the worst days of the "killing fields" demonstration, around 300 people had been dying annually of overdose in British Columbia, mainly in Vancouver. By 2019, that number was at 981.[26] Although VANDU and others had flooded the streets with naloxone, had created pop-up overdose prevention sites beyond Insite, and the health authorities had slightly increased heroin and hydromorphone prescribing, they hadn't been able to bring these resources to scale.

People who used Insite regularly were still much safer: no one was dying of overdose there. And no one who was enrolled in the heroin or hydromorphone prescribing programs was dying of overdose, either. But those programs weren't anywhere near able to meet the numbers in need. That's why Hastings Street looked the way it did when I visited—and it was also why a VANDU member whom I interviewed there was running for a seat on the City Council.

"Spike" Peachey had been one of the participants in Vancouver's heroin prescribing trials and was still receiving a prescription when we met.

He has long, dark brown hair and a mustache—and despite the heroin, at times seemed to almost vibrate with pain. His story was another that was full of heartbreaking reversals. He'd overcome an abusive childhood, kicked an earlier bout of addiction through abstinence, and become a successful computer programmer—only to be denied ongoing pain care after an accident that broke his legs, pelvis, hips, ribs, back, and skull.

After his medication was cut off, he returned to heroin, winding up on the street. While homeless, he used Insite to protect himself while injecting. But what really helped him get back on his feet was prescription heroin.

"It saved my life," he told me. The study in which he participated found that over the course of just six months, participants reduced their street drug use from several times a day to several times a month, if at all. It practically eliminated their participation in crime: they went from engaging in criminal acts nearly every other day down to once a month or less.

For him, recovery was a harm reduction experience of gradual improvement. "It didn't change immediately because I was in such a depression that it took several years of first being medicated and then just living in a stable environment," he said. He was part of VANDU's fight to ensure that heroin prescriptions were continued for trial participants, which was especially unnerving for him after his prior experience of being cut off from pain treatment.

Today, Peachey has an apartment and a new career training doctors about the stigma associated with addiction and pain. "Now I see a future. I have a life. I know that I have something to offer. I know that I have something very valid to offer," he said. It is impossible to listen to him and not be moved to do better.

In the sea of chaos around them, the Crosstown Clinic, where VANDU members and others get their heroin, and Insite are islands of safety. Outside, Hastings Street bustles with all that drug energy, interspersed with people just trying to get to work and the encroaching emblems of gentrification. But within Insite, nurses discreetly monitor people as they calmly inject in their mirrored stations. It is nothing like the rushed, sloppy technique you see people use outside, where, even if arrest is unlikely, there's still always a chance of an unwanted interruption and the potential loss of the experience people have risked so much to seek.

As Election Day in Canada approached during my visit, it struck me that Insite's injection booths actually look more like voting booths than anything else, which nicely reflects the messy democratic process that it took to obtain them.

Every injection taken at any one OPS is a chance to avoid Russian roulette with street drugs—and Insite and the pop-up sites VANDU and other activists have created nearby during the fentanyl crisis have reported hundreds of overdose reversals. But in the face of a poisoned drug supply, it's hard for them to keep up.

However, the confluence of VANDU's activism and COVID-19 may finally allow Vancouver to make change at the scale that is needed. When the pandemic struck, Vancouver's activists didn't hesitate to fight once again for their people. They had already been arguing that people who are addicted need access to safer drugs—not just a safe place to use potentially toxic substances.

The coronavirus added urgency to their pleas. During a pandemic, not only are people who use drugs at risk from the drugs themselves, they are also at risk of getting and spreading the disease while doing illegal transactions—and that also increases risk for everyone else around them. The pandemic itself had made the idea of harm reduction visible beyond the drugs field: early on, it was raised as a strategy to deal with the fact that it is unrealistic to expect people to completely avoid social contact for months on end. With pandemic isolation almost certain to increase harms like overdose, excess drinking and eating, and other potentially compulsive behaviors, it was an idea whose time had clearly come.

And so, because it is not illegal for Canadian doctors to prescribe drugs like opioids and stimulants to treat addiction, they began to do so. In March of 2020, the provincial health minister overseeing addiction care for British Columbia published safer supply guidelines for physicians and urged them to provide prescriptions to more patients.[27] That month, prescribing expanded to reach 600 people—and the number more than doubled by June.[28] By September, the policy had gone nationwide—with Prime Minister Justin Trudeau saying that he was "moving forward aggressively" on safe supply.[29] Because the pandemic itself had significantly increased stress—as well as creating variance in drug purity that itself can increase risk—overdoses had already risen substantially across the country by then.

Thanks to the activists of Vancouver, however, Canada was once again at the vanguard of harm reduction and compassionate care.

twenty-one

The American Challenge

OUISE VINCENT WAS FAST ASLEEP WITH HER TEENAGE DAUGHTER, SELENA, dozing next to her when a SWAT team in full combat gear burst into her bedroom. At the time, in September of 2013, Vincent was living in her mother's gracious suburban house in Greensboro, North Carolina. She was recovering from a crushed pelvis and a leg injury that she'd suffered in a hit-and-run accident—and running an underground syringe exchange program. Her mom, a seventy-year-old retired high school history teacher, still got up early every day to make breakfast. She was puttering around in the kitchen at 5:30 a.m. when the police arrived, so at least the family was spared having their door smashed to bits.

Louise has pale skin, long, almost-black hair, a husky, weathered voice, and an upbeat and comforting mien. The accident that disabled her had occurred on a country road, near the drug rehab where she'd worked as a counselor after completing its program. Though many who knew her past assumed that she must have been injured in a drug-fueled escapade, she'd actually been completely sober when she was run over and left to die on the side of the road. Fortunately, someone had found her. She remembers little other than crawling in a field—and waking up in a hospital.

The September after the crash, she was living at her mom's house, trying to recuperate and raise her daughter. The night before the SWAT raid, Selena, who was biracial and had a dazzlingly warm smile, had wanted some comfort. As she'd done much earlier in life, she snuggled up to her mom and eventually drifted off to asleep.

But now, the officers had their AR-15s drawn. They were shouting, using laser sights, and sweeping the bewildered women with blinding lights as they entered the bedroom. While the police were yelling and arresting Vincent, her mother dragged their dog, which was a large but friendly pit bull, downstairs. (This was another small mercy. Dogs are commonly shot during SWAT raids, with police fatally injuring around 500 pups a year during these arrests.[1])

Incredibly, around 20,000 SWAT raids are carried out annually[2]—and they kill and wound hundreds of innocent people, including children.[3] Most target drug crime, even when there is no evidence that violence has been involved. The March 2020 raid that killed paramedic Breonna Taylor is only one of the best known of many resulting catastrophes—but she is far from alone. Nearly two-thirds of these police home invasions target minorities, according to a study by the American Civil Liberties Union—and 79 percent are carried out to execute a search warrant, rather than deal with an active shooter or hostage situation that might genuinely require such a show of force.

Perhaps not surprisingly, the SWAT team was originally created by the same L.A. police chief who publicly advocated shooting casual drug users.[4] The use of such militarized tactics is another of the many ways that the war on drugs places a higher priority on its goal of supply reduction than it does on human life.

Vincent doesn't know why she was targeted in such an extreme way. She had been arrested previously for her needle exchange work. For at least a decade, she had run what was probably the largest underground syringe program in the South. But her prior encounters with law enforcement were nothing like this. The warrant cited "medical refuse" in her garbage—however, there were no syringes or controlled substances. She was also demonstrably being treated by a visiting nurse because of her injuries. The police also noted her past conviction for cocaine sales. She suspects a racist neighbor may have played a role as well: he frequently called the police if she had Black friends visiting, claiming, without evidence, that they were selling drugs. She also knows that if she herself had been Black, the raid might have had a much deadlier outcome.

Thankfully, however, no one was physically injured. And, despite their high-tech gear and the undoubtedly costly assault on Vincent's home, the cops' mission was fruitless. No one at the house was dealing, and no drugs were found. After being arrested and fighting through numerous legal hassles, Vincent was not convicted.[5] She continues to provide needles, naloxone, and support, all while working to politically organize current and former drug users.

The raid did have one salutary effect, however. It radicalized Vincent's mother, who had previously seemed to think that her daughter was exaggerating her claims of injustice, police brutality, racism, and other excesses related to drug policy. After years of feeling as though her pain and her life's work were being dismissed, Vincent felt heard. Finally, her mom was starting to understand why she was so driven to take on this cause.

Vincent's experience illustrates just some of the difficulties faced even now by harm reductionists, especially in the American South. In a climate of such heavy-handed law enforcement, trying to organize drug users is far more difficult than in Canada and Europe. Her story makes clear just how big a challenge they face. While criminalization is certainly a huge obstacle everywhere, the American drug war is among the most vicious and pervasive, creating hurdles in nearly every system supposedly meant to "help." Government—federal, state, and local—rarely wants to hear the voices of drug users—let alone pay them, even small sums, to provide perspective the way Canada and much of the European Union does. This makes creating and sustaining organizations led by users profoundly difficult.

Nonetheless, despite all of this, today Vincent is executive director of the North Carolina Survivors Union, which is basically an American version of the Dutch junkiebond—minus the government support. It both provides services like needle exchange and organizes users to fight for better policies. In 2019, the organization's annual budget was nearly half a million dollars, with funding from foundations like the Comer Family Foundation and George Soros's Open Society Institute, as well as from a manufacturer of hepatitis C drugs, which aims to promote treatment and prevention of that disease.[6]

Vincent also helps lead the affiliated national drug user activist organization, which is called the Urban Survivors Union (although it now includes rural and suburban chapters as well). In her case, the term "survivor" is an understatement and more than apt: she has persisted and succeeded despite the almost unspeakable damage the drug war has done to her and her family. These days, the group has at least forty-one local affiliates, up from five when it started, each with dozens to hundreds of members. Overall, it has over 3,000 members.

In North Carolina, the organization occupies a low-slung brick building in Greensboro. Vincent jokes that visitors don't know what to expect: some actually think that they sell drugs and call her up to try to buy them; others walk in suspecting that they will find some kind of drug-fueled orgy. "The police have tried to raid it," she said. "They're often very disappointed that we're just typing on the computer. I mean, there's the idea that we were just in here, clothes off, jumping from the [metaphorical] chandeliers."

The space has a warm, funky, welcoming atmosphere, with mismatched furniture including a well-worn brown leather couch. The wall behind it is painted with a black-and-white cityscape of twisty towers, with the words "Dare to Be Different" written within. Also prominent is a Grateful Dead lightning skull logo. There's a counter where people can check in and ask questions; a refrigerator with free sodas and snacks. Scattered throughout are posters with slogans like "Love is the Drug/There is no recovery from death/Support harm reduction," and "Nothing about us without us."

Throughout the day, people come in to get needles and naloxone, and some stick around to wait for support group meetings or just hang out. One man, a veteran, asks if someone could accompany him to the VA hospital because he is not feeling safe enough to get there on his own. One of the volunteers walks out with him to help.

It's illegal for NCSU to knowingly allow injecting in the bathroom—and there's a sign on the door to that effect. However, it's also nearly impossible to completely prevent, so they have a door that opens outward and locks from the outside rather than the reverse. This way, if someone does OD, they will not need to break down the door to be able to save a life.

VINCENT'S RUN-IN WITH THE SWAT TEAM WAS FAR FROM HER FIRST ENCOUN-
ter with the brutality of the drug war, and it would not be her last. Raised
by academic parents, she had a happy, middle-class childhood until ado-
lescence hit, along with what she later learned was bipolar disorder. "However mental illness works, whatever light switch got kicked on in my brain,
it happened then," she said. At twelve or thirteen, she began using drugs,
and within months, her parents sent her away to an abusive wilderness
program, with filthy, punishing conditions and humiliation as "therapy."
For many years, her family's response to her problems was almost always
tough love and rejection.

By 2006, she was a single mother. After various rehabs, medications,
and diagnoses, she managed to complete college and began working toward getting a master's in public health. At the time, she was abstinent
and militant in her support for twelve-step programs. She now sees her
rigidity as a reaction—she says she felt she had to convince others that it
was the "one true way" in order to keep herself convinced, especially as
she learned about other approaches in her reading and classes.

Nonetheless, she tentatively supported the idea of needle exchange.
Wanting to find out more about it, she contacted the North Carolina Harm
Reduction Coalition. That group had received grants to promote—but was
not legally able to provide—syringe exchange in the state. Through them,
she met harm reductionist Thelma Wright. And yes, Thelma and Louise
then became a team.

Soon Wright had arranged for Vincent to attend a syringe exchange
conference organized by Seattle's Dave Purchase. She also visited the needle exchange in Atlanta, which is the largest aboveground program in the
South. After that, there was nothing ambivalent at all about her embrace
of harm reduction. She was home.

"I'd never seen a real needle exchange operating. I'd only read about
it and talked about it. It was all just sort of ideas," Vincent said. But what
she saw in one of the most distressed areas of Atlanta, a neighborhood
known as the Bluff, convinced her. "I really saw love and grace. And in that
moment, all the questions I had just went away."

Wright hired Vincent almost immediately after they met. "It was an im-
pulse hire," Vincent jokes. Together, they began running an underground

syringe exchange in North Carolina, starting in around 2008. Wright, who is Black, and Vincent, who is white, were able to reach across user communities that are sometimes isolated, even from each other.

WHILE THERE HAVE BEEN MANY ATTEMPTS TO START A NATIONAL USERS' UNION or a network of them in the United States—going back at least to the first harm reduction conference in 1996—it has been difficult to sustain them. The one that Vincent now helps lead—the Urban Survivors Union (USU)—was born as a local group in Seattle in 2009.

It went national starting at a meeting in Denver in October 2013, which was where Vincent first got involved. When she arrived in the Mile High City in her wheelchair, she was barely hanging on—it was not long after the SWAT raid on her mom's house. And she was in constant pain due to her leg injury, which wasn't healing properly.

But the support she got there from her fellow user activists is what sustained her—and it's what still carries her now. Among them, she feels welcome and at home. "We love you for who you are and we understand who you are," is how she describes their embrace and the sense she continues to take from it of the importance of bringing this hope to others.

Vincent would require all the support she could get from this community she was helping to create. For one, her doctor was refusing to provide adequate pain treatment—even though her injury was visibly profoundly painful and she did not misuse the small doses that she was allowed. "He was being really hateful," she said of the physician's response to her desperate pleas for mercy. In a misguided attempt to "protect" her abstinent recovery from risk related to drug exposure, she was left in agony that destroyed it.

Vincent descended into a pitiless, unrelenting depression, eventually buying heroin again. The shame that she felt over doing so meant that she sometimes refused to seek medical attention even as her wounded leg worsened. At other points, it was Vincent who was rejected by doctors and expelled from care: her mental illness sometimes made her unreliable about keeping appointments.

By the time she was able to re-engage with the medical system and get methadone treatment, she'd developed an antibiotic-resistant infection that caused her to lose one eye, and nearly her life. Then, in 2016, her leg had to be amputated—again, a surgery that could have been prevented if she'd been given appropriate and compassionate care for her injury consistently from the start.

Her daughter Selena's life also swerved out of control as Louise's health declined. Like Louise, Selena had begun showing symptoms of bipolar disorder as puberty hit—and, similarly, she had also started using drugs. Louise knew intimately how risky this could be, and it worried her tremendously. But she certainly wasn't going to use the "tough love" approach that hadn't helped her and, in fact, had made her own teenage life hell. At the same time, she knew how impulsive and reckless she had been at Selena's age. She thought a respite, somewhere safe, even if temporary, might buy some time for her to grow.

Consequently, she was much relieved when she was able to persuade her daughter to go to a rehab. Together, they chose what seemed like the nicest facility they could afford, which was on the West Coast. "Finally, I could relax for a minute. She was safe,"[7] Louise recalled thinking.

But then, in one of the cruelest twists of fate imaginable, Selena died from an overdose while in rehab. The center—unlike Louise's program, which had trained Selena in overdose prevention—did not stock naloxone. "If someone else in rehab had overdosed with her there, she could have saved them. She had the knowledge and skills," Vincent said, with fury and pain evident in her voice. Instead, the phantom fear that stocking naloxone at a rehab might "enable" relapse had enabled yet another death. Selena was only nineteen years old.

When Louise first heard this unbearable news, she broke down. She couldn't imagine how she could endure it. She certainly wanted to check out, at the very least temporarily. However, when she called the friend who usually sold her heroin, he refused to supply her. "Girl, I don't think this is safe for you," she recalls him saying, "I don't want you to die." And so she made it through that night. And then the next.

The ensuing weeks were much harder to take. Vincent knew no one would blame her if she "accidentally" overdosed. But, as she put it, "The

work wouldn't let me stop. I had created a monster that required feeding."
Harm reduction, for her, was bigger than addiction—and a balm for grief.

For one, she knew that the local needle exchange wouldn't be able
to continue without interruption without her. She also knew that if she
stopped providing naloxone, preventable overdose deaths would rise.
She'd already heard from many people she'd given it to about how they'd
used it to save lives. And she herself had, by then, reversed many ODs;
one had even been captured in a cell phone video, which had aired on
CNN's *Sanjay Gupta, MD* show.[8] In the clip, she helps revive a woman
who is seen coming back from a close brush with death that had left her
ashen and barely breathing.

Vincent agonized. Her daughter's death filled her with self-hate. She
knew it was irrational to blame herself, but she couldn't help feeling she
should have been able to do something more to prevent it. Still, even if
she hadn't been able to save her daughter, she clearly had saved other
people's children. And she could continue to do so, if she could only keep
going.

Over time, through her grief, she came to see that after years of feeling
rejected, isolated, unwanted, and unloved, she had finally found her place.
At the organization she'd created, she had community, purpose, and passion. She still hurt. She would never get over losing Selena, but this was
something to live for. She would survive this, too.

As of 2019, the NCSU had distributed nearly 3,500 naloxone kits—
and 1,629 people reported back that they had used their kits to save a life.
The group has distributed more than 500,000 needles—most of which
are returned or otherwise properly disposed of.[9] They also have support
groups, such as an "Any Positive Change" group where people can share
experiences and get help with improvements they want to make in any
aspect of their lives, not limited to drugs.

In fact, at the one I visited, no one talked about substance use at all;
the conversation centered on relationships and loss. Around ten people
attended, with one talking about how a friend died in the gutter outside
his own home, because his family was practicing tough love and had told

him to leave. Although some people were visibly intoxicated, no one was disrespectful, and everyone followed the rules about when to speak. It felt soothing. It had the same kind of welcoming warmth that I'd felt in many twelve-step meetings.

NCSU has also been successful in its activism: along with allies, they lobbied for legislation that legalized needle exchange in North Carolina in 2016, finally allowing them to do what they had done underground for eight years, without fear of arrest. They also won legislation that prevents police from charging people with drug possession if residue is found in syringes, so long as they tell the police that they are carrying needles.

Vincent, NCSU, and USU have also led numerous public information and media efforts, fighting back against stigma and dehumanization. One of their cleverest efforts is an initiative against prosecutions for what has become known as "drug-induced homicide." In these cases, people who have sold, given, or even just shared drugs with someone who has overdosed are charged with murder.

The rise in these prosecutions is a sign that support for the war on drugs isn't entirely dead yet. Although most of the political rhetoric during the opioid crisis has called for reduced incarceration and shorter sentences, these new state laws and increased use of pre-existing laws take policy in the opposite direction. A May 2018 investigation by the *New York Times* found more than 1,000 drug-induced homicide arrests or prosecutions were carried out between 2015 and 2018, with the number of these cases doubling between 2015 and 2017 alone.[10]

It's like a bait and switch: while drug reformers and harm reductionists are pushing to reduce or eliminate mandatory minimum sentences for possession and dealing, these prosecutions provide a way to keep the prisons full by calling the crime that garners the long prison term murder, rather than dealing or possession. And of course, there's no evidence that locking the same people up for long periods of time under a different label could make lengthy prison terms effective. We already know that sentencing users and dealers to fifteen to life for drug crimes doesn't work; changing the name of their crime isn't going to fix that.

In fact, this specific policy probably makes the situation even worse. That's because these prosecutions also undo any real protection provided by "Good Samaritan" laws, which are intended to exempt people from prosecution for drug possession if they call for help during an overdose. Being spared prosecution for drug possession but remaining eligible to be charged with murder instead isn't exactly going to make people more likely to seek needed help.

USU aims to stop these prosecutions, with its "Reframe the Blame" campaign. Pointing out that the vast majority of overdose victims have also sold drugs to friends or shared them, the group suggests that these prosecutions simply make two tragedies out of one, without doing anything at all to reduce harm or addiction. The heart of the campaign is a form the group created, humorously labeled a "Do Not Prosecute" order. Modeled on efforts to allow dying people to take charge of their medical care, this is an advance directive aimed instead at law enforcement. It says that, in the case of the signatory's accidental overdose death, they do not want their friends or dealers prosecuted.

"The idea originated with drug users sitting around talking, saying, 'I love my friends and I love the people I hang out with and I don't want anybody going to jail because of my behavior . . . How can I make sure this doesn't happen?'" said Vincent. Introduced in 2018, it has gotten media coverage from *VICE* to the *New Yorker,* and more than 5,000 people have now signed on.

User activism, like the rest of harm reduction, is finally starting to take off now in a way that it never has before in America. "We're doing beautiful, beautiful things," Vincent said. "We have drug users who are building services and growing, and I am growing and I'm growing with my friends and partners. And that is not a place I ever thought I'd be, but we have to do more. We cannot fight for harm reduction and not fight for racial justice. We cannot fight for harm reduction and not fight for disability justice. We cannot fight for harm reduction, and not have an intersectional response. We cannot do this alone."

Vincent also recognizes how important being involved in activism has been to her mental health and ability to manage her drug use. "I've had so many people I love die," she said. "My daughter died of overdose. I can't imagine what I would do if I wasn't fighting the drug war. And if I wasn't involved in a drug user movement. This is absolutely what creates and keeps my connection to life and gives purpose."

She adds, "The drug user rights movement is about human connection and resiliency to me. So it's about fighting back. It's about us. It's about people understanding and seeing the truth and refusing to just buy the lie. I think it really is about taking control and changing the narrative. Drug user rights are human rights."[11]

twenty-two

Redoing the Future

NEW YORK IMPOSED ITS COVID-19 LOCKDOWN ON MARCH 20, 2020, as we caught our first glimpse of the virus's vicious potential. All non-essential businesses were shut, schools and universities closed, and everyone was ordered to stay home whenever possible. We hoarded toilet paper and lentils. We cheered our health care workers nightly at seven p.m. with shouts and percussion. We were sad that we couldn't harmonize from balcony to balcony like the Italians did—or at least I was. Sirens screamed across most of the city, but in my neighborhood, which is filled with medical centers, it was often eerily quiet. There was no traffic, and therefore no need for ambulances to screech to get cars to move aside.

No one yet knew exactly how the virus spread—and the emphasis at first was on cleaning surfaces and handwashing, rather than wearing masks. But soon it became obvious that we could not sustain a lifestyle in which we had to presume every single item and person outside our household was a deadly threat. We needed to know what activities actually did carry the highest risk and what measures best reduced that danger. We needed to know when to be most vigilant and when we could ease up a bit. Basically, we needed harm reduction.

And, to my delight—in a time of very little delight—the concept began to be discussed almost everywhere. No longer framed as "controversial," harm reduction was mainly presented as an accepted part of public health—and one that could allow both individuals and policy makers to manage what was already starting to feel unmanageable. For example, a

May op-ed in the *Washington Post* described the origins of harm reduction in HIV prevention for injectors, noting that it faces "the reality that if a behavior with harmful consequences is going to happen regardless, steps should be taken to reduce the risk for both individuals and others around them." The author, Dr. Leana Wen, former health commissioner of Baltimore, argued that, similarly, people will need harm reduction tools to allow them to make better choices around COVID risks.[1]

In *The Atlantic* at around the same time, Harvard epidemiologist Julia Marcus wrote that requiring people to abstain from most social contact indefinitely is not realistic—and that harm reduction makes more sense. "Risk is not binary," she explained. "And an all-or-nothing approach to disease prevention can have unintended consequences."[2] Requiring perfection in COVID risk-taking behavior can backfire, just as it does with other types of abstinence, as people simply give up entirely on attempting to reduce risk. Alan Marlatt's "abstinence violation effect" has been amply demonstrated across multiple types of behavior. Not surprisingly, once people believe that they've already blown it, they tend to stop bothering with further efforts to protect themselves. With the coronavirus, this could be deadly—and as with HIV, not only to one person, but to others they might infect.

In September, former ACT UP member and now assistant professor of epidemiology at Yale Gregg Gonsalves interviewed Anthony Fauci, who has led the National Institute for Allergy and Infectious Disease since the early days of AIDS. The two former sparring partners—scientist and activist-turned-scientist—discussed managing COVID risks. Explaining that he was visualizing his experience over the years with HIV, Fauci said, "I'm flashing in my mind . . . [on] how difficult it is for society to accept harm reduction . . . And then when you accept it, you realize, why didn't I do this before?"

That's a question nearly everyone in the movement has long asked. At many times, it has seemed as though no progress was being made—or, worse, that we were taking three steps back for every tiny move forward. And yet when you look at the trajectory over the last thirty-two years— since Edith Springer first met Liverpool's Allan Parry and brought the harm reduction movement to America in 1988—the advances are clear. A philosophy and strategy developed by drug users and researchers for drug users, however improbably, had gone global—and proved to be a gift to public health.

The change is both qualitative and quantifiable. In 1988, without even studying the issue, Congress had voted overwhelmingly to ban federal funding for syringe exchange on moral grounds. At the time, only six tiny programs were known to be operating in the entire country: three underground sites run by Jon Parker on the East Coast; the underground exchange in San Francisco; Dave Purchase's Tacoma health department–approved program; and New York City's doomed pilot study. All faced organized national opposition claiming that they "sent the wrong message" during a war on drugs supported by 90 percent of the population.[3]

As of 2019, however, there were nearly 300 exchanges across the country[4]—and the federal ban has been lifted, at least with regard to paying for all services and items needed other than the syringes themselves. Now known as "syringe service programs"—to emphasize that they do more than exchange needles—they are mainly seen as just another evidence-based public health tool. In conjunction with states' legalization of nonprescription needle sales and possession, syringe service programs are believed to be responsible for the 80 percent reduction in new HIV infections among drug users that occurred between the late eighties and the mid 2000s.[5]

Aside from the silly ban on funding the actual needles, federal agencies like the CDC and NIDA support and promote these programs as a key part of an effective response to blood-borne disease, opioid addiction, other injection drug use, and overdose. While there is often NIMBY opposition, even archconservative Indiana governor and later Trump vice president Mike Pence has been forced to accept them to protect health. Consequently, many state and local health agencies now have employees or even departments with the phrase "harm reduction" in their titles or job descriptions.

Another indicator of progress is the spread of naloxone. In 1988, it was prescription-only and rarely used outside of medical settings. Despite its lifesaving potential, no one was pushing change. But by 2019, thanks to Dan Bigg and many others, at least 600 groups were distributing it across the country. It is also available by mail order and from many health departments and can be purchased at pharmacies. Forty-nine states have now legalized over-the-counter naloxone sales—and the market for the drug is estimated at $290 million annually. As I write in early 2021, the FDA is considering a requirement that naloxone be co-prescribed with opioid prescriptions, regardless of whether they are written for pain or for addiction treatment.[6]

Moreover, there is near universal endorsement of naloxone availability among parent groups and state, national, and local health authorities. Cops often carry and use it frequently. While occasional cranks call for cutting off people who have had multiple overdoses, demagoguing the issue isn't the clear win that attacking needle exchange was for politicians. Blocking a lifesaving tactic to "send a message" is no longer a cheap way to prop up the culture war. Today, there is wide and organized resistance that cannot be silenced or dismissed as "pro drug." People with addiction are starting to be seen as part of "us," not "them."

The undoing of the drug war can also be seen in the rise of cannabis legalization. Recreational sales and use are now legal in fifteen states, which makes the drug legal for a full third of the American population. Thirty-five states now permit medical marijuana. In 2020 alone, New Jersey, Arizona, Montana, and South Dakota fully legalized, and Mississippi opted to allow medical marijuana.[7] It is hard to imagine that New York, Pennsylvania, and Connecticut will let their neighbors monopolize one of the few new bright spots for tax revenue for long. Indeed, the governors of all three states are pushing for legalization in 2021. If they succeed, this would bring the total to 40 percent of Americans with legal access.

If the tipping point for federal legalization hasn't already been reached, it's coming soon. National support for cannabis legalization is at an all-time high: 68 percent, according to Gallup's fall 2020 poll, up from just 12 percent in 1970. And, for the first time ever, the House voted, 228–164, to remove marijuana from the "Schedule One" category that makes it illegal on the federal level. In their remarks on their civil rights achievements for the year, House Democrats proudly listed the passage of this legislation, further cementing the alliance between racial justice and drug policy reform that Michelle Alexander had helped inspire. While President Joe Biden favors only decriminalization of possession, Democratic Senate Majority Leader Chuck Schumer is pushing for full legalization. The winds are in their favor.

Criminalization of other substances is also starting to be undone. In 2020, Washington, D.C., ended criminal penalties for possession of psychedelic drugs like LSD and psilocybin. Meanwhile, a program that allows police to end repeat arrests for drug possession, sex work, and shoplifting—known as Law Enforcement Assisted Diversion (LEAD)—is now in fifty-one jurisdictions in twenty-one states, including the cities of Los Angeles, New Orleans, and Atlanta, with many more sites planned. Co-created by a long-time harm reductionist, LEAD essentially decriminalizes drugs for its participants, while providing voluntary access to services like housing and treatment. It also explicitly introduces police to harm reduction ideas.[8]

But it was the state of Oregon that made the most significant legal change in the U.S. in 2020. It went far beyond decriminalizing marijuana and psychedelics—and way past LEAD's programs, which offer decriminalization only to some. Via a ballot initiative supported by the Drug Policy Alliance, Oregon entirely decriminalized possession of personal use amounts of all drugs within the state. People caught with small quantities of cocaine, heroin, or other substances no longer face criminal penalties. Instead, they can choose between accepting a one-time assessment of treatment and other health needs at an independent center designed to do such evaluations or paying a $100 fine.

The policy is modeled on that of Portugal, which decriminalized all drugs and significantly expanded treatment in 2001. Soon the country saw dramatic reductions in HIV infections and AIDS cases, and overdose deaths, as well as some decline in teen use. Adult use increased slightly—but no more than it did in comparable European countries that did not decriminalize.[9]

Notably, in Oregon's new system, "treatment" is broadly construed—options include harm reduction programs like syringe exchange, as well as access to other resources, like housing and employment assistance. However, even if someone rejects further participation, there is no punishment, nor are people penalized if they try treatment and decide to leave. It is the most progressive drug policy enacted in recent American history—and goes far beyond the still-criminalized frameworks of earlier reform initiatives in California and Arizona. Other states are already considering similar moves.

Oregon's legislation also provides funding for treatment and for the new assessment centers, which will be overseen by a group that includes drug users and other affected people themselves, as well as experts. It requires that treatment provided be evidence based. This initiative is a significant win for harm reduction—and it passed with 58 percent of the vote.[10]

Even better, in the aftermath of Joe Biden's election victory, nearly every major media analysis noted that while the country remains deeply divided on many issues, drug policy reform is a rare area of bipartisan agreement. All of the 2020 drug reform initiatives, in both red and blue states, passed—typically by margins greater than those of the presidential candidate who won the state.

Thanks to harm reduction, decriminalization of drug possession has gone from being seen as a fringe idea that "sends the wrong message" to, increasingly, being considered a matter of common sense. These days, no one can make a good argument for caging people for substance possession, especially when faced with these harsh realities: jail doesn't treat addiction successfully; within jail, treatment is rarely available; incarceration increases overdose death risk; arrest is not a good way to determine who most needs care; and criminalization wastes enormous amounts of money that might otherwise fund effective help.

Illustrating this trend, in 2018, the Chief Executives Board of the agencies of the United Nations endorsed decriminalization—following a report from its usually hardline anti-drug agency which said that possession arrests do not help and can cause harm.[11] Moreover, in 2020, the U.N. removed marijuana from its category of dangerous drugs without medical uses, though it continues to ban recreational use. We are truly starting to undo the toxic idea of "drugs"—and the vicious war that targeted certain users of some substances. But much more change is needed.

Kassandra Frederique, who started as an intern at the Drug Policy Alliance in 2009 and became its executive director in 2020, led the fight for the Oregon initiative. The first Black woman to run DPA, Frederique described experiencing the rise of Black Lives Matter as she fought for decriminalization on the state level. "It was really exciting," she said. "Everyone's talking about divestment, and 'We shouldn't spend all this money on criminal justice, we need to spend it on healthcare.' And we're like, 'We're doing this! We're doing this in Oregon!' And then to win . . ."

In fact, the embrace of harm reduction by Black Lives Matter and its extraordinary presence on the streets throughout the year is another crucial development in the history of the movement. From the start, BLM has recognized that the war on drugs is central to the way that police currently dodge charges of racism to justify their violence. The horrific death of George Floyd in Minneapolis on May 25, 2020—which galvanized the largest activist movement in recent history—could not be a clearer example. In behavior that shocks the conscience, Officer Derek Chauvin murdered Floyd by kneeling on his neck for nearly nine minutes. During these agonizing moments, his accomplice, Officer Tou Thao actually joked with bystanders. "This is why you don't do drugs, kids," he said.[12]

Let that remark in those circumstances sink in for a minute. Without invoking explicit racism, Thao was attempting to rationalize Chauvin's life-threatening violence, framing it as "anti-drug" and therefore acceptable. To make the connection even more blatant, when attorneys for the police tried to defend their actions, again they blamed drugs. Chauvin, the lawyers claimed, didn't actually kill Floyd. It was the fentanyl and methamphetamine in his blood that had done it—causing an overdose or some other deadly pharmacological response, which, by sheer coincidence, occurred at the same time that the Black man was under the cop's knee.[13] Implicit in this statement and others related to Floyd's history of illegal drug use is the idea that it disqualifies him as a person—and that, as someone who took drugs, he deserved maltreatment, even death.

The use of drug war tropes to dehumanize people and deflect recognition of racism has been a central element in nearly all of the police killings of Black people that have provoked recent outrage; most notably, the SWAT raid that killed Breonna Taylor. The twenty-six-year-old EMT did not use or sell drugs but was killed in an absurdly overzealous attempt to take down her ex-boyfriend. Around the same time that her home was being invaded, her ex was quietly arrested elsewhere without incident—and without such a show of force, despite the fact that he was the presumed target. Meanwhile, she was shot to death as her current partner tried to defend her from assailants who hadn't clearly identified themselves as police and did not seek immediate help for their victims.

Black Lives Matter stood up in protest. And this movement will not accept a "drug exception to the Constitution." It refuses to allow the lives of Black people, regardless of drug use, to be devalued. BLM's multiracial demonstrations across the country and the visibility these actions gave to police killings have also spread the word about harm reduction. This activism, along with horrifying videos of deaths like Floyd's, has made real inroads into white indifference. Many whites who had not previously recognized systemic racism began to see the depth of the injustice it creates as well as the enabling role of the drug war.

To reform the system, BLM activists worked with other groups in a coalition called the Movement for Black Lives to create and promote legislation that it aptly labeled the "BREATHE Act." Sponsored by Congresswomen Ayanna Pressley and Rashida Tlaib, it calls for national drug decriminalization. The BREATHE Act would shift funds away from police and prisons to health-focused responses to mental illness and addiction. It would ban no-knock SWAT raids, increase harm reduction services, and abolish the DEA, among many other measures. It is a radical break with the past. Drug arrests are "a nexus of policing in America," said Frederique, adding that, "If we want to fundamentally take away one of the tools that police used to exploit communities of color, we have to decriminalize drugs."

The work of harm reduction activists, Michelle Alexander, and others to connect drug policy reform to other movements for legal reform and racial justice has coalesced during the rise of the Movement for Black Lives. Led by Black people, this powerful alliance will likely fuel positive change for many years to come.

THE INFLUENCE OF HARM REDUCTION IS NOW BEING SEEN ACROSS MANY OTHER aspects of American culture. In a potent symbolic development, the 1980s organization that was born as the advertising industry's anti-drug effort, the Partnership for a Drug-Free America, has now become the Partnership to End Addiction. Previously known for its stigma-generating spots—notably, the frying egg image captioned, "This is your brain on drugs. Any questions?"—it was once among the staunchest pillars of the drug war and sometimes literally showed people who use drugs as demons in its ads. But today, it advises parents on compassionate ways of preventing and treating addiction. This reflects an enormous shift. The goal is no longer the impossible ideal of a world without consciousness-altering substances, but instead, to try to fight the genuine damage associated with addiction.

On a much lighter note, pop culture also reflects the rise of harm reduction. In the hit 1994 film *Pulp Fiction*, a gangster's moll played by Uma Thurman was revived from a heroin overdose by a ludicrous underground procedure in which adrenaline was injected straight into her heart with a preposterously large needle. This unfortunately created a new street myth about overdose reversal—rather than illustrating the genuinely dramatic results of the real treatment.

More recently, however, twenty-first-century films like one of Tyler Perry's *Madea* sequels and TV series like HBO's teen drug drama *Euphoria* accurately portray—in positive ways—the use of naloxone to reverse overdose. Meanwhile, crime dramas have gone from drug war porn like *Miami Vice* (1984–1989) to the gritty realism of *The Wire* (2002–2008), which actually included a plotline about a neighborhood-level attempt at legalization and harm reduction. The disgraceful reality show *Cops*, which often glorified officers making low-level drug arrests, ran for thirty-two seasons starting in 1989. It was finally canceled this year, basically by Black Lives Matter.

But as is often the case with reform movements, harm reduction's rise has not been linear. Along the way, there have also been some stunning setbacks. One of the saddest was seen in Liverpool, which went from leading the world movement in the late eighties to being made to follow the British conservative government's abstinence-focused "recovery agenda," in 2010.[14] Although Merseyside's downfall probably began when John Marks started getting international media attention for his radical prescribing way back in the nineties, the situation became much worse in the late 2000s, when the Tories returned to power.

Overall, Great Britain went from being far more progressive than America in most aspects of drug policy to being so regressive that medical marijuana access is highly limited and recreational legalization isn't even really on the radar. Incredibly, Scotland, which has long had an uneasy relationship with harm reduction, now has an overdose death rate that is as high by some measures as that in the U.S. Since 2015, a rise in homelessness and increased cocaine injecting has also resulted in dozens of new HIV infections in Glasgow.[15] Fortunately, a new generation of activists is fighting back, pushing the government to allow supervised injection at overdose prevention sites.

But sadly, by its very nature, harm reduction will never be able to save everyone. After all, the idea begins with the pragmatic acceptance that while harm can be minimized, eradicating risk-taking is impossible and probably not even desirable. And so, during the fentanyl era—when many harm reductionists who had survived the AIDS years were only just beginning to address the resultant trauma—another spate of deaths began. In the U.S., fentanyl and similar synthetics, which were once seen only occasionally and in a few geographic regions, have now spread across the entire country. And these street drugs are exponentially more likely to cause overdose death compared to heroin or medical opioids.

One of the most tragic losses was that of Dan Bigg, who died from an overdose in 2018. He was at home, apparently attempting to cope with his chronic insomnia. He seemed fine at the time his wife went to bed. But while the early days of naloxone distribution were filled with triumph, street synthetics present a much more difficult challenge than heroin and most prescription opioids. They can kill rapidly, leaving far less time for successful intervention. Bigg died that night from a mixture of drugs that included a type of fentanyl. He was found dead the next morning.[16]

As gay men who survived the AIDS crisis learned, sometimes the impact of trauma is not apparent for many years. Frequently, the damage only becomes visible when people face new, severe stresses. For example, many gay men who hadn't previously had drug problems turned to methamphetamine in middle age, in part as a response to all of the loss they'd experienced. A similar phenomenon—especially in people who have been in the field for many years—may now be occurring among harm reductionists trying to deal with fentanyl.

Although only some were lost to overdose or HIV-related illness, the early deaths of pioneer harm reductionists like Bigg, Yolanda Serrano, John Paul Hammond, Dave Purchase, Alan Marlatt, John Watters, Imani Woods, Keith Cylar, Renee Edgington, and far too many others have made the field's genuine and significant successes bittersweet for many survivors.

The fentanyl crisis has also made overdose reversal much more challenging. Treating a fentanyl overdose not only requires a quicker response, but often, a higher dose of naloxone. To make matters worse, sometimes, fentanyl temporarily paralyzes the victim's chest, which interferes with rescue breathing. All of this makes helping far more stressful than it used to be. In many places, rescuers are being traumatized by the sheer volume of overdoses, the constant fear of not getting there in time, and the loss of those who they are unable to reach. Some are even faced with horrifying choices when there are multiple overdoses but only a limited amount of naloxone.

This has bolstered the fight for overdose prevention sites (OPS) where medical care and abundant naloxone are readily available. And there is some good news here. While the fierce opposition to needle exchange in the eighties and nineties meant that cities that allowed them typically did so quietly and grudgingly, today there is actually a race among at least a half dozen cities to be the first to open one in the U.S. These include New York City and Ithaca in New York, as well as Seattle, San Francisco, and Denver. In many of them, leading politicians have spoken out in support—in huge contrast to their outright opposition or silence on syringe exchange.

Nationally, President Biden has said that he supports harm reduction, but he has not taken a position on overdose prevention sites. But, in one more sign of progress, the 2020 Democratic presidential debates were almost a mirror image of those in the nineties, with candidates this time trying to show how reformist they are, rather than how reactionary. All but Biden came out for total marijuana legalization, all spoke out against mass incarceration, and both Elizabeth Warren and Bernie Sanders advocated for overdose prevention sites. The Democratic party no longer reflexively favors the drug war—and President Biden's compassionate response to his son's addiction suggests that he, too, may at last be ready for change.

But the winner of the American OPS race so far is Philadelphia. In 2020, the City of Brotherly Love won a lawsuit filed against it by the U.S. Department of Justice, which claimed that allowing supervised injection would violate the 1986 "crackhouse" law—ironically, one of Joe Biden's signature drug war measures. That legislation bans landlords and renters from allowing drug use on their properties. Prosecutors argued that this meant that health officials could not supervise injections to prevent overdose, either.[17]

Fortunately, the judge disagreed. Unfortunately, this decision was reversed on appeal. But now that Biden is president, his attorney general will have the option of simply dropping the lawsuit, which would allow Philadelphia to move forward. Activists are pressing for them to do just that.

And if they succeed, many other cities are likely to follow suit. One observer joked that the real race to open an overdose prevention site is for second place: that is, to be able to start up without having to deal with all the legal and media hassles connected with being first.

Moreover, not all of the effects of the pandemic on harm reduction have been negative. In the U.S., concern about spreading disease forced the federal government to at least temporarily lift regulations that serve as barriers to medication treatment with methadone and buprenorphine. Starting in the spring of 2020, many patients became more readily able to receive monthly or biweekly prescriptions, rather than having to show up at a clinic daily. Critically, new prescriptions are now allowed to be initiated by telemedicine—including over the phone, not just by internet—rather than in person. This has been liberating for both current and new patients, as well as for their doctors.

Harm reductionists have long called for making these medications far more easily available. They are continuing to push to make the changes in regulations permanent and to allow even more flexibility. While access to easier care has been spotty, and some patients are now facing issues related to financial problems with clinics caused by COVID, the data gathered here shows that these relaxed rules work may finally be enough to lead to national change.

Further, in additional welcome changes spurred by the COVID pandemic, many jurisdictions reduced or even stopped drug possession arrests. Some states also freed thousands of people already charged with nonviolent offenses from jails and prison, as it became clear that lockups can seed infection to whole communities. Many cities banned evictions and also expanded "housing first" policies for homeless people, offering free hotel rooms along with harm reduction services to curb the spread of the virus. Again, the implementation of these policies has been uneven— and some places that reduced incarceration and homelessness regressed later in the pandemic. But, like the eased medication requirements, these changes show that drastic decarceration and better housing policies are possible, and research on these efforts can provide a framework for future expansion.

Most encouragingly of all, however, Canada, pushed by VANDU and other drug user activists, has gone even further. In many of its provinces, people with addiction can now be prescribed strong opioids and stimulants to replace their street drugs—and there is support from the national government for others to follow suit. Studies are ongoing, and it is likely that this form of harm reduction will expand and take hold up north. Recently, Vancouver also moved to ask the national government to allow it to decriminalize all drug possession.

SO HOW DO WE CONTINUE TO UNDO DRUGS AND ADVANCE HARM REDUCTION? What efforts are needed to effectively fight the overdose crisis, without causing further damage? Where should we go from here—and how can we genuinely help? And what is the future of harm reduction beyond drugs?

As always, we need to start with the essence of harm reduction, which is compassion and respect for the inherent dignity and value of human life. At a bare minimum, policies to change risky behavior cannot be more harmful than the behavior they seek to alter; we can't continue to hurt people in the aid of helping them or others. And we simply cannot go on allowing only some folks the privilege of being able to reduce risk when they take substances—while targeting others for prison or even death for using equally or less risky drugs. It's just not fair.

In the long term, this means that we need to completely revise or ideally eliminate the Controlled Substances Act and its nonsensical "schedules," which give the veneer of science to a set of prohibitions and regulations that is, in reality, arbitrary and steeped in racist history. It makes no sense to allow law enforcement officials to have the final say over the nature of a "legitimate medical purpose" or to be the arbiters of which drugs are banned entirely.[18] Nor is it rational to continue with policy that maintains that the only acceptable recreational drugs ever permissible for all eternity are those allowed to be marketed after 1914 by Western governments (that is, alcohol, caffeine, and nicotine). But that's what current law does.

Recognizing that someone can get pleasure from a new substance or that it has risks is not the same as determining whether it has any acceptable medical or recreational use: we'd better hope the cure for cancer isn't any fun, otherwise it might be immediately "scheduled" once discovered by the Drug Enforcement Administration. This would delay research, perhaps indefinitely. As soon as the DEA declares that a drug is not medically useful, it becomes highly restricted, and research is often practically or financially impossible, as we've seen in the fight for medical marijuana (which, incidentally, may have some cancer-fighting and anti-Alzheimer's properties).

At the same time, there is no pathway at all for approval of new nonmedical drugs, only backdoors like labeling them as "supplements," which are not tested for safety or efficacy and are in general poorly regulated. One example here is kratom, an herb with opioid-like effects that is now used by many pain and addiction patients to replace prescription or street drugs. From its long history of use in Asia, kratom clearly has a far lower risk of overdose—which means that banning it now would increase harm— but it is not ideal to have a drug suddenly available to millions without real testing. And even with supplements, the DEA retains the authority to ban them at any time without conducting research on what effects this might have, which it almost did with kratom before users fought back.

Harm reduction says we must undo all of this and create policy based on scientific evidence of what best preserves life and health. It reveals

the racism and injustice in our ideas about "drugs" and provides a better
way forward. It turns many moral questions into empirical ones: if you
can prove that a policy—regardless of what it is—saves more lives than it
blights, then it can be seen as a form of harm reduction. At the same time,
the philosophy does require accepting that people will always seek some
ways to alter consciousness and that there is no way to "arrest our way out
of this" or eliminate this human trait. Indeed, trying to do so is incompatible with human dignity and freedom.

To create national policy that would reduce harm, then, we need to
recognize that the Controlled Substances Act is not fit for its purpose and
that no public good comes from giving law enforcement agencies control over medical and scientific questions.[19] Also critical to this effort is
reversing the results of the Supreme Court's 1919 *Webb* decision, which
declared that maintaining the "comfort" of someone with addiction is
outside the realm of legitimate medicine. Later regulations and decisions
have since codified this into law, and they must be repealed.

Under current legal doctrine, doctors who want to treat pain are under
constant threat—ever aware that if police determine that their prescribing
makes them an outlier or if authorities decide that their patients are mere
"addicts," every one of their actions suddenly becomes a crime, regardless
of their intent. And it's just as bad in addiction medicine. To ensure that
they do not accidentally violate these laws, doctors often feel that they
have to prove that they are doing more than simply "maintaining addicts"
when they use controlled substances to treat addiction. Only two medications are allowed in these efforts—methadone and buprenorphine—even
though there is no real pharmacological reason to deny access to others.

An entire bureaucracy is devoted to surveilling methadone patients
and ensuring that they attend counseling or at least engage in some activity that is beyond medication, regardless of data that show that medication
by itself reduces mortality. Essentially, anyone with contact with these
drugs is assumed to be a criminal first, not a doctor or a patient. People
using opioid medication to treat addiction and their doctors are subject to
the most onerous regulation in medicine, which, not surprisingly, means
that physicians tend to steer away from these areas. Patients are allowed
to risk paralysis, brain damage, and even death in choosing other medical

treatments—but they are allowed no such power when it comes to balancing the risk between addiction and pain.

We do not treat any other medications in this bizarre way.

To end this disastrous mistake, the entirety of medical regulation of controlled substances must be shifted to an agency like the FDA, which is scientific and can develop more sensible pathways to both medical and nonmedical drug approval and better ways of actually regulating sales. The FDA should develop regulations for nonmedical drug approvals and should determine how to classify or "schedule" the risks of drugs scientifically, not based on a series of moral panics. It should end the use of vague and unscientific terms like "abuse potential" and "physical and psychic [sic!] dependence," which remain in regulations related to controlled substances. And it should always be required to assess drug risks on a harm reduction basis; that is, in context. In other words, regulators must consider questions like: If we ban this substance, will the substitute that some people will inevitably find be more or less harmful? And what would be the least harmful way to manage the problem?

While it's certainly true that both the FDA and the DEA failed to prevent the current opioid catastrophe, at least the FDA actually has the expertise and training to have the potential to do better with more resources. Law enforcement agencies like the DEA do not. The DEA has total control over the medical opioid supply: it sets manufacturing quotas for each drug. Since it utterly failed to use that power appropriately during this crisis, any value it might have over the FDA in managing these medications seems null. Moreover, prosecuting doctors for overprescribing does not reduce harm, and—in the absence of actual criminality like selling doses for dollars or trading sex for drugs—any genuine problem can be solved by simply taking away medical licenses, rather than criminal prosecution. Given its complete failure to control either the medical or the illegal supply of drugs, the DEA should be abolished as the Movement for Black Lives recommends.

To make effective harm reduction policy instead, health agencies like the FDA and the Centers for Disease Control need a new approach. They must recognize that they can only manage what they measure: if they incentivize the wrong metrics, they will get the wrong outcomes. Our current strategy, for example, has been extremely efficacious at reducing the number and dose level of opioid prescriptions, which is its measure for success. Since 2011, the total amount of opioids prescribed has fallen by at least 60 percent, with much of the reduction coming from cutting off patients who take high doses.[20] But when measured by outcomes related to harm that people actually care about—like the number of overdose and suicide deaths, addiction rates, and quality of life for people in pain—it could not be a worse failure.

Harm reduction, instead, focuses on these real-world effects and "side effects." For example, when a doctor is suspected of overprescribing, harm reduction regulators wouldn't simply stop her from practicing and leave her patients stranded, as is currently done. Instead, they'd require that "bridge" prescriptions be provided to prevent withdrawal and that other available and affordable practitioners are found to ensure care for all patients, regardless of whether they have addiction, pain, or both. These patients must be treated as such: not forced to accept alternative care when what they were already receiving was working for them.

Under a harm reduction regime, doctors would also explicitly be permitted to prescribe for people who are addicted in order to allow those who are not ready, willing, or able to stop to have a safer medical supply. Pain patients who need high-dose treatment and their doctors would have a legal safe haven so that they don't have to live in fear of police or regulators who make decisions based on prescription numbers, not individual needs. This would be liberating to everyone in medicine: if doctors don't have a class of patients that they are legally required to police to determine whether they are in pain or addicted, it would not be acceptable to treat anyone "like an addict" or drug seeker. With no class of patients that are legally and culturally designated as acceptable targets of contempt, everyone would benefit, even pain patients who did get misclassified as addicted. The moralistic jurisprudence of *Webb* and its legacy of pain would finally be nullified.

Of course, as a general philosophy, harm reduction also has enormous potential for improving the way we make decisions about risk far beyond drug policy. We're already seeing the idea being used to cope with COVID-19, and it has spurred creative thinking in many areas of public health. As noted earlier, it can expand the scope of anorexia treatment to reach people who are not ready or able to make complete change; similarly, it can be used in other types of eating disorder treatment, and even just for the general population seeking to become healthier by changing diet and exercise.

Getting the small fries with a Big Mac can be a form of "any positive change"—and can lead to bigger improvements, just as small changes in drug use can. One obstetrician-gynecologist on Twitter spoke about using harm reduction approaches with pregnant patients who have gestational diabetes and can't or won't make big dietary and exercise changes overnight; she also sees prenatal care in general as both a form of harm reduction and a forum for it.

And for women who cannot quit drinking during pregnancy, researchers are studying supplementation with a nutrient call choline that may reduce the permanent damage that alcohol can cause to the developing fetal brain. While choline also helps when given after these babies are born, rodent studies suggest it would have a much bigger effect if given during pregnancy—and there are other substances that also show promise. Of course, such strategies will certainly be controversial and raise fears about "enabling." But given the enormous and lifelong damage done to children with fetal alcohol spectrum disorders (FASD) during prenatal development, it is an important new area for harm reduction. It's estimated that 2 to 5 percent of the North American population has FASD, which makes it more common than autism.[21]

Also controversial, while growing, is the use of e-cigarettes and other safer forms of nicotine delivery as harm reduction for tobacco. The potential for success for harm reduction here is already clear from the case of Sweden, which, in recent years, promoted an oral form of tobacco called snus and now has the lowest rate of daily smoking in Europe, as well as the lowest rate of lung cancer in men.[22] Although it makes many public health officials queasy to support anything but the utter abolition of nicotine use, harm reduction offers a far more realistic path to better health. And, while more research is needed on the long-term risks associated with e-cigarettes, it is already clear that, when regulated appropriately, they are less dangerous than the old-fashioned kind.

Harm reduction also offers hope in coping with climate change: many practices like recycling, buying less, eating more vegan and vegetarian meals, and reducing long-distance travel can be approached in a gradual way. This can not only have a big impact on a population level by itself, but can also lead to greater change over time—in contrast with scolding and telling people that the only way to help is to radically reform immediately, which often just leads to rebellion or not bothering to try at all.

Bike lanes and measures to create more walkable cities can be harm reduction in urban planning; reducing social media use rather than quitting entirely is another example. Education in prison and other strategies that improve health can be harm reduction for incarcerated people. And many criminal legal system reforms, while not optimal in themselves, are harm reduction in context and can be steps toward greater change. For example, the restorative justice movement—which seeks to provide accountability for perpetrators and healing for victims without resorting to methods like incarceration—has specifically incorporated harm reduction thinking in its approach. Moreover, restorative justice itself can be seen as a harm reduction alternative to the current system.

Some harm reductionists do object to some of the broader ways that the term is now being used. For example, during the 2020 elections, many Democrats talked about voting as a form of harm reduction: even though their preferred candidates were no longer options, they would still vote because the alternative would do greater harm to their constituencies. This was missing the point, these critics argued. Choosing a candidate who is less harmful doesn't necessarily encompass the broader lessons of radical compassion, antiracism, and elevating the voices of people at risk that the movement values, they claimed, seeing this as a false analogy or incorrect elaboration of the idea.

Debate over these kinds of questions will likely persist, both within and around harm reduction. In many areas outside of drug policy, determining whether a small step is the beginning of a greater change or a sidestep that allows greater transformation to be avoided is not easy. With addiction and many kinds of individual behavior change we have data: clean needles and heroin prescribing and other gradual measures do not prevent or preclude bigger changes; they often enable them. But in terms of social and political change, it's not as clear-cut.

These arguments also raise another issue that successful radical political movements eventually face. That is, their goals require changes in conventional culture and politics. But when such victories are achieved, inevitably, the rough edges get sanded down. Adulterated forms of the message proliferate, ideas are co-opted, that cool band that only you and your weirdo friends loved is now embraced by the conformist masses. Monique Tula, executive director of what is now known as the National Harm Reduction Coalition, puts it this way: "In order to influence culture, you have to become mainstream."

And for harm reduction, which was born among outsiders, punks, freaks, and hippies, doing so can entail loss and compromise. Since the start, radical harm reductionists have warned about the problem of co-optation: elements of this dispute can be seen in ongoing clashes over the role of active users in organizations and similar debates related to professionalization and medicalization. Keeping the renegade spirit of the early illegal needle exchangers alive and centering active users are critical. But the legal victories and greater cultural acceptance that allowed syringe exchange to come up from the underground matter at least as much.

HISTORIANS HAVE LONG OBSERVED AMERICA'S SUCCESSION OF PANICS OVER various drugs, which crackdowns on supply have always failed to solve. In fact, when feared drugs recede, it is rarely because law enforcement has made them hard to get. Instead, change comes when younger users—who have seen damage done to older siblings and parents—decide to try a different high.

This process leads to fairly predictable cycles of around ten years each, in which stimulants alternate in popularity with depressants. For example, the sixties saw a great deal of amphetamine use; in the seventies, kids learned that "speed kills," and heroin use spiked. The eighties swung back to stimulants: this time, powder and then crack cocaine. The nineties was the time of "heroin chic" models and addicted grunge musicians;

the early 2000s began with rural methamphetamine outbreaks, followed by the rise of OxyContin and other prescription opioids. These days, young people aren't nearly as likely to initiate either prescription opioid or heroin use as their older siblings and parents were—but methamphetamine use is again rising. Once people are addicted, of course, their use tends to involve multiple substances and is less influenced by trends and fashion, but the overall pattern is clear.

If we want to do better than continually replacing our old demon drugs with new ones, we need harm reduction. We must recognize that prevention must target common factors that predispose people to addiction, not the media's latest claims about the new and "most addictive drug ever." People who become addicted tend to share at least one of the following three features—often, all of them. First, they are likely to have been born with an outlying temperament, which typically reflects a risk for mental illness and often leads to difficulties with socializing. Second, they frequently suffer high levels of childhood trauma, which is often the catalyst that transforms latent predispositions into active disorders. Finally, they may be faced with a future that seems hopeless to them. If we mitigate the pain caused by these experiences in youth, we can reduce the odds that any risks they do take with drugs will lead to addiction.

We also need to accept that cutting supply (when that can actually be achieved, which is not often) leads to substitution; it almost never ends existing addictions or prevents new ones from occurring. If we're going to try to reduce specific supplies, then, this must be done in a conscientious way that does not simply shift people from safer medical drugs to more dangerous street substances. We can make substitution trends work for harm reduction, rather than against it. But that can only happen if we acknowledge the existence of substitution and work to ensure that policies tend to move people, say, from chaotic opioid use to kratom or marijuana or maintenance opioids, rather than from prescription opioids to heroin contaminated by fentanyl.

We live in a world where creative chemists can rapidly design new psychoactive substances when others become hard to get and where the internet can make them almost immediately available around the world.

We live as a social species that has always enjoyed various ways of altering consciousness, whether for pleasure, comfort, or relief. Given these facts—and a greater understanding of the racist and political purposes of the drug war—ending criminalization is the only rational way to proceed. Through harm reduction, we can undo the ideology that underpins damaging policies and make way for a future that is healthier, happier, and more humane for everyone.

Acknowledgments

I'M NOT SURE HOW MANY SYNONYMS THERE ARE FOR GRATITUDE OR WAYS TO express my thanks to those who have helped this book be born. I hope there are at least dozens, because so many, many people made important contributions. To start, I want to thank the Liverpudlians who made harm reduction into an international movement, especially Russell Newcombe, Peter McDermott, Alan and Lyn Matthews, and Pat O'Hare—as well as Jean Paul Grund and his fellow organizers and researchers from the Netherlands. Additional gratitude to U.K. physicians and health leaders John Strang and John Ashton.

Next, I'd like to thank Edith Springer—the Goddess of Harm Reduction herself—for bringing the movement to America and helping spread to the word to so many. I greatly appreciate your wisdom and encouragement. Allan Clear, executive director of the Harm Reduction Coalition from 1995 to 2016, provided critical insight, support, and material, as did Mark Kinzly and Paul Cherashore—much thanks to all!

Deepest gratitude as well to the members of the Harm Reduction Working Group, especially Ricky Bluthenthal, Charles Collins, Pat Garrett, Mark Gerse, Sara Kershnar, Gerald LeNoir, Joyce Rivera, Scott Stokes, and Kevin Zeese. I'd also particularly like to acknowledge Heather Edney and Lisa Moore. And extra special thanks to Stephanie Comer, both for funding and guiding the movement and for helping me document it.

I'm further grateful to many Bay Area harm reductionists and experts, including Sheigla Murphy, Craig Reinarman, Les Pappas, John Newmeyer, Jennifer Lorvick, Hilary McQuie, Rose May Dance, Trish Case, Rev. Cecil Williams, Janice Mirikitani, Paul Harkin, Tracey Helton, Marsha Rosenbaum, Dee Dee Stout, Patt Denning, Jeanne Little, Phil Coffin, and, of course, Maureen Gammon, without whom I might never have been here to write this book.

New York folks who deserve exceptional thanks include Tracie Gardner, Charles King, Chuck Eaton, Andrew Tatarsky, Louis Jones, Bart Majoor, Ronald Johnson, Stephen Dansiger, Ernie Drucker, Tony Scro, and Denise Paone. On the ACT UP gratitude list are Jill Harris (extra special thanks for the records), Dan Keith Williams, Donald Grove, Monica Pearl, Deb Levine, and Glenn Backes.

For help on the history of the Chicago Recovery Alliance, I'm grateful to Sarz Maxwell, Greg Scott, Karen Bigg, Cheryl Hull, Suzanne Carlberg-Racich, Peter Moinichen, and Maya Doe-Simkins. And for the Seattle-Tacoma portions, as well as other insights, I'd like to thank Sue Purchase, George Parks, Judith Gordon, Alisa Solberg, and Kris Nyrup.

For assistance related to parent activism, I'm grateful to Gretchen Burns Bergman, Carole Katz Beyer, Denise Cullen, Denise Mariano, and Julia Negron. Other scholars and researchers who were immensely helpful include Don Des Jarlais, Alex Kral, Sam Friedman, Kurt Schmoke, Caroline Jean Acker, Susan Collins, Andrea Efthimiou, Samuel Roberts, Robert Heimer, Charles Kaplan, William Miller, Virginia Berridge, Nick Heather, Katie Witkiewitz, Steffanie Strathdee, Seema Clifasefi, Kathie Kane-Willis, Amirah Sequeira, Jeff Ondocsin, Jon Zibbell, and Emily Dufton.

Special thanks to Johann Hari, Nancy Campbell, and Susan Chambre, who shared previously unpublished interviews and support. And further props to Amy Bianco, who provided essential background and context related to Siobhan Reynolds, whom I dearly wish were here to tell me again what I am getting wrong. (Of course, any errors here are mine alone.) For other records help, I'd like to thank Mohamad (Adam) Brooks at Columbia and Tal Nadan at the New York Public Library. Sarah Schulman and the ACT UP Oral History Project are also much appreciated.

I also want to send my gratitude to Donald MacPherson, for his help with the Vancouver section, and to Karen Ward, Spike Peachey, Garth Mullins, Ann Livingston, Dean Wilson, Mark Tyndall, Travis Lupick, Darwin Fisher, Chris Van Veen, and Scott MacDonald.

Miscellaneous but heartfelt thanks as well to Corinne Carey, Daniel Raymond, Paula Santiago, Doug Gary, Joy Rucker, Jenn Awa, Roberto Elser, Alessandra Ross, Michael Botticelli, Jason Farell, Chad Sabora, Tim Santamour, Emanuel Sferios, and especially Louise Vincent.

Ethan Nadelmann, co-founder and executive director of the Drug Policy Alliance from 2000 to 2017, provided crucial insight and background; I also want to thank Howard Josepher for his thoughts here. Extreme gratitude to Kassandra Frederique, current leader of DPA, for her acumen and sagacity. And much appreciation to Monique Tula, who became executive director of what is now called the National Harm Reduction Coalition in 2016, and gave not only welcome access to records, but also cogent analysis.

My first reader and brilliant friend Alissa Quart deserves more thanks than I can offer, for editing and advice and comfort. My sister, Kira Smith, did a fantastic job as a research assistant, especially with the many, many endnotes and transcripts. Thanks as well to CLK Transcription. Additional appreciation to Anne Giles and Randy Epstein for their excellent editorial advice. I also extend infinite thanks to my husband, Ted Johnson, for his love and support as I wrestled with the complexities of harm reduction.

And of course, extra-special super-duper thanks to my fabulous editor Renée Sedliar, who much improved this book and always boosted my spirits and accommodated my process. My agent, Andrew Stuart, has also been wonderful throughout the development of *Undoing Drugs*: thank you all!

Notes

INTRODUCTION

1. Frank Newport, "Record-High 50% of Americans Favor Legalizing Marijuana Use," Gallup, October 17, 2011, https://news.gallup.com/poll/150149 /record-high-americans-favor-legalizing-marijuana.aspx. Max Frankel, "Plots for Hire: Media Mercenaries Join the War on Drugs," *New York Times Magazine*, February 6, 2000.

CHAPTER ONE: FACING AIDS

1. Don C. Des Jarlais et al., "HIV 1 Infection among IV Drug Users in Manhattan, New York City, from 1977 through 1987," *Journal of the American Medical Association* 26, no. 7 (1989): 1009–1012, DOI:10.1001/jama.1989 .03420070058030.

2. Randy Shilts, *And the Band Played On: Politics, People and the AIDS Epidemic* (New York: Penguin, 1988, updated paperback edition), 103–104.

3. Ricardo E. Barreras, "New York City's Needle Exchange Policy and the Intersection of Science, Activism and Politics: A Case Study of Activist Research and Social Change" (PhD diss., City University of New York, NY 2004).

4. Barreras, "New York City's Needle Exchange Policy."

5. Des Jarlais, "HIV 1 Infection among IV Drug Users."

6. Richard A. Serrano and Jane Fritsch, "Yeah, I Mean It! Gates Says of Idea to Shoot Drug Users," *Los Angeles Times*, September 8, 1990, https://www.latimes .com/archives/la-xpm-1990-09-08-me-478-story.html.

7. Kathy Dobie, "Yolanda Serrano," *Ms.*, January/February 1989. Robert Sullivan, "Yolanda Serrano, 45, Organizer of Anti-AIDS Needle Exchanges," *New York Times*, October 22, 1993, https://www.nytimes.com/1993/10/22/obituaries /yolanda-serrano-45-organizer-of-anti-aids-needle-exchanges.html.

8. Dobie, "Yolanda Serrano."

9. Sullivan, "Yolanda Serrano."

10. Dobie, "Yolanda Serrano."

11. Sullivan, "Yolanda Serrano."

12. Julio Martinez headed New York's Department of Substance Abuse Services from 1979 to 1989. Tony Scro, interview by author, New York, 2020.

13. Will Di Novi, "Across the 'Bridge of Pain': How Rikers Island Jail Became America's Most Infamous Penitentiary," *Pacific Standard*, July 27, 2015.

14. Sheldon Landesman, interview by Ronald Bayer, Columbia Center for Oral History, New York, 1995.

15. Stephen Follansbee, interview by Sally Smith Hughes, The AIDS Epidemic in San Francisco: "The Response of Community Physicians, 1981–1984," Regional Oral History Office, The Bancroft Library University of California Berkeley, California, 1996, p. 63, https://digitalassets.lib.berkeley.edu/rohoia/ucb/text/aidsepidinsanfran02hughrich.pdf.

16. Dobie, "Yolanda Serrano."

17. Eric Margolis, "Evaluating Outreach in San Francisco," *Community-Based AIDS Prevention: Studies of Intravenous Drug Users and Their Sexual Partners*, National Institute on Drug Abuse, 1991.

18. Sheigla Murphy, interview by author, 2019.

19. "A Timeline of HIV and AIDS," HIV.gov, accessed October 19, 2020, https://www.hiv.gov/hiv-basics/overview/history/hiv-and-aids-timeline.

20. Unless otherwise noted, Murphy's story and quotes in this chapter are from the author's interview with her.

21. "Study Finds Sharing Is a Necessity, Not a Ritual," *AIDS Policy Law* 10, no. 18 (1995): 8, https://pubmed.ncbi.nlm.nih.gov/11362830/.

22. John A. Newmeyer, "Why Bleach? A Development of a Strategy to Combat HIV Contagion among San Francisco Intravenous Drug Users," *Needle Sharing Among Intravenous Drug Abusers: National and International Perspectives*, National Institute on Drug Abuse Monograph 80 (1988). Geoffrey A. Froner, "Injection of Sodium Hypochlorite by Intravenous Drug Users," *Journal of the American Medical Association* 258, no. 3 (1987): 325, DOI:10.1001/jama.1987.03400030041022.

23. Newmeyer, "Why Bleach?"

24. Les Pappas, interview by author, 2019.

CHAPTER TWO: UNDOING POWERLESSNESS

1. Michael Soyka, "New Developments in the Management of Opioid Dependence: Focus on Sublingual Buprenorphine-Naloxone," *Substance Abuse and Rehabilitation* 6 (January 6, 2015): 1–14, DOI:10.2147/SAR.S45585.

2. Neil Woods and J. S. Rafaeli, *Drug Wars: The Terrifying Inside Story of Britain's Drug Trade* (London: Ebury Press, 2018), 125–132. (This quote and quote from second patient above.)

3. Johann Hari, *Chasing the Scream* (New York: Bloomsbury, 2016), 208.

4. Woods and Rafaeli, *Drug Wars*, 127.

5. Woods and Rafaeli, *Drug Wars*, 133.

6. W. M. Compton, Y. F. Thomas, F. S. Stinson, and B. F. Grant, "Prevalence, Correlates, Disability, and Comorbidity of DSM-IV Drug Abuse and Dependence in the United States: Results from the National Epidemiologic Survey on Alcohol and Related Conditions," *Arch Gen Psychiatry* 64, no. 5 (May 2007): 566–576, DOI:10.1001/archpsyc.64.5.566.

7. Author interview with John Marks, 1993.

8. John-Paul Grund and Joost Breeksema, "Coffee Shops and Compromise: Separated Illicit Drug Markets in the Netherlands," *Lessons for Drug Policy Series* (July 2013), accessed October 20, 2020, https://www.opensociety foundations.org/publications/coffee-shops-and-compromise-separated-illicit -drug-markets-netherlands.

9. Known as MDHG (in Dutch, the acronym spells Medical Social Service of Heroin Users), these groups included professionals and former users as well as active users. They helped support the Junkiebonden and had some overlapping membership, but were separate organizations. Wouter M. de Jong, "AIDS and Self-Organization of Drug Users in the Netherlands," in *The Effectiveness of Drug Abuse Treatment: Dutch and American Perspectives*, eds. Jerome J. Platt, Charles D. Kaplan, and Patrica McKim (Malabar, FL: R. E. Krieger, 1990), 303–313, https://archive.org/details/effectivenessofd0000unse. Also author's interview with Jean Paul Grund, 2019, and emails.

10. Author interview with Jean Paul Grund, 2019. de Jong, "AIDS and Self-Organization of Drug Users."

11. John Marks, "Opium, the Religion of the People," *Lancet* 22, no. 1 (June 22, 1985): 1439–1440, DOI:10.1016/s0140-6736(85)91857-4.

12. John Strang and Michael Gossop, eds., *Heroin Addiction and the British System: Volume 1, Origins and Evolution* (London: Routledge, 2005), 31. Mike Ashton, "Doctors at War," *Druglink*, (July/August 1986).

13. Matthias Pierce et al., "Impact of Treatment for Opioid Dependence on Fatal Drug-Related Poisoning: A National Cohort Study in England," *Addiction (Abingdon, England)* 111, no. 2 (2016): 298–308, DOI:10.1111/add.13193.

14. Toby Seddon, "Prescribing Heroin: John Marks, the Merseyside Clinics and Lessons from History," *International Journal of Drug Policy* 78, https://doi .org/10.1016/j.drugpo.2020.102730. Peter McDermott, *Heroin Addiction and the British System: Volume 1, Origins and Evolution*, eds. John Strang and Michael Gossop (London: Routledge, 2005). Additional information on Liverpool history and people from author interviews with Alan Matthews, Russell Newcombe, Peter McDermott, Pat O'Hare, Ethan Nadelmann, and John Ashton in 2019.

15. Roy Robertson and Alison Richardson, "Heroin Injecting and the Introduction of HIV/AIDS into a Scottish City," *Journal of the Royal Society of Medicine* 100,

no. 11 (2007): 491–494, DOI:10.1177/014107680710001108. Mandy Rhodes, "Choose Life—Dr Roy Robertson, the Front Line of Harm Reduction," *Holyrood*, last modified March 26, 2019, https://www.holyrood.com/inside-politics/view,choose-life-dr-roy-robertson-the-front-line-of-harm-reduction_10074.htm.

16. Robertson and Richardson, "Heroin Injecting and the Introduction of HIV/AIDS."

17. J. R. Robertson et al., "Epidemic of AIDS Related Virus (HTLV-III/LAV) Infection Among Intravenous Drug Abusers," *British Medical Journal* 292 (1986): 527–530, https://doi.org/10.1136/bmj.292.6519.527. Rhodes, "Choose Life."

18. Francis X. Clines, "Via Addict Needles, AIDS Spreads in Edinburgh," *New York Times*, January 4, 1987, https://www.nytimes.com/1987/01/04/world/via-addict-needles-aids-spreads-in-edinburgh.html.

19. Andrew Moss, "AIDS and Intravenous Drug Use: The Real Heterosexual Epidemic," *British Medical Journal (Clinical Research Ed.)* 294, no. 6569 (1987): 389–390, DOI:10.1136/bmj.294.6569.389.

CHAPTER THREE: UNDOING ADDICTION

1. McDermott, *Heroin Addiction and the British System*, 152.

2. The speaker was Glenn Margo, director of health promotion for San Francisco's health department. Author interview with John Ashton.

3. "The Birth of Harm Reduction" (circa 1986), YouTube video, posted by UK Harm Reduction, November 3, 2016, https://www.youtube.com/watch?v=7LTpFBEv_m0&t=9s.

4. The first staffer to exchange needles was almost certainly Alan Matthews. Author interview with Alan Matthews. Author interview with Russell Newcombe.

5. "The Birth of Harm Reduction."

6. Woods and Rafaeli, *Drug Wars*, 135.

7. Allan Parry, "Needle Swop in Mersey," *Druglink* (January/February 1987), 7, https://www.drugwise.org.uk/druglink-article-1987-needle-swop-in-mersey-by-allan-parry/.

8. Allan Parry, "The Rise and Fall of the Mersey Harm Reduction Strategy," Invia un amico, Stampa, July 1, 1994.

9. Allan Parry testimony, *Congressional Hearings before the Subcommittee on Health and the Environment of the Committee on Energy and Commerce*, House of Representatives, 101st Congress, April 24, 1989, Needle Exchange Programs, Serial no. 101-70, p. 202, https://books.googleusercontent.com/books/content
?req=AKW5QadWxYwu45YSWgkljhdNVqHZS6ChIPk5JhWCZPgPDR
rHmsU10PgOgtWeEgP-0F9pOQNLQqwwPdWtNZ6g55NQfbcVWv8ULX3
MuHHRaJ9CESN9IW6T-m77lZvoeqGV7zrzS3270-J9tTBxd-BdwpTn4
X9utpUYuyTgG_Ox5-igCCjbMEyCG9i1BDkpLwvFc4Lj5ewhrBvX3u
USsrUr9ZDEHrD0kvxxr4q6h8ii953TAGkwCkBE1_tOtuZgFuyFuA3
HskRIADkd.

10. Russell Newcombe interview by author, 2019, all quotes in this section.

11. Dave Walsh, "Liverpool 47 Plaque: 'Better to Break the Law, than Break the Poor,'" *The Socialist*, October 10, 2018, https://www.socialistparty.org.uk /issue/1013/28059.

12. John Ashton and Howard Seymour, *New Public Health* (London: Open University Press, 1988), vii.

13. John Ashton interview by author, 2019. Pat O'Hare, "Merseyside, the First Harm Reduction Conferences, and the Early History of Harm Reduction," *International Journal of Drug Policy* 18, no. 2 (2007): 141–144, https://doi.org /10.1016/j.drugpo.2007.01.003.

14. Howard Seymour, "The Liverpool Model: A Population Based Approach to Harm Reduction," *International Journal of Drug Policy* 8, no. 4 (1997): 201–206.

15. Parry, "The Rise and Fall of the Mersey Harm Reduction Strategy."

16. Allan Parry, "Drug Politics in Liverpool: A Personal Account, Part 2," *Druglink* (July/August 1991): 16–18, https://www.drugwise.org.uk/wp-content /uploads/JulyAugust91.pdf.

17. Russell Newcombe, "High Time for Harm Reduction," *Druglink* (January/ February 1987): 10–11, https://www.drugwise.org.uk/wp-content/uploads /JanFeb8721.pdf.

18. Disclosure: I had a romantic relationship with Peter McDermott.

19. Author interview with Peter McDermott, 1993.

20. Author interview with John Marks, 1993.

21. Marks was influenced by psychologist John Booth Davies, who wrote a book called *The Myth of Addiction* (London: Routledge, 1992). Author interview with John Marks, 1993.

22. Author interview with Peter McDermott, 1993.

23. McDermott, *Heroin Addiction and the British System*, 152.

24. Leading figures in the development of harm reduction in Liverpool in the local health authority include most notably John Ashton and Howard Seymour. John R. Ashton and Howard Seymour, "Public Health and the Origins of the Mersey Model of Harm Reduction," *International Journal of Drug Policy*, no. 21 (2010): 94–96. Also, author interviews with Peter McDermott and Pat O'Hare, 2019.

25. Ashton interview, 2019.

26. Steve Lohr, "Liverpool Journal: There's No Preaching, Just the Clean Needles," *New York Times*, February 29, 1988, https://www.nytimes.com/1988/02/29 /world/liverpool-journal-there-s-no-preaching-just-the-clean-needles.html.

CHAPTER FOUR: THE GODDESS OF HARM REDUCTION

1. Manuscripts and Archives Division, The New York Public Library, "Edith Springer workshop," *The New York Public Library Digital Collections*, 1995, http:// digitalcollections.nypl.org/items/57839d69-43ed-4af4-9d7c-9c3936c13824.

2. Author interviews with Edith Springer, 2019 and 2020.

3. Springer was employed by the Narcotics and Drugs Research Institute, NDRI, which Don Des Jarlais led.

4. The physician was Stephan Sorrell. Author interview with Edith Springer.

5. No one is clear about this: Springer said that she thought that ADAPT could have come up with the idea independently, but she's not sure. Interviews with Don Des Jarlais and other NDRI sources suggest there was contact between NDRI and MidCity. Other interviews and material on ADAPT provide no further clarity.

6. The co-creator of "Eroticizing Safer Sex" was Luis Palacios-Jimenez. Springer interviews, 2019 and 2020.

7. Sourcing in this section via author interview with Springer unless otherwise noted.

8. Edith Springer interviewed by Dan Bigg and Donald Grove, video, date unknown.

9. Kenneth Anderson, "Islamic World Takes Same Drugs We Do: It Just Has Different Rules about Them," AlterNet.org, last modified December 22, 2014, https://www.alternet.org/2014/12/drugs-islamic-world-same-substances-different-rules/.

10. Musto provides a good overview. David F. Musto, *The American Disease: Origins of Narcotic Control* (New York: Oxford University Press, expanded edition, 1987, first published 1973 by Yale University Press).

11. Dan Baum, "Legalize It All," *Harper's*, April 2016, https://harpers.org/archive/2016/04/legalize-it-all/.

12. "NEGRO COCAINE EVIL.: Mississippi Judge Urges Grand Jury to Punish Druggists," *New York Times*, March 20, 1905, https://www.nytimes.com/1905/03/20/archives/negro-cocaine-evil-mississippi-judge-urges-grand-jury-to-punish.html. Edward Williams, "NEGRO COCAINE 'FIENDS' ARE A NEW SOUTHERN MENACE: Murder and Insanity Increasing among Lower Class Blacks Because They Have Taken to 'Sniffing' Since Deprived of Whisky by Prohibition," *New York Times*, February 8, 1914, https://www.nytimes.com/1914/02/08/archives/negro-cocaine-fiends-are-a-new-southern-menace-murder-and-insanity.html.

13. Musto, *The American Disease*, 31.

14. Musto, *The American Disease*, 43.

15. Musto, *The American Disease*, 65.

16. Becky Little, "How Prohibition Fueled the Rise of the Ku Klux Klan," last modified February 19, 2019, https://www.history.com/news/kkk-terror-during-prohibition.

17. Hari, *Chasing the Scream*, 15.

18. Edith Springer interviewed by Dan Bigg and Donald Grove, date unknown.

19. Author interview with Edith Springer, 2020.

20. *Taking Drugs Seriously: A Film about the Radical Drugs and AIDS Policy in Liverpool*, directed by Nancy Platt (1990; Liverpool, England: BBC 2 Open Space).

CHAPTER FIVE: ACT UP AND THE JOHNNY APPLESEED OF NEEDLES

1. The musician was Stephen Dansiger, now a PhD psychologist. It was re-leased by SOL, a singles-only label put out by Bob Mould of Hüsker Dü and Steve Fallon, the owner of the famed nightclub Maxwell's in Hoboken. Author interview with Dansiger, 2019.

2. Bruce Lambert, "AIDS Battler Gives Needles Illicitly to Addicts," *New York Times*, November 20, 1989, https://www.nytimes.com/1989/11/20/nyregion /aids-battler-gives-needles-illicitly-to-addicts.html.

3. Springer was employed by the Narcotics and Drugs Research Institute. Don Des Jarlais became a world leader in AIDS and IV drug use research there and provided support for syringe exchange.

4. John Curtis, "What the Needles Said," *Yale Medicine*, Summer 2001, https://medicine.yale.edu/news/yale-medicine-magazine/what-the-needles-said/.

5. The researcher who brought up San Francisco's bleach program was proba-bly either Doug Goldsmith or Sam Friedman.

6. Natasha Geiling, "The Real Johnny Appleseed Brought Apples—and Booze—to the American Frontier," *Smithsonian Magazine*, November 10, 2014, https://www.smithsonianmag.com/arts-culture/real-johnny-appleseed-brought -applesand-booze-american-frontier-180953263/.

7. The health commissioner was David Sencer. Warwick Anderson, "The New York Needle Trial: The Politics of Public Health in the Age of AIDS," *American Journal of Public Health* 81, no. 11 (1991): 1506–1517, https://doi.org/10.2105 /AJPH.81.11.1506.

8. The New York City Department of Health reported 7,989 new infections in IV drug users between 1985 and 1988, but they suspect this is a significant undercount, because it was not mandatory for physicians to report new infections (many people got tested anonymously, like I did) and some people didn't reveal how they believed they had been infected. Kira Smith, email from New York City Department of Health.

9. Bruce Lambert, "Drug Group to Offer Free Needles to Combat AIDS in New York City," *New York Times*, January 8, 1988, https://www.nytimes.com /1988/01/08/nyregion/drug-group-to-offer-free-needles-to-combat-aids-in-new -york-city.html.

10. Michel Marriott, "Needle Plan Fails to Attract Addicts, so It's Revised," *New York Times*, January 30, 1989, https://www.nytimes.com/1989/01/30/nyregion /needle-plan-fails-to-attract-drug-addicts-so-it-s-revised.html. Stephen C. Joseph, *Dragon within the Gates: The Once and Future AIDS Epidemic* (New York: Car-roll & Graf, 2018), 226.

11. Edith Springer interview by Allan Clear on Harm Reduction Coalition podcast 43, October 6, 2011.

12. Marriott, "Needle Plan Fails to Attract Addicts."

13. Judge Laura Drager, decision in Needle Eight case.

14. Richard Elovich interview by Sarah Schulman, New York, N.Y., May 14, 2007, http://www.actuporalhistory.org/interviews/images/elovich.pdf.

15. Susan Chambre, *Fighting for Our Lives: New York's AIDS Community and the Politics of Disease* (New Brunswick: Rutgers University Press, 2006), 131.

16. Elovich interview by Sarah Schulman. All Elovich quotes from that interview unless otherwise specified.

17. Catherine Woodard, "Needle Giveaway to Invite Arrest," *New York Newsday*, March 2, 1990.

CHAPTER SIX: THE TRIAL OF THE NEEDLE EIGHT

1. Joseph, *Dragon within the Gates*.

2. John H. Kennedy, "Man Who Gives Out Needles Is Acquitted," *Boston Globe*, January 10, 1990.

3. Joseph, *Dragon within the Gates*, 166.

4. Carla AbouZahr and Ties Boerma, "Health Information Systems: The Foundations of Public Health," *Bulletin of the World Health Organization* 83, no. 8 (2005): 578–583, https://www.questia.com/library/journal/1G1-136121211/health-information-systems-the-foundations-of-public.

5. Steven Johnson, *The Ghost Map: The Story of London's Most Terrifying Epidemic—and How It Changed Science, Cities, and the Modern World* (New York: Riverhead, 2007), 163. "150th Anniversary of John Snow and the Pump Handle," CDC, last modified September 2, 2004, https://www.cdc.gov/mmwr/preview/mmwrhtml/mm5334a1.htm.

6. The defense was led by ACT UP lawyers Jill Harris, Mike Spiegel, and David Patterson. No transcript exists, but there are videotapes of some of the witness testimony. Author attended most but not all of the trial. Manuscripts and Archives Division, The New York Public Library, Gay Men's Health Crisis Records, "Needle Exchange Trial Original footage," New York Public Library Digital Collections, accessed October 29, 2020, http://digitalcollections.nypl.org/items/22966e1c-d4a2-4165-927d-b06a5ce21256.

7. Diane E. Logan and G. Alan Marlatt, "Harm Reduction Therapy: A Practice-Friendly Review of Research," *Journal of Clinical Psychology* 66, no. 2 (2010): 201–214, DOI:10.1002/jclp.20669. J. Hartmann-Boyce et al., "Electronic Cigarettes for Smoking Cessation," *Cochrane Database of Systematic Reviews* 10 (October 14, 2020), DOI:10.1002/14651858.CD010216.pub4. Ashley N. Gearhardt et al., "Binge Eating Disorder and Food Addiction," *Current Drug Abuse Reviews* 4, no. 3 (2011): 201–207, DOI:10.2174/1874473711104030201. The

behavior change technique is known as "motivational interviewing." See https://www.psychotherapy.net/data/uploads/51194e1c160b2.pdf. B. L. Burke, H. Arkowitz, and M. Menchola, "The Efficacy of Motivational Interviewing: A Meta-analysis of Controlled Clinical Trials," *J Consult Clin Psychol* 71, no. 5 (October 2003): 843–861, DOI:10.1037/0022-006X.71.5.843. PMID: 14516234.

8. Andrew Kirtzman, "Needle Distribution Defended," *New York Daily News*, April 10, 1991.

9. Emily Sachar, "AIDS Activists on Trial for Providing Needles," *Newsday*, April 9, 1991.

10. Maia Szalavitz, "DOH Waffles on Needle Hygiene," *Village Voice*, May 22, 1990.

11. Bruce Lambert, "The Free-Needle Program Is Under Way and Under Fire," *New York Times*, November 13, 1988, https://www.nytimes.com/1988/01/08/nyregion/drug-group-to-offer-free-needles-to-combat-aids-in-new-york-city.html.

12. "The Tuskegee Timeline," CDC, last modified March 2, 2020, https://www.cdc.gov/tuskegee/timeline.htm.

13. Jacques Normand, David Vlahov, and Lincoln E. Moses, *Preventing HIV Transmission: The Role of Sterile Needles and Bleach* (Washington, D.C.: National Academies Press, 1995).

14. Lambert, "The Free-Needle Program Is Under Way and Under Fire."

15. Joseph, *Dragon within the Gates*, 201.

CHAPTER SEVEN: EXPOSING RACISM IN THE DRUG WAR

1. Duncan Osborne, "Needle Exchange Trial Unites Old Foes in the Common Goal of AIDS Prevention," *Outweek*, April 17, 1991.

2. Affidavit of Dan Keith Williams, dated June 14, 1990, and filed in the Needle Eight Case.

3. Dan Keith Williams interview by Jim Hubbard, New York, N.Y., March 26, 2004, http://www.actuporalhistory.org/interviews/images/williams.pdf.

4. Dan Keith Williams interview by Jim Hubbard.

5. Note: In 1991, Williams was accused of stealing $16,000 from ACT UP, which he says he actually spent on needles and other supplies, but without appropriate authorization. He was confronted in an emotional meeting and apologized. No charges were filed. Williams had an alcohol problem at the time, as well as untreated bipolar disorder. See Published and near Print Material, Media (1 of 3), December 1990–June 1991. MS ACT UP: The AIDS Coalition to Unleash Power: Series X. Published and near Print Material Box 141, Folder 7. New York Public Library. Archives of Sexuality and Gender. See also Dan Keith Williams interview, ACT UP oral history.

6. Brittney Cooper, "Stop Poisoning the Race Debate: How 'Respectability Politics' Rears Its Ugly Head—Again," *Salon*, last modified March 18, 2015,

https://www.salon.com/2015/03/18/stop_poisoning_the_race_debate_how
_respectability_politics_rears_its_ugly_head_again/.

7. Michelle Alexander, *The New Jim Crow: Mass Incarceration in the Age of Colorblindness* (New York: New Press, 2010), 17.

8. Carol Mueller, "Ella Baker and the Origins of Participatory Democracy," in Jacqueline Bobo et al., eds., *The Black Studies Reader* (New York: Routledge, 2004), 79–89. Troy Duster, *The Legislation of Morality* (New York: Free Press, 1970).

9. "AP Impact: After 40 Years, $1 Trillion, US War on Drugs Has Failed to Meet Any of Its Goals," Fox News, last updated November 17, 2004, https://www.foxnews.com/world/ap-impact-after-40-years-1-trillion-us-war-on-drugs-has-failed-to-meet-any-of-its-goals.

10. Dan Baum, *Smoke and Mirrors: The War on Drugs and the Politics of Failure* (Boston: Back Bay Books, 1997), 13.

11. "US Sentencing Commission Implements Crack Law," Families Against Mandatory Minimums, last modified March 4, 2016, https://web.archive.org/web/20120303203150/http:/www.famm.org/FederalSentencing/USSentencing Guidelines/USSentencingGuidelinesUpdates/USSentencingCommission ImplementsCrackLaw.aspx. United States Sentencing Commission, "Chapter Four: Racial, Ethnic, and Gender Disparities in Federal Sentencing Today," in *Fifteen Years of Guidelines Sentencing* (2004), 113–135, https://www.ussc.gov/sites/default/files/pdf/research-and-publications/research-projects-and-surveys/miscellaneous/15-year-study/15_year_study_full.pdf.

12. Lisa Weil, "Drug-Related Evictions in Public Housing: Congress' Addiction to a Quick Fix," *Yale Law & Policy Review* 9, no. 161 (1991), https://digitalcommons.law.yale.edu/cgi/viewcontent.cgi?referer=https://www.google.com/&httpsredir=1&article=1202&context=ylpr. Alexander, *The New Jim Crow*, 52.

13. Lorelei Laird, "Ex-offenders Face Tens of Thousands of Legal Restrictions, Bias and Limits on Their Rights," *ABA Journal*, last modified June 13, 2013, https://www.abajournal.com/magazine/article/ex-offenders_face_tens_of_thousands_of_legal_restrictions. Austin Jenkins, "From Drugs to Prison to Law School, Woman Faces One Extra Hurdle to Become a Lawyer," KNKX, last modified May 11, 2017, https://www.knkx.org/post/drugs-prison-law-school-woman-faces-one-extra-hurdle-become-lawyer.

14. Alexander, *The New Jim Crow*, 53.

15. Cecil Williams, *No Hiding Place: Empowerment and Recovery for Our Troubled Communities* (New York: Harper Collins, 1992), 4.

16. Alexander, *The New Jim Crow*, 222.

17. Cathy J. Cohen, *The Boundaries of Blackness: AIDS and the Breakdown of Black Politics* (Chicago: University of Chicago Press, 1999), 334.

18. Cohen, *The Boundaries of Blackness*, 346.

19. Ernest Quimby and Samuel R. Friedman, "Dynamics of Black Mobilization against AIDS in New York City," *Social Problems* 36, no. 4 (October 1989).

20. Harlon L. Dalton, "AIDS in Blackface," *Daedalus* 118, no. 3 (1989): 205–227.

21. Craig Reinarman and Harry G. Levine, eds., *Crack in America: Demon Drugs and Social Justice* (Berkeley: University of California Press, 1997), 32.

22. Adam Walinsky, "Crack as a Scapegoat," *New York Times*, September 16, 1986, https://www.nytimes.com/1986/09/16/opinion/crack-as-a-scapegoat.html.

23. Reinarman and Levine, *Crack in America*, 32, 24, 20.

24. Maia Szalavitz, "The Demon Seed That Wasn't," City Limits, last modified February 15, 2004, https://citylimits.org/2004/02/15/the-demon-seed-that-wasnt/.

25. Author interview with Lisa Moore, 2019.

26. Dan Keith Williams interview by Jim Hubbard.

CHAPTER EIGHT: HOUSING WORKS

1. Benjamin Shepard and Ronald Hayduk, eds., *From ACT UP to the WTO: Urban Protest and Community Building in the Era of Globalization* (London: Verso, 2002), 354.

2. Dan Keith Williams interview by Jim Hubbard.

3. "New York City Group Leads the Way toward a More Optimistic Future for ASOs," Relias Media, last modified July 1, 2004, https://www.reliasmedia.com/articles/7082-new-york-city-group-leads-the-way-toward-a-more-optimistic-future-for-asos.

4. Shepard and Hayduk, *From ACT UP to the WTO*, 355.

5. Shepard and Hayduk, *From ACT UP to the WTO*, 358.

6. Charles King interview by Sarah Schulman, New York, N.Y., January 20, 2010, http://www.actuporalhistory.org/interviews/images/king.pdf.

7. The two other founders of Housing Works were Eric Sawyer and Virginia Shubert. Housing Works, "Housing Works Annual Report 2015," https://s3.amazonaws.com/housingworks-site/documents/HW_Inc_AnnualReport_2015_v4.pdf.

8. The Minority Task Force on AIDS, which was alone among Black-led groups in supporting needle exchange early on in New York. Interview with Ronald Johnson, former executive director.

9. Author interviews: Charles King, 2019; Louis Jones, 2019 and 2020. See also Stephanie Golden, "Harlem's Holistic AIDS Alternative," *Yoga Journal* (January/February) 1993. Nancy Kelly McGowan Mackenzie, "A Community Response to the Needs of Drug Users," *Health/PAC Bulletin* 23, no. 4 (Winter 1993).

10. Deborah Padgett, Benjamin Henwood, and Sam Tsemberis, *Housing First: Ending Homelessness, Transforming Systems and Changing Lives* (Oxford: Oxford University, 2016), viii, ix.

11. Gregory Scruggs, "Once a National Model, Utah Struggles with Homelessness," Reuters, last modified January 10, 2019, https://www.reuters .com/article/us-usa-homelessness-housing/once-a-national-model-utah-struggles -with-homelessness-idUSKCN1P41EQ.

12. Richard Cho, "Four Clarifications about Housing First," United States Intragency Council on Homelessness, last modified June 18, 2014, https://www .usich.gov/news/four-clarifications-about-housing-first/.

CHAPTER NINE: THE HEIRESS AND THE BIKER

1. Email from Stephanie Comer.

2. All quotes from Stephanie Comer are from author interview, unless otherwise noted.

3. "AIDS & Addicts: Toxic Wetlands," *The MacNeil/Lehrer NewsHour*, August 6, 1991. Comer interview.

4. Don Des Jarlais was a key collaborator. H. Hagan, D. C. Des Jarlais, D. Purchase, T. Reid, and S. R. Friedman, "The Tacoma Syringe Exchange," *Journal of Addictive Disease* 10, no. 4 (1991): 81–88, DOI:10.1300/J069v10n04_06. PMID: 1777501.

5. Author interview with Alisa Solberg, 2019.

6. Susan Sherman and Dave Purchase, "Point Defiance: A Case Study of the United States' First Public Needle Exchange in Tacoma, Washington," *International Journal of Drug Policy* 12, no. 1 (2001): 45–57, DOI:10.1016/S0955 -3959(00)00074-8. Matt Driscoll, "From 13,000 in Tacoma to 100 Million Nationwide, Needle Exchange Proves Worth over 30 Years," *News Tribune*, September 14, 2018, https://www.thenewstribune.com/news/local/news-columns -blogs/matt-driscoll/article218298450.html#adnrb=900000.

7. Jane Gross, "Needle Exchange for Addicts Wins Foothold against AIDS in Tacoma," *New York Times*, January 23, 1989, https://www.nytimes.com/1989 /01/23/us/needle-exchange-for-addicts-wins-foothold-against-aids-in-tacoma .html?module=inline.

8. Kate Shatzkin, "A Coming of Age for Needle Exchange—Tacoma, a Pioneer in AIDS Prevention, Host of 3-Day Meeting," *Seattle Times*, October 12, 1990. Portland's needle exchange was founded and run by Kathy Oliver.

9. Edward H. Kaplan was the researcher who came up with the idea of studying the needles themselves, working with Robert Heimer, professor of epidemiology and pharmacology at Yale.

10. Mireya Navarro, "Yale Study Reports Clean Needle Project Helps Check AIDS," *New York Times*, August 1, 1991, https://www.nytimes.com/1991/08/01 /nyregion/yale-study-reports-clean-needle-project-helps-check-aids.html.

11. Richard Weinmeyer, "Needle Exchange Programs' Status in US Politics," *AMA Journal of Ethics*, last updated March 2016, https://journalofethics.ama-assn.org/article/needle-exchange-programs-status-us-politics/2016-03.

12. Founded in 1986 by law professor Arnold Trebach and attorney and activist Kevin Zeese, it was DPF that first brought European harm reduction supporters from the U.K. and the Netherlands to the U.S. and connected them with legislators and public health officials. DPF had likely funded the trip on which Allan Parry first meet Edith Springer, for example—and it helped arrange for him and Dave Purchase to testify in front of Congress in favor of needle exchange in 1989. The group also supported both Parker and Purchase directly, most notably with a shared $50,000 award for their work, which was granted in 1990. Drug Policy Alliance, "Past Winners," Reform Conference, accessed October 22, 2020, https://www.reformconference.org/achievement-awards/past-winners.

13. "Majority Now Supports Legalizing Marijuana," Pew Research Center, last updated April 4, 2013, https://www.pewresearch.org/politics/2013/04/04/majority-now-supports-legalizing-marijuana/.

14. Sherman, "Point Defiance."

CHAPTER TEN: ANY POSITIVE CHANGE

1. Dan Bigg interview with Nancy Campbell, shared with author.

2. Author interview with Dan Bigg, date unknown.

3. Zachary Siegel, "The Patron Saint of Harm Reduction," The Fix, last modified December 21, 2014, https://www.thefix.com/content/patron-saint-harm-reduction.

4. Narcotics Anonymous World Service Board of Trustees, "Bulletin #29: Regarding Methadone and Other Drug Replacement Programs," Narcotics Anonymous, accessed October 22, 2020, https://na.org/?ID=bulletins-bull29.

5. Pierce et al., "Impact of Treatment for Opioid Dependence on Fatal Drug-Related Poisoning." Maia Szalavitz, "The Wrong Way to Treat Opioid Addiction," *New York Times*, January 17, 2018.

6. Dee-Dee Stout, *Coming to Harm Reduction Kicking and Screaming* (Bloomington, Ind.: Authorhouse, 2009), 145.

7. All of the Bigg quotes in this section are from Nancy Campbell's interview with him.

8. Dan Bigg, interviewed by Siena Comer, April 2018. Shared with author by Stephanie Comer.

9. The Betty Ford Institute Consensus Panel, "What Is Recovery? A Working Definition from the Betty Ford Institute," *Journal of Substance Abuse Treatment* 33, no. 3 (2007): 221–228, DOI:10.1016/j.jsat.2007.06.001.

CHAPTER ELEVEN: REFINING HARM REDUCTION

1. Campbell interview with Bigg.

2. Imani Woods, "My Journey to Harm Reduction," *Harm Reduction Communication* 4 (Spring 1997), https://issuu.com/harmreduction/docs/hrc_1997_spring.

3. Dont Rhine, "Below the Skin: AIDS Activism and the Art of Clean Needles Now," *Xtra* 15, no. 3 (2013), https://www.x-traonline.org/article/below-the-skin-aids-activism-and-the-art-of-clean-needles-now.

4. Mark Bowden, "Outraged over Indifference to AIDS, Act Up Is Rewriting the Rules of Protest," *Philadelphia Inquirer*, June 5, 2011, https://www.inquirer.com/philly/health/Outraged_over_indifference_to_AIDS_Act_Up_is_rewriting_the_rules_of_protest.html.

5. Dave Purchase, "Do Unto Others: The Huwomanity of Harm Reduction," *Harm Reduction Communication* 4 (1997): 1, https://issuu.com/harmreduction/docs/hrc_1997_spring.

6. Will Hall, "Harm Reduction Guide to Coming off Psychiatric Drugs and Withdrawal," https://willhall.net/comingoffmeds/.

CHAPTER TWELVE: UNDOING OVERDOSE

1. Author interview with Dan Bigg, date unknown.

2. James Enoch et al., *Taking Back What's Ours* (London: INPUD Secretariat, 2020), https://www.inpud.net/en/taking-back-whats-ours-oral-history-movement-people-who-use-drugs.

3. Nancy Campbell, *OD: Naloxone and the Politics of Overdose* (Cambridge: MIT Press, 2020), 89.

4. Author interview with John Strang, 2019.

5. Campbell interview with Bigg.

6. Author interview with Sarz Maxwell, 2019.

7. Campbell, *OD: Naloxone and the Politics of Overdose*, 163.

8. Author interview with Maxwell, also emails.

9. Sarz Maxwell et al., "Prescribing Naloxone to Actively Injecting Heroin Users: A Program to Reduce Heroin Overdose Deaths," *Journal of Addictive Diseases* 25, no. 3 (2006), DOI:10.1300/J069v25n03_11.

10. Maxwell et al., "Prescribing Naloxone to Actively Injecting Heroin Users." Later, overdose deaths in Chicago would rise dramatically as the city had one of the first outbreaks of fentanyl contamination of heroin, which almost certainly would have been worse without CRA's naloxone distribution.

11. Eliza Wheeler et al., "Community-Based Opioid Overdose Prevention Programs Providing Naloxone—United States, 2010," *Morbidity Mortality Weekly Report* 61, no. 6 (2012), https://www.ncbi.nlm.nih.gov/pmc/articles/PMC4378715/.

12. Maia Szalavitz, "Do DIY Anti-Overdose Kits Help?" *Time*, last modified May 29, 2009, http://content.time.com/time/health/article/0,8599,1901794,00 .html.

13. Author interview with Greg Scott in Chicago.

CHAPTER THIRTEEN: UNDOING TREATMENT

1. Patt Denning interview by David Van Nuys, Wise Counsel podcast, November 12, 2008, https://www.centersite.net/common/rss/podcasts/wisecounsel /audio/20081115_wisecounsel_patt_denning_harm_reduction.mp3.

2. Author interview with Patt Denning, 2019.

3. Van Nuys, Denning interview.

4. M. Lieberman et al., *Encounter Groups: First Facts* (New York: Basic Books, 1973), 174.

5. Van Nuys, Denning interview.

6. Paul M. Roman and J. A. Johnson, *National Treatment Center Study Summary Report: Public Treatment Centers* (Athens: Institute for Behavioral Research, University of Georgia, 2004).

7. Maia Szalavitz, *Help at Any Cost: How the Troubled-Teen Industry Cons Parents and Hurts Kids* (New York: Riverhead, 2006), 26–33.

8. Meredith Huey Dye et al., "The Availability of Integrated Care in a National Sample of Therapeutic Communities," *The Journal of Behavioral Health Services and Research* 39, no. 1 (2012): 17–27, DOI:10.1007/s11414-011-9251-1.

9. Maia Szalavitz, "Hazelden Introduces Antiaddiction Medications into Recovery for First Time," TIME.com, Nov. 5, 2012, https://healthland.time.com /2012/11/05/hazelden-introduces-antiaddiction-medications-in-recovery-for -first-time/.

10. Andrew Tatarsky, via email.

CHAPTER FOURTEEN: COME AS YOU ARE

1. G. Alan Marlatt, "Highlights of Harm Reduction: A Personal Report from the First National Harm Reduction Conference in the United States," in *Harm Reduction: Pragmatic Strategies for Managing High-Risk Behaviors*, ed. G. Alan Marlatt (New York: Guilford Press, 2002).

2. The acronym BAR stood for "Behavioral Alcohol Research."

3. William R. Miller, "Loss of Control Drinking in Alcoholics," *Alcohol Health & Research World* 19, no. 1 (1995): 36–37.

4. Author interview with George Parks, 2020.

5. Author interview with Doug Gary, 2019, and email.

6. Purchase, "Do Unto Others."

7. Marlatt, "Highlights."

8. Marlatt, "Highlights."

9. "Alcohol Facts and Statistics," National Institute on Alcohol Abuse and Alcoholism, last modified February 2020, https://www.niaaa.nih.gov/publications /brochures-and-fact-sheets/alcohol-facts-and-statistics.

10. G. Alan Marlatt, "The Controlled Drinking Controversy: A Commentary," *American Psychologist* 38, no. 10 (1983): 1097–1110, DOI:10.1037//0003 -066x.38.10.1097.

11. Marlatt, "Controlled Drinking."

12. Ironically, while AA's position is that true alcoholics can never learn controlled drinking, its founders were not opposed to potential members experimenting: official literature suggests that people who are "not convinced" of their powerlessness should make an attempt at moderation and come back to meetings if they fail. *Alcoholics Anonymous, Twelve Steps and Twelve Traditions* (New York: Alcoholics Anonymous World Services, June 1988 edition), 23.

13. There's an even more bizarre footnote to this case. The woman who led the charge against the Sobells, Mary Pendery, was later murdered by her lover, a person with a severe alcohol use disorder, whom she had treated. See Stanton Peele, "How the Disease Theory of Alcoholism Killed Mary Pendery, and Harm Reduction Could Have Saved Her," last updated May 30, 2011, http://www .peele.net/blog/110530.html.

14. Marlatt, "Controlled Drinking."

15. Maia Szalavitz, "Twelve Steps Back," Brill's Content, last modified June 17, 2004, http://www.doctordeluca.com/Documents/Brill's_12-Steps-Back _Jan01.htm.

16. Szalavitz, "Twelve Steps Back."

17. Author interview with George Parks, 2020.

18. Author interview with George Parks, 2020.

19. Ido Hartogsohn, "Constructing Drug Effects: A History of Set and Setting," *Drug Science, Policy and Law* 3 (2017), https://doi.org/10.1177 /2050324516683325. Luke Bainbridge, "A Second Summer of Love," *Guardian*, last updated April 20, 2008, https://www.theguardian.com/music/2008/apr/20 /electronicmusic.culture. Also, author interview, Peter McDermott, date unknown.

CHAPTER FIFTEEN: NOTHING ABOUT US WITHOUT US

1. Edney quotes this section from Heather Edney interview with author, 2019, unless otherwise noted.

2. Heather Edney and Brooke Lober, "junkphood," accessed October 23, 2020, https://www.heatheredney.com/junkphood.

3. Maia Szalavitz, "The Mysterious Consequences of Repeatedly Overdosing on Opioids," *Vice*, last updated June 5, 2019, https://www.vice.com/en/article /wjv474/the-mysterious-consequences-of-repeatedly-overdosing-on-opioids.

4. Maia Szalavitz, "Genetics: No More Addictive Personality," *Nature* 522, no. 7557 (June 25, 2015): S48–49, DOI:10.1038/522S48a.

5. Quotes in this section from Paul Cherashore, "A Dog and Pony Show? Users in the Harm Reduction Movement," *Harm Reduction Communication* 8 (Spring 1999): 4, 5, https://issuu.com/harmreduction/docs/hrc_1999_spring, and from Paul Cherashore, written copy of speech, shared with author.

CHAPTER SIXTEEN: UNDOING TOUGH LOVE

1. Author interview with Gretchen Burns Bergman, 2019. Unless otherwise noted, this is the source of her quotes throughout this chapter.

2. Emil J. Chiauzzi and Steven Liljegren, "Taboo Topics in Addiction Treatment: An Empirical Review of Clinical Folklore," *Journal of Substance Abuse Treatment* 10 (1993): 303–316, http://www.profkramer.com/assets/chiauzzi-1993.pdf.

3. Facts in this paragraph from: "Criminal Justice Facts," The Sentencing Project, accessed October 23, 2020, https://www.sentencingproject.org/criminal-justice-facts/#:~:text=Since%20the%20official%20beginning%20of,1980%20to%20452%2C964%20in%202017. "The Use of Incarceration in the United States," American Society of Criminology (November 2000), https://www.asc41.com/policies/ASC_Policy_Paper_The_Use_of_Incarceration_in_the_United_States_2001.pdf. "Policy and Prejudice: Paradoxes of U.S. Drug Policies," Stanford University, accessed May 19, 2020, https://web.archive.org/web/20200519133616/https://web.stanford.edu/class/e297c/poverty_prejudice/paradox/htele.html. "The Effective National Drug Control Strategy 1999," Common Sense for Drug Policy, accessed October 23, 2020, http://www.csdp.org/edcs/. "AP Impact: After 40 Years, $1 Trillion, US War on Drugs Has Failed to Meet Any of Its Goals," Fox News, last updated November 17, 2004, https://www.foxnews.com/world/ap-impact-after-40-years-1-trillion-us-war-on-drugs-has-failed-to-meet-any-of-its-goals.

4. Eric K. Sterling, "U.S. Drug Policy," Institute for Policy Studies, last updated November 1, 1999, https://ips-dc.org/us_drug_policy/. H. Jalal et al., "Changing Dynamics of the Drug Overdose Epidemic in the United States from 1979 through 2016," *Science* 361, no. 6408 (September 21, 2018), DOI:10.1126/science.aau1184. PMID: 30237320.

5. Disclosure: I received the Soros Justice Fellowship from the Open Society Foundation to complete and publicize my last book, *Unbroken Brain*. The organization was originally called the Open Society Institute, https://fconline.foundationcenter.org/fdo-grantmaker-profile/?key=OPEN012.

6. In 2000, DPF would merge with Nadelmann's think tank, the Lindesmith Center, to become the Drug Policy Alliance under his leadership.

7. *Medical Marijuana Referenda Movement in America: Hearing before the Subcommittee on Crime of the Committee on the Judiciary, House of Representatives*, 105th Congress (1997) (transcript of the ads, Steve Mitchell, former police officer and assistant U.S. attorney): 180, https://books.google.com/books?id=zKnHSp17c0gC&dq=john+sperling+arizona+proposition+200+drugs&source=gbs_navlinks_s.

8. Nick Gillespie, "Prescription: Drugs," *Reason*, February 1, 1997, https://reason.com/1997/02/01/prescription-drugs/.

9. Bill Moyers, *Moyers on Addiction, Close to Home* (PBS, 1998), online video, https://billmoyers.com/series/moyers-on-addiction-close-to-home-1998/. Note: I was series researcher and associate producer for this show.

10. "The Internet News Audience Goes Ordinary," Pew Research Center, last updated January 14, 1999, https://www.pewresearch.org/politics/1999/01/14/the-internet-news-audience-goes-ordinary/.

11. This is the earliest capture of the drug czar website, which is late 1998: https://web.archive.org/web/19980101000000*/whitehousedrugpolicy.gov. Erowid went online in 1995: https://erowid.org/general/about/about_article5.shtmlhttps://erowid.org/general/about/about_article5.shtml.

12. Gretchen B. Bergman, "Mothers Protest Prohibition—Again," Alternet, September 30, 2011.

13. Emily Dufton, *Grass Roots: The Rise and Fall and Rise of Marijuana in America* (New York: Basic Books, 2017), 132, 107–118, 89–93,168.

14. Cable Neuhaus, "David and Phyllis York Treat Problem Teenagers with a Stiff Dose of 'Toughlove,'" *People*, last updated November 16, 1981, https://people.com/archive/david-and-phyllis-york-treat-problem-teenagers-with-a-stiff-dose-of-toughlove-vol-16-no-20/.

15. Martin Sheen, "Prop. 36 Would Devastate the Drug Court System," *Los Angeles Times*, August 7, 2000, https://www.latimes.com/archives/la-xpm-2000-aug-07-me-201-story.html.

16. "Proposition 36 Victory," Drug Policy Alliance, accessed October 24, 2020, https://www.drugpolicy.org/departments-and-state-offices/california/proposition-36-victory.

17. "Proposition 36 Victory."

18. Maia Szalavitz, "Former Addict: What Indiana Can Learn from New York about Needle Exchanges," *Time*, last updated April 5, 2016, https://time.com/3769693/clean-needle-programs-hiv/.

19. "Former Clinton Drug Czar on the Fight between Science and Politics," The Takeaway, last updated April 9, 2015, https://www.wnyc.org/story/pres-clintons-former-drug-czar-perils-science-and-politics/. Note: whoever booked Barry McCaffrey as an expert on using science to do drug policy was either a brilliant ironist or hilariously ill-informed.

There were indeed several Canadian studies that seemed to show that needle exchange didn't stop the spread of HIV, but their authors showed that other factors were responsible for these outliers, namely pre-existing differences in risk between poorer needle exchange users and wealthier nonusers in a country where syringe sales are legal.

Julie Bruneau and Martin T. Schechter, "The Politics of Needles and AIDS," *New York Times*, April 9, 1998, https://www.nytimes.com/1998/04/09/opinion/the -politics-of-needles-and-aids.html?searchResultPosition=1.

20. Mark Schoofs and Rachel Zimmerman, "Clinton Says He Regrets Decision against Needle-Exchange Program," *Wall Street Journal*, July 12, 2002. Peter Lurie and Ernest Drucker, "An Opportunity Lost: HIV Infections Associated with Lack of a National Needle-Exchange Programme in the USA," *Lancet* 349, no. 9052 (1997): 604–608, https://doi.org/10.1016/S0140-6736(96)05439-6.

21. Tim Rhodes and Dagmar Hedrich, eds., *Harm Reduction: Evidence, Impacts, and Challenges* (Luxembourg: Publications Office of the European Union), 39, https://www.emcdda.europa.eu/system/files/publications/555/EMCDDA -monograph10-harm_reduction_final_205049.pdf.

22. Benedikt Fischer et al., "Heroin-Assisted Treatment (HAT) a Decade Later: A Brief Update on Science and Politics," *Journal of Urban Health* 84, no. 4 (2007): 552–562, https://www.ncbi.nlm.nih.gov/pmc/articles/PMC2219559/.

23. The history of the backlash against harm reduction in Merseyside is complex and highly contested. What is known is that within two years, 41 out of 450 of Marks's patients died after losing access to his prescriptions. Peter Carty, "Drug Abuse: The End of the Line," *Guardian*, December 10, 1997. Toby Seddon, "Prescribing Heroin: John Marks, the Merseyside Clinics and Lessons from history," *International Journal of Drug Policy* 78 (April 2020): 1–7, https://doi .org/10.1016/j.drugpo.2020.102730.

24. Maia Szalavitz, "The U.S. Government Stopped Other Countries from Legalizing Weed for Generations," *Vice*, last updated July 2, 2018, https://www.vice.com/en/article/kzkmnw/the-us-stopped-other-countries-from -legalizing-weed-for-generations.

CHAPTER SEVENTEEN: UNDOING PAIN CARE

1. Maia Szalavitz, "Dr. Feelscared," *Reason*, August/September 2004, https:// reason.com/2004/08/01/dr-feelscared-2/.

2. "AG Corbett, Erie County DA Foulk Announce Charges against Erie County Doctor for Illegally Prescribing Drugs," Office of Pennsylvania Attorney General Tom Corbett, last updated June 1, 2005, http://www.doctordeluca.com /Library/WOD/HeberleCharged-Poster05.pdf.

3. "Erie Doctor Draws Support for Defense against Painkiller Charges," The Associated Press State & Local Wire, August 6, 2005.

4. David Bruce, "Patients Defend Doctor, Bemoan Loss of Painkilling Drugs," *Erie Times-News*, May 3, 2005.

5. Transcript of behind-the-scenes footage by Amy Bianco of Siobhan Reynolds ABC *Nightline* interview in April 2005.

6. Art Van Zee, "The Promotion and Marketing of OxyContin: Commercial Triumph, Public Health Tragedy," *American Journal of Public Health* 99, no. 2 (2009): 221–227, https://www.ncbi.nlm.nih.gov/pmc/articles/PMC2622774/.

7. Allen G. Breed, "Hillbilly Heroin Holds Appalachia in Its Grip of Death and Addiction," *Los Angeles Times*, June 17, 2001, https://www.latimes.com /archives/la-xpm-2001-jun-17-mn-11349-story.html.

8. Silvia Deandrea, "Prevalence of Undertreatment in Cancer Pain: A Review of Published Literature," *Annals of Oncology* 19, no. 2 (2008): 1985–1991, https://www.ncbi.nlm.nih.gov/pmc/articles/PMC2733110/#bib7.

9. Facts in this paragraph: Gery P. Guy et al., "Vital Signs: Changes in Opioid Prescribing in the United States, 2006–2015," *Morbidity and Mortality Weekly Report* 66, no. 26 (2017): 697–704, https://www.ncbi.nlm.nih.gov/pmc /articles/PMC5726238/. "Vital Signs: Overdose of Prescription Opioid Pain Relievers—United States, 1999–2008," *Morbidity and Mortality Weekly Report* 60, no. 43: 1487–1492, figure 2, https://www.cdc.gov/mmwr/preview/mmwrhtml /mm6043a4.htm#fig2. "Overdose Death Rates," National Institute on Drug Abuse, "National Drug Overdose Deaths 1999–2018" (PowerPoint), https:// www.drugabuse.gov/drug-topics/trends-statistics/overdose-death-rates.

10. Rachel N. Lipari and Arthur Hughes, "How People Obtain the Prescription Pain Relievers They Misuse," *The CBHSQ Report*, January 12, 2017. Center for Behavioral Health Statistics and Quality, Substance Abuse and Mental Health Services Administration, Rockville, MD, https://www.samhsa.gov/data /sites/default/files/report_2686/ShortReport-2686.html.

11. R. F. Catalano, H. R. White, C. B. Fleming, and K. P. Haggerty, "Is Nonmedical Prescription Opiate Use a Unique Form of Illicit Drug Use?" *Addictive Behaviors* 36, nos. 1–2 (2011): 79–86, https://doi.org/10.1016/j .addbeh.2010.08.028.

12. Mark C. Bicket et al., "Prescription Opioids Commonly Unused After Surgery: A Systematic Review," *JAMA Surgery* 152, no. 11 (2017): 1066–1071, DOI:10.1001/jamasurg.2017.0831.

13. Meredith Noble et al., "Opioids for Long-Term Treatment of Noncancer Pain," Cochrane Systematic Review, last modified January 20, 2010, https://www .cochranelibrary.com/cdsr/doi/10.1002/14651858.CD006605.pub2/full.

14. Jalal et al., "Changing Dynamics."

15. Bianco, *Nightline* pre-taping with Siobhan Reynolds, April 2005.

16. Szalavitz, "Dr. Feelscared."

17. From the draft of a book proposal by Siobhan Reynolds, shared by Amy Bianco.

18. Another case the same year, *U.S. v. Doremus*, also ruled against such prescribing. Musto, *The American Disease*, 132. *Webb v. United States*, 370 U.S. 249, 96 (1919), https://supreme.justia.com/cases/federal/us/249/96/.

19. Musto, *The American Disease*, 132. "Understanding Medical Regulation in the United States," Federation of State Medical Boards, https://www.fsmb.org/siteassets/education/pdf/best-module-text-intro-to-medical-regulation.pdf.

20. Duster, *The Legislation of Morality*, 15.

21. "Drug Misuse and Addiction," National Institute on Drug Abuse, last updated July 2020, https://www.drugabuse.gov/publications/drugs-brains-behavior-science-addiction/drug-misuse-addiction.

22. U.S. Dept. of Justice, Drug Enforcement Administration, Diversion Control Division, Title 21 United States Code Controlled Substances Act, Subchapter I, Part A, Section 802, https://www.deadiversion.usdoj.gov/21cfr/21usc/802.htm.

23. Reynolds draft book proposal.

24. U.S. Dept. of Justice, Drug Enforcement Administration, Diversion Control Division, Title 21 Code of Federal Regulations, Part 1306.04, https://www.deadiversion.usdoj.gov/21cfr/cfr/1306/1306_04.htm.

25. Jacob Sullum, "William Hurwitz Sentenced to Less Than Five Years," *Reason*, July 16, 2007, https://reason.com/2007/07/16/william-hurwitz-sentenced-to-l/.

26. Szalavitz, "Dr. Feelscared."

27. Maia Szalavitz, "The Doctor Wasn't Cruel Enough: How One Physician Escaped the Panic over Prescription Drugs," *Reason*, June 2, 2006, https://reason.com/2006/06/02/the-doctor-wasnt-cruel-enough/.

28. Erica Goode, "Stronger Hand for Judges in the 'Bazaar' of Plea Deals," *New York Times*, March 22, 2012, https://www.nytimes.com/2012/03/23/us/stronger-hand-for-judges-after-rulings-on-plea-deals.html.

29. "Presumed Guilty: Research the System," PBS, accessed October 26, 2020, https://www.pbs.org/kqed/presumedguilty/3.2.1.html. Justin A. Julian, Kristin A. Toy, and David. H. Sohn, "Medical-Legal Risks of Prescribing Pain Medications," Huffington Post, last updated September 17, 2017, https://www.huffpost.com/entry/medical-legal-risks-of-prescribing-pain-medications_b_59c908cee4b0b7022a646c36. Cites https://apps2.deadiversion.usdoj.gov/CasesAgainstDoctors/spring/main?execution=e1s1, which is not being updated. More cases can be found here: "Criminal Cases Against Doctors," U.S. Department of Justice, Drug Enforcement Administration, Diversion Control Division, accessed October 26, 2020, https://www.deadiversion.usdoj.gov/crim_admin_actions/.

30. Radley Balko, "The Worst Kind of Ham Sandwich: The Vindictive Grand Jury Investigation of Pain-Relief Advocate Siobhan Reynolds," Slate, last modified December 21, 2010, https://slate.com/news-and-politics/2010/12/the-vindictive-grand-jury-investigation-of-pain-relief-advocate-siobhan-reynolds.html.

31. Felice J. Freyer, "Doctors Are Cutting Opioids, Even if It Harms Patients," *Boston Globe*, last modified January 3, 2017, https://www.bostonglobe.com/metro/2017/01/02/doctors-curtail-opioids-but-many-see-harm-pain-patients/z4Ci68TePafcD9AcORs04J/story.html. Maia Szalavitz, "When the Cure Is Worse than the Disease," *New York Times*, February 9, 2019, https://www.nytimes.com/2019/02/09/opinion/sunday/pain-opioids.html.

32. Tami L. Mark and William Parish, "Opioid Medication Discontinuation and Risk of Adverse Opioid-Related Health Care Events," *Journal of Substance Abuse Treatment* 103 (2019): 58–63, https://doi.org/10.1016/j.jsat.2019.05.001.

33. Szalavitz, "When the Cure Is Worse than the Disease." M. I. Demidenko et al., "Suicidal Ideation and Suicidal Self-Directed Violence Following Clinician-Initiated Prescription Opioid Discontinuation among Long-Term Opioid Users," *General Hospital Psychiatry* 47 (July 2017): 29–35, DOI:10.1016/j.genhosppsych.2017.04.011.

34. Jocelyn James et al., "Mortality after Discontinuation of Primary Care–Based Chronic Opioid Therapy for Pain: A Retrospective Cohort Study," *Journal of General Internal Medicine* 34 (2019): 2749–2755, https://doi.org/10.1007/s11606-019-05301-2.

35. Abby Alpert et al., "Supply-Side Drug Policy in the Presence of Substitutes: Evidence from the Introduction of Abuse-Deterrent Opioids," National Bureau of Economic Research Working Paper 23031, January 2017, https://www.nber.org/papers/w23031.pdf.

CHAPTER EIGHTEEN: UNDOING OVERDOSE, PART 2

1. Elizabeth Merrall et al., "Meta-Analysis of Drug-Related Deaths Soon after Release from Prison," *Addiction* 105, no. 9 (2010): 1545–1554, DOI:10.1111/j.1360-0443.2010.02990.x.

2. Tracey Green et al., "Fatal Overdoses after Implementing Medications for Addiction Treatment in a Statewide Correctional System," *JAMA Psychiatry* 75, no. 4 (April 1, 2018): 405–407, DOI:10.1001/jamapsychiatry.2017.4614.

3. William White, "Loved Ones GRASPing for Help: An Interview with Denise and Gary Cullen," accessed October 28, 2020, http://www.williamwhitepapers.com/pr/GRASPing%20for%20Help%20Denise%20and%20Gary%20Cullen.pdf.

4. Wheeler, "Community-Based Opioid Overdose Prevention Programs."

5. "Naloxone Overdose Prevention Laws," Prescription Drug Abuse Policy System, last updated July 1, 2017, http://pdaps.org/datasets/laws-regulating-administration-of-naloxone-1501695139.

6. "Car Crash Deaths and Rates—Injury Facts," National Safety Council, accessed October 26, 2020, https://injuryfacts.nsc.org/motor-vehicle/historical-fatality-trends/deaths-and-rates/#:~:text=In%202018%2C%20the%20death%20rate,per%20100%20million%20miles%20driven.

For drunk driving specifically:

"Alcohol-Impaired Driving Fatalities 1982–2018," Responsibility.org, accessed October 26, 2020, https://www.responsibility.org/wp-content/uploads /2020/02/FAAR_3974_State-of-Drunk-Driving-Fatalities_Shareable_JPGS-V2 -Pg09.jpg.

Also:

"Car Crash Deaths and Rates" Injury Facts, National Safety Council, accessed October 26, 2020, https://injuryfacts.nsc.org/motor-vehicle/historical -fatality-trends/deaths-and-rates/#:~:text=In%202018%2C%20the%20death %20rate,per%20100%20million%20miles%20driven.

7. "NCHS Releases New Monthly Provisional Estimates on Drug Overdose Deaths," National Center for Health Statistics, last updated September 11, 2019, https://www.cdc.gov/nchs/pressroom/podcasts/20190911/20190911.htm.

8. Wheeler, "Community-Based Opioid Overdose Prevention Programs."

9. Unless otherwise noted, quotes and background on Denise Cullen are from author interviews in 2015 and 2019.

10. Holly Hedegaard, Arialdi Minino, and Margaret Warner, "Drug Overdose Deaths in the United States, 1999–2018," NCHS Data Brief 356, National Center for Health Statistics (2020), https://www.cdc.gov/nchs/data/databriefs /db356-h.pdf. "Naloxone Overdose Prevention Laws," Prescription Drug Abuse Policy System, last updated July 1, 2017, http://pdaps.org/datasets/laws -regulating-administration-of-naloxone-1501695139.

11. "Role of Naloxone in Opioid Overdose Fatality Prevention," transcript of hearing by the Food and Drug Administration, Center for Drug Evaluation and Research, Office of the Assistant Secretary for Health, National Institute on Drug Abuse, Centers for Disease Control and Prevention, April 12, 2012.

12. The mother who testified was Marilee Murphy Odendahl, who has also become a harm reduction activist.

13. "Drug Overdose Immunity and Good Samaritan Laws," National Conference of State Legislatures, last updated June 5, 2017, https://www.ncsl.org /research/civil-and-criminal-justice/drug-overdose-immunity-good-samaritan -laws.aspx.

14. The Drug Free America Foundation was initially a front group for a tough love rehab and "gay conversion" center called Straight Inc. After all of its teen programs were forced to close, it began sending representatives to the U.N. to try to remove references to harm reduction. Straight had been so punishing that lawsuits and regulators eventually targeted it for child abuse in all eight states where it operated between 1976 and 1993. It pioneered many of the abusive tactics used in other "gay conversion" programs. Kathryn Otter, one of the Needle Eight, was atrociously maltreated in a copycat rehab run by one of its former leaders. Maia Szalavitz, *Help at Any Cost* (New York: Riverhead, 2006), 53, 60.

CHAPTER NINETEEN: UNDOING DIVISIONS

1. Alexander, *The New Jim Crow*, 3.

2. Author interview and emails with Ricky Bluthenthal, 2019, 2020.

3. Unless otherwise noted, quotes from Michelle Alexander are from *The New Jim Crow*.

4. Notably, two Black women within the movement, Deborah Peterson Small and Nkechi Taifa, along with many others. All Tracie Gardner quotes from author interviews, 2019, 2020.

5. Steve Howard, "George Shultz on Legalizing Drugs," *Los Angeles Times*, November 26, 1989, https://www.latimes.com/archives/la-xpm-1989-11-26-op-153-story.html. Mark Perry, "Milton Friedman Interview from 1991 on America's War on Drugs," last modified August 6, 2015, https://www.aei.org/carpe-diem/milton-friedman-interview-from-1991-on-americas-war-on-drugs/.

6. Coalition for Safety, "Public Partners," accessed January 10, 2021, https://www.coalitionforpublicsafety.org/partners.

7. "One Year after the First Step Act: Mixed Outcomes," The Sentencing Project, last updated December 2019, https://www.sentencingproject.org/publications/one-year-after-the-first-step-act/.

8. "Syringe Exchange Programs—United States, 2008," *Morbidity and Mortality Weekly Report* 59, no. 45: 1488–1491, https://www.cdc.gov/mmwr/preview/mmwrhtml/mm5945a4.htm/Syringe-Exchange-Programs-United-States-2008#tab1. David Showalter, "Federal Funding for Syringe Exchange in the US: Explaining a Long-Term Policy Failure," *International Journal of Drug Policy* 55 (2018): 95–104, DOI:10.1016/j.drugpo.2018.02.006.

9. Gregg Gonsalves and Forrest Crawford, "How Mike Pence Made Indiana's HIV Outbreak Worse," last updated March 3, 2020, https://www.politico.com/news/magazine/2020/03/02/how-mike-pence-made-indianas-hiv-outbreak-worse-118648.

10. Showalter, "Federal Funding for Syringe Exchange in the US."

11. Christopher Ingraham, "Michigan Becomes the 10th State to Allow Recreational Marijuana," *Washington Post*, November 7, 2018, https://www.washingtonpost.com/business/2018/11/07/michigan-becomes-th-state-allow-recreational-marijuana/. Justin McCarthy, "Two in Three Americans Now Support Legalizing Marijuana," Gallup, October 22, 2018, https://news.gallup.com/poll/243908/two-three-americans-support-legalizing-marijuana.aspx.

12. "Michael Botticelli Plenary," YouTube video, from 10th National Harm Reduction Conference, October 23, 2014, posted by National Harm Reduction Coalition, October 31, 2014, https://www.youtube.com/watch?v=J3Uqsx9rI2E.

CHAPTER TWENTY: REDOING ORGANIZING

1. Maia Szalavitz, "A Tale of Two Cities in the Grips of the Opioid Crisis," *Nation,* updated February 21, 2019, https://www.thenation.com/article/archive/opioid-epidemic-sif-harm-reduction/.

2. B. Pauly et al., "Impact of Overdose Prevention Sites during a Public Health Emergency in Victoria, Canada," *PLoS ONE* 15, no. 5 (2020), https://doi.org/10.1371/journal.pone.0229208.

3. Mike Howell, "Downtown Eastside: Canada's 'Most Famous Junkie' Comes Clean," *Vancouver Courier*, February 27, 2014, https://www.vancouverisawesome.com/courier-archive/news/downtown-eastside-canadas-most-famous-junkie-comes-clean-2969404.

4. Hari, *Chasing the Scream*, 200.

5. Travis Lupick, *Fighting for Space* (Vancouver: Arsenal Pulp Press, 2018), 77–80.

6. Travis Lupick, "The Vancouver Area Network of Drug Users Looks Back on 20 Years Fighting for Human Rights," Straight, last modified September 4, 2017, https://www.straight.com/news/959286/vancouver-area-network-drug-users-looks-back-20-years-fighting-human-rights.

7. Stephanie Strathdee et al., "Needle Exchange Is Not Enough: Lessons from the Vancouver Injecting Drug Use Study," *AIDS* 11, no. 8 (1997): 59–65, https://journals.lww.com/aidsonline/Fulltext/1997/08000/Needle_exchange_is_not_enough__lessons_from_the.1.aspx. Also, author interview with Strathdee, 2019; unless otherwise noted, Strathdee quotes and background are from this interview.

8. Statistics Canada, Focus on Geography Series, 2016 Census, Province of British Columbia, Total population by Aboriginal identity and Registered or Treaty Indian status, British Columbia, 2016 Census.

9. Author interview with Donald MacPherson, 2019.

10. Michael V. O'Shaughnessy et al., "Deadly Public Policy: What the Future Could Hold for the HIV Epidemic among Injection Drug Users in Vancouver," *Current HIV/AIDS Reports* 9 (2012): 394–400, https://doi.org/10.1007/s11904-012-0130-z.

11. Dean Wilson, presentation at Stimulus Conference held by Canadian Drug Policy Coalition, Edmonton, Canada, October 4, 2018.

12. Hari, *Chasing the Scream*, 188–195.

13. Lupick, *Fighting for Space*, 107–112.

14. Eugenia Oviedo-Joekes et al., "The North American Opiate Medication Initiative (NAOMI): Profile of Participants in North America's First Trial of Heroin-Assisted Treatment," *Journal of Urban Health* 85, no. 6 (2008): 812–825, DOI:10.1007/s11524-008-9312-9.

15. Ambrose Uchtenhagen, "Heroin-Assisted Treatment in Switzerland: A Case Study in Policy Change," *Addiction* 105 (2010): 29–37, DOI:10.1111/j .1360-0443.2009.02741.x.

16. "Four Pillars Drug Strategy," City of Vancouver, accessed October 26, 2020, https://vancouver.ca/people-programs/four-pillars-drug-strategy.aspx.

17. Lupick, *Fighting for Space*, 182.

18. Ann Livingston presentation at Stimulus Conference held by Canadian Drug Policy Coalition, Edmonton, Canada, October 4, 2018.

19. Hari, *Chasing the Scream*, 199.

20. The expert was Ethan Nadelmann, who was at the time the executive director of the Lindesmith Center. That center later merged with the Drug Policy Foundation to become the Drug Policy Alliance. Author interview, Ethan Nadelmann.

21. Joanne Csete, *From the Mountaintops: What the World Can Learn from Drug Policy Change in Switzerland* (New York: Open Society Foundation, 2013), 19. R. B. Haemmig, "Harm Reduction in Bern: From Outreach to Heroin Maintenance," *Bulletin of the New York Academy of Medicine* 72, no. 2 (1995): 371–379, https://www.ncbi.nlm.nih.gov/pmc/articles/PMC2359428/. Dagmar Hedrich, *European Report on Drug Consumption Rooms* (Luxembourg: Office for Official Publications of the European Communities, 2004), http://webcache.googleusercontent.com/search?q=cache:3n3Up7m4eJsJ:www .emcdda.europa.eu/attachements.cfm/att_2944_EN_consumption_rooms_report .pdf+&cd=5&hl=en&ct=clnk&gl=us.

22. Uchtenhagen, "Heroin-Assisted Treatment in Switzerland." Haemmig, "Harm Reduction in Bern."

23. The other organizers were Vancouver's Portland Hotel Society, which did "housing first" before it had a name. See generally Lupick, *Fighting for Space*.

24. Lupick, *Fighting for Space*, 144, 257.

25. Szalavitz, "A Tale of Two Cities in the Grips of the Opioid Crisis."

26. "Illicit Drug Toxicity Deaths in BC, January 1, 2010 to September 30, 2020," British Columbia Coroners Service, accessed October 26, 2020, https:// www2.gov.bc.ca/assets/gov/birth-adoption-death-marriage-and-divorce/deaths /coroners-service/statistical/illicit-drug.pdf.

27. Eva Uguen-Csenge, "B.C. Releases Plan to Provide Safe Supply of Drugs during COVID-19 Pandemic," CBC News, last modified March 27, 2020, https://www.cbc.ca/news/canada/british-columbia/safe-supply-drug-plan-covid -1.5511973.

28. "Hundreds of British Columbians Are Accessing Province's 'Safe Supply' of Drugs," CBC News, last modified June 1, 2020, https://www.cbc.ca /news/canada/british-columbia/safe-supply-bc-drug-overdose-covid-public -health-emergency-1.5594197.

29. Darryl Dyck, "Trudeau Says Focus Is on Safe Supply, Not Decriminalization as Overdose Deaths Spike," *Globe and Mail*, last modified September 2, 2020, https://www.theglobeandmail.com/canada/british-columbia/article-trudeau-says-focus-is-on-safe-supply-not-decriminalization-as/.

CHAPTER TWENTY-ONE: THE AMERICAN CHALLENGE

1. John W. Whitehead, "The Growing Epidemic of Cops Shooting Family Dogs," Counterpunch, last modified March 22, 2019, https://www.counterpunch.org/2019/03/22/the-growing-epidemic-of-cops-shooting-family-dogs/.

2. Dara Lund, "Cops Do 20,000 No-Knock Raids a Year. Civilians Often Pay the Price When They Go Wrong," Vox, last modified May 15, 2015, https://www.vox.com/2014/10/29/7083371/swat-no-knock-raids-police-killed-civilians-dangerous-work-drugs.

3. Kevin Sack, "Door-Busting Raids Leave a Trail of Blood," *New York Times*, March 18, 2017, https://www.nytimes.com/interactive/2017/03/18/us/forced-entry-warrant-drug-raid.html.

4. Terry Gross, "Militarization of Police Means U.S. Protesters Face Weapons Designed for War," NPR *Fresh Air*, last modified July 1, 2020, https://www.npr.org/2020/07/01/885942130/militarization-of-police-means-u-s-protesters-face-weapons-designed-for-war. This features journalist Radley Balko, whose work in this area is indispensable.

5. Unless otherwise noted, quotes from Vincent in this chapter are from author interview with Louise Vincent, 2019.

6. "NCSU 2019 Annual Report," North Carolina Urban Survivors Union, accessed October 26, 2020, https://sway.office.com/GELnYglMcPS6LBbE?ref=website.

7. Jonathan Michels, "Harm Reduction Is Compassion, Harm Reduction Is Love: Louise's Story," last modified May 14, 2017, https://scalawagmagazine.org/2017/05/harm-reduction-is-compassion/.

8. Sanjay Gupta, "Reversing an OD" (CNN, 2014), from Internet Archive, MPEG video, https://archive.org/details/CNNW_20140601_113000_Sanjay_Gupta_MD/start/60/end/120.

9. "NCSU 2019 Annual Report.

10. Rosa Goldensohn, "They Shared Drugs. Someone Died. Does That Make Them Killers?" *New York Times*, May 25, 2018, https://www.nytimes.com/2018/05/25/us/drug-overdose-prosecution-crime.html.

11. Quote here and in previous paragraph from James Enoch et al., *Taking Back What's Ours* (London: INPUD Secretariat, 2020), https://www.inpud.net/en/taking-back-whats-ours-oral-history-movement-people-who-use-drugs.

CHAPTER TWENTY-TWO: REDOING THE FUTURE

1. Leana Wen, "We're Retreating to New Strategy on Covid-19. Let's Call It What It Is," *Washington Post*, May 13, 2020, https://www.washingtonpost.com/opinions/2020/05/13/were-retreating-new-strategy-covid-19-lets-call-it-what-it-is/.

2. Julie Marcus, "Quarantine Fatigue Is Real," *Atlantic*, last modified May 11, 2020, https://www.theatlantic.com/ideas/archive/2020/05/quarantine-fatigue-real-and-shaming-people-wont-help/611482/.

3. Associated Press, "Poll Finds 90% Favor Keeping Drugs Illicit," *New York Times*, September 15, 1988, https://www.nytimes.com/1988/09/15/us/poll-finds-90-favor-keeping-drugs-illicit.html.

4. Barrot H. Lambdin et al., "Overdose Education and Naloxone Distributions within Syringe Service Programs—United States, 2019," *Morbidity and Mortality Weekly Report* 69, no. 33 (2020): 1117–1121, https://www.cdc.gov/mmwr/volumes/69/wr/mm6933a2.htm.

5. Don C. Des Jarlais et al., "Syringe Service Programs for Persons Who Inject Drugs in Urban, Suburban, and Rural Areas—United States, 2013," *Morbidity and Mortality Weekly Report* 64, no. 48 (December 11, 2015): 1337–1341.

6. Eliza Wheeler et al., "Opioid Overdose Prevention Programs Providing Naloxone to Laypersons—United States, 2014," *Morbidity and Mortality Weekly Report* 64, no. 23 (2015), https://www.cdc.gov/mmwr/preview/mmwrhtml/mm6423a2.htm; http://www.pdaps.org/datasets/laws-regulating-administration-of-naloxone-1501695139. The exception is Nebraska: https://www.biopharmadive.com/news/teva-narcan-generic-fda-approval-co-prescription/553148/.

7. "State Medical Marijuana Laws," National Conference of State Legislatures, last updated November 10, 2020, https://www.ncsl.org/research/health/state-medical-marijuana-laws.aspx. Zachary Siegel, "2020 Election Results Prove America's War on Drugs Is Finally Ending," NBC News.com Think, last updated November 9, 2020, https://www.nbcnews.com/think/opinion/2020-election-results-prove-america-s-war-drugs-finally-ending-ncna1247141.

8. Author interview with Kris Nyrop, 2018. Also LEAD website, https://www.leadbureau.org/.

9. Alex Stevens, Caitlin Elizabeth Hughes, Shann Hulme, and Rebecca Cassidy, "Depenalization, Diversion, and Decrimininalization: A Realist Review and Programme Theory of Alternatives to Criminalization for Simple Drug Possession," *European Journal of Criminology* (November 2019), https://doi.org/10.1177/1477370819887514.

10. "Oregon Measure 110 Election Results: Decriminalize Some Drugs and Provide Treatment," *New York Times*, December 4, 2020, https://www.nytimes.com/interactive/2020/11/03/us/elections/results-oregon-measure-110-decriminalize-some-drugs-and-provide-treatment.html.

11. Colleen Cowles, *War on Us: How the War on Drugs and Myths about Addiction Have Created a War on All of Us* (St. Paul, Minn.: Fidalgo Press, 2019), 194–195.

12. Seth W. Stoughton, Jeffery J. Noble, and Geoffrey P. Alpert, "George Floyd's Death Shows Exactly What Police Should Not Do," *Washington Post*, May 29, 2020, https://www.washingtonpost.com/outlook/george-floyd-police-training /2020/05/29/0aca572e-a127-11ea-b5c9-570a91917d8d_story.html.

13. Jon Collins, "Ex-Cops' Attorneys Attribute Floyd's Death to Drugs, Foreshadowing Central Theme at Trial," Minnesota Public Radio, last updated September 10, 2020, https://www.mprnews.org/story/2020/09/10/excops-attorneys -attribute-floyds-death-to-drugs-foreshadowing-central-theme-at-trial.

14. William D. Floodgate, "From Maintenance to Recovery: Exploring the Reorientation towards Recovery in British Drug Policy during a Time of Reform and Economic Austerity," doctoral dissertation, University of Manchester, 2017, https://www.research.manchester.ac.uk/portal/files/66046259/FULL_TEXT .PDF.

15. Jillian Deutsch, "Glasgow Faces 'Perfect Storm' with HIV Spike," *Politico*, last updated February 16, 2020, https://www.politico.eu/article/glasgow -scotland-hiv-epidemic-drug-addicts/.

16. Maia Szalavitz, "Dan Bigg Is a Harm-Reduction Pioneer and His Overdose Doesn't Change That," *Vice*, last updated October 24, 2018, https://www .vice.com/en/article/7x3yag/dan-bigg-overdose-harm-reduction.

17. Zachary A. Siegel, "Biden's 'Crack House' Crusade," *The Appeal*, last updated September 11, 2019, https://theappeal.org/joe-biden-crack-house-statute/.

18. "Drugs of Abuse," U.S. Department of Justice Drug Enforcement Administration, 2017, https://www.dea.gov/sites/default/files/drug_of_abuse.pdf.

19. The DEA is required to consult the Department of Health and Human Services, which has medical researchers assess the medical value of substances when it makes scheduling decisions. However, it has the ultimate power to make the decision, regardless. (See previous note for reference.)

20. "Prescription Opioid Use in the U.S. Has Declined by 60% from 2011 Peak, According to New Report from the IQVIA™ Institute for Human Data Science," *IQVIA*, last updated December 17, 2020, https://www .iqvia.com/en/newsroom/2020/12/prescription-opioid-use-in-the-us-has -declined-by-60-from-2011-peak-according-to-new-report-from-the. Maia Szalavitz, "Forcing Pain Patients off Their Meds Won't End the Opioid Crisis," *Vice*, last updated August 21, 2018, https://www.vice.com/en/article/7xqa44/forcing -pain-patients-off-their-meds-will-not-end-the-opioid-crisis.

21. J. R. Wozniak et al., "Four-Year Follow-up of a Randomized Controlled Trial of Choline for Neurodevelopment in Fetal Alcohol Spectrum Disorder," *J Neurodevelop Disord* 12, no. 9 (2020), https://doi.org/10.1186/s11689-020- 09312-7.

22. C. E. Gartner, W. D. Hall, S. Chapman, and B. Freeman, "Should the Health Community Promote Smokeless Tobacco (Snus) as a Harm Reduction Measure?" *PLoS Medicine* 4, no. 7 (2007): e185, https://doi.org/10.1371/journal.pmed.0040185. J. Foulds et al., "Effect of Smokeless Tobacco (Snus) on Smoking and Public Health in Sweden," *Tobacco Control* 12 (2003): 349–359, https://www.statista.com/statistics/433390/individuals-who-currently-smoke-cigarettes-in-european-countries/.

Index